# PRAISE
## *VISIONARY LEADERSHIP IN HEALTHCARE*

"*Wei & Horton-Deutsch have used their voices—and those of an immensely talented pool of coauthors—to write a book that actually leads us toward developing and sustaining visionary leadership and supplies us with the necessary passion to engage. This text belongs on the bookshelf of all thoughtful and compassionate leaders and will be the go-to resource for our emerging healthcare leader colleagues!*"

–Judith F. Karshmer, PhD, PMHCNS-BC, FAAN
Dean and Professor, Edson College of Nursing and Health Innovation
Chief Wellness Officer
Arizona State University

"*The pandemic has proven to be a pivotal time in the history of healthcare. Nursing leaders are heeding the mindful call to lead from head, heart, and hands to set the course for the future of nursing and create a caring health ecosystem to transform humanity.* Visionary Leadership in Healthcare *will be an invaluable resource for the healthcare community and facilitate our kuleana (responsibility) to lead with inspiration, hope, and resilience.*"

–Kelly M Johnson, PhD, RN, NEA-BC
Senior Vice President, System Chief Nurse Executive, and Chief Nursing Officer
The Queen's Medical Center

"*Visionary Leadership in Healthcare redefines leadership as an expression of love and caring. This robust book spans the breadth of leadership theory and translates it into practice based on trust, caring, and compassion. With contemporary narratives and reflective questions for each chapter, this book is a relevant way forward for the practice of caring conscientiousness for all healthcare leaders. A must-read for all nursing academics teaching leadership practice and all executive healthcare leaders to reach a more reflective, intentional leadership presence.*"

–Karen Drenkard, PhD, RN, NEA-BC, FAAN
Associate Dean and Professor
George Washington University School of Nursing

"This volume is an important addition to the library of core sources for nursing leadership practice, particularly when that leadership is guided by Caring Science. Nursing, as a values-led profession, requires leaders that are grounded in their core values and led by purpose. This book helps the reader move toward greater engagement, openness, equity, inclusiveness, and authenticity—truly a values-based caring style of leader. I appreciate the case studies and reflective questions to help the reader move from absorbing knowledge to application. The section on nurturing healthy and healing work environments is so timely for addressing the global effects of the COVID-19 pandemic and its impact on caregivers, particularly nursing. I look forward to adding this work to my personal library and using it to help guide a next generation of nursing leaders in their growth and development."

–Gay Landstrom, PhD, RN, NEA-BC, FAONL, FACHE
Senior Vice President and Chief Nursing Officer, Trinity Health


"Drs. Holly Wei and Sara Horton-Deutsch, known for their professional work in Caring Science and the promotion of transformational relationships, have honored healthcare professions with their new book, Visionary Leadership in Healthcare. A must-read!"

–Dale E. Beatty, DNP, RN, NEA-BC, Caritas Coach
Chief Nurse Executive, Vice President of Patient Care Services
Stanford Health Care

# VISIONARY LEADERSHIP
# in Healthcare

Excellence in Practice, Policy, and Ethics

Holly Wei, PhD, RN, NEA-BC, FAAN
Sara Horton-Deutsch, PhD, RN, PMHCNS, FAAN, ANEF

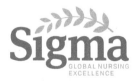

*Sigma Theta Tau International Honor Society of Nursing (Sigma) is a nonprofit organization whose mission is developing nurse leaders anywhere to improve healthcare everywhere. Founded in 1922, Sigma has more than 135,000 active members in over 100 countries and territories. Members include practicing nurses, instructors, researchers, policymakers, entrepreneurs, and others. Sigma's more than 540 chapters are located at more than 700 institutions of higher education throughout Armenia, Australia, Botswana, Brazil, Canada, Colombia, Croatia, England, Eswatini, Ghana, Hong Kong, Ireland, Israel, Italy, Jamaica, Japan, Jordan, Kenya, Lebanon, Malawi, Mexico, the Netherlands, Nigeria, Pakistan, Philippines, Portugal, Puerto Rico, Scotland, Singapore, South Africa, South Korea, Sweden, Taiwan, Tanzania, Thailand, the United States, and Wales. Learn more at www.sigmanursing.org.*

Sigma Theta Tau International
550 West North Street
Indianapolis, IN, USA 46202

To request a review copy for course adoption, order additional books, buy in bulk, or purchase for corporate use, contact Sigma Marketplace at 888.654.4968 (US/Canada toll-free), +1.317.687.2256 (International), or solutions@sigmamarketplace.org.

To request author information, or for speaker or other media requests, contact Sigma Marketing at 888.634.7575 (US/Canada toll-free) or +1.317.634.8171 (International).

ISBN:          9781646480210
EPUB ISBN: 9781646480227
PDF ISBN:   9781646480234

First Printing, 2022

**Publisher:** Dustin Sullivan
**Acquisitions Editor:** Emily Hatch
**Cover Designer:** Michael Tanamichi
**Interior Design/Page Layout:** Becky Batchelor
**Indexer:** Larry D. Sweazy

**Managing Editor:** Carla Hall
**Publications Specialist:** Todd Lothery
**Project Editor:** Carla Hall
**Copy Editor:** Erin Geile
**Proofreader:** Todd Lothery

Library of Congress Cataloging-in-Publication Data

Names: Wei, Holly, 1966- author. | Horton-Deutsch, Sara, author. | Sigma
   Theta Tau International, issuing body.
Title: Nurse-led visionary leadership in healthcare : excellence in
   practice, policy, and ethics / Holly Wei, Sara Horton-Deutsch.
Description: Indianapolis, IN : Sigma Theta Tau International, [2022] |
   Includes bibliographical references and index. | Summary: "The world is
   constantly changing, and during a time of great challenges, our
   healthcare systems must evolve-moving beyond an illness narrative and
   toward one that focuses on health and healing. In doing so, our
   leadership styles must evolve as well. Nurse-Led Visionary Leadership in
   Healthcare informs, expands, and empowers nurse leaders to envision and
   transform the current healthcare system using an evolved worldview to
   achieve a global, life-sustaining perspective. Lead authors and editors,
   Holly Wei and Sara Horton-Deutsch model their call to move away from
   hierarchical leadership to more engaged, open, equitable, inclusive,
   authentic, and caring leadership styles"-- Provided by publisher.
Identifiers: LCCN 2022001595 (print) | LCCN 2022001596 (ebook) | ISBN
   9781646480210 (paperback) | ISBN 9781646480227 (epub) | ISBN
   9781646480234 (pdf) | ISBN 9781646480241 (epub)
Subjects: MESH: Leadership | Nurse's Role | Nursing, Supervisory | Nurse
   Administrators | Nursing--organization & administration
Classification: LCC RT86.4 (print) | LCC RT86.4 (ebook) | NLM WY 105 |
   DDC 610.7306/9--dc23/eng/20220209
LC record available at https://lccn.loc.gov/2022001595
LC ebook record available at https://lccn.loc.gov/2022001596

# DEDICATION

This book is dedicated to developing visionary, adaptive, and relational health professionals and leaders around the world to unleash more of the power of each person to facilitate and influence the transformation of healthcare.

# ACKNOWLEDGMENTS

We genuinely acknowledge all those engaged in pursuing a leadership journey with a shared vision of creating a world they would like to see and who are willing to engage in deep dialogue and collaboration to influence and transform healthcare collectively.

We offer special gratitude to all those at Sigma who provided support and guidance throughout the submission of this book and their shared commitment to this vital topic.

# AVAILABLE BOOK RESOURCES

This textbook has an accompanying Learner Activities Workbook and Facilitator Guide. The Learner Activities Workbook includes reflective questions and narratives for each chapter. Learners can use the reflective questions and narratives to guide their reading, thinking, and group discussions or activities. The Facilitator Guide includes the following materials for each chapter:

- Reflective questions and guiding answers

- Narratives and guiding responses

- Quizzes and answers

- Instructor PowerPoint slides (www.sigmanursing.org/visionary-leadership-in-healthcare or scan the QR code below).

Both the Learner Activities Workbook and the Facilitator Guide are available as free downloads from the Sigma Repository (http://hdl.handle.net/10755/22206) and available to purchase as print books from your favorite online retailer. Simply search the book title in your favorite online store, adding "workbook" or "guide" to narrow your search.

**Instructor PowerPoint Slides**

**Free Ancillaries**

# ABOUT THE LEAD AUTHORS

**Holly Wei, PhD, RN, NEA-BC, FAAN,** is a Professor and Assistant Dean for the PhD program at the University of Louisville School of Nursing. Her overarching research focuses on healthcare organizational culture, leadership development, clinician well-being, stress genomic biomarkers, and patient care quality. She is known nationally and internationally for her nursing practice models and a Convergent Care Theory. Multiple healthcare systems have used Wei's nursing models to guide practice and promote organizational culture and patient care with significant improvements in nursing practice and patient care quality.

Wei's scholarly work has reached and influenced the nursing profession in academia and clinical nursing practice globally. In the past five years, Wei had over 50 peer-reviewed publications and delivered over 70 presentations, including radio and TV interviews, influencing tens of thousands of nurses globally. Some of her articles are among the top-read, top-downloaded, and top-cited articles of journals. Wei is an Associate Editor of the *International Journal for Human Caring*. She sits on two boards of directors and two journals' editorial board positions, including *Advances in Nursing Science*.

Wei has received numerous prestigious awards throughout her career. Recently, she received the International Leininger Caring-Culture Award, Board of Governors Distinguished Professor for Teaching, DAISY Extraordinary Faculty, Nurse Educator of the Year, Scholar-Teacher Award, Outstanding Research Scholar Award, and Nursing Research Award. These awards affirm her significant contributions and influences in nursing leadership and practice regionally and globally.

**Sara Horton-Deutsch, PhD, RN, PMHCNS, FAAN, ANEF,** is a Caritas Coach and a Professor and the Director of the Kaiser Permanente/USF Partnership at the University of San Francisco, where she mentors the next generation of nursing leaders through the lens of Caring Science and values-based leadership. She also serves as a Faculty Associate with the Watson Caring Science Institute. In 2021, she co-created and initiated the Caritas Leadership Program, a uniquely customized six-month program guiding participants through executive Caring Science leader dialogues, interactive circles, and participant transformation projects. She is also a founding partner of Better Together Healing, LLC, a holistic practice partnership specializing in an integrative approach to heal the self, build collaborations, and create healthy and bounded communities. As a therapeutic practitioner and Caritas leadership coach, she collaborates with healthcare professionals and organizations seeking balance and growth who are open to engaging in innovative approaches to healing. Her comprehensive approach includes certifications in professional coaching and training through the Leadership Circle and Working with Resilience, providing comprehensive profiles and assessments to raise the conscious practice of leadership and build regenerative success at work.

Horton-Deutsch holds a research fellowship at the University of South Africa School of Human Sciences, where she encourages critical discourse and collaborates with faculty to enhance research and scholarship. Her research foci are on leadership development, reflective practice, and creating healing and healthy work environments. She has co-edited four textbooks. Her work has been published in three books with Sigma: *Reflective Practice: Transforming Education and Improving Outcomes* (2012 & 2017), *Reflective Organizations: On the Front Lines of QSEN & Reflective Practice Implementation* (2015), and *Caritas Coaching: A Journey Toward Transpersonal Caring for Informed Moral Action in Healthcare* (2018).

Her most recent awards, honors, and fellowships include 2020–2021 Experienced Academic Nurse Leadership Academy Faculty Mentor, Sigma; 2018–2019 Faculty Fellowship in Ignatian Tradition, University of San Francisco; 2016–2024 Invited Research Fellow, University of South Africa, Johannesburg, South Africa; 2016–2017 Nurse Faculty Leadership Academy, Faculty Mentor, Sigma; 2014 Fellow, American Academy of Nursing; 2013 Fellow, Academy of Nursing Education; Fellow, National League for Nursing.

# CONTRIBUTING AUTHORS

Full author biographies can be found at the end of each chapter.

**Stephanie Wilkie Ahmed, DNP, NP-BC,** is Associate Chief Nursing Officer and Watson Caring Science Scholar in Residence in the University of Miami Health System.

**Mary Jo Assi, DNP, RN, NEA-BC, FAAN,** is Associate Chief Nursing Officer and Partner, Strategic Consulting, at Press Ganey.

**Nancy M. Ballard, PhD, RN, NEA-BC,** is Assistant Professor at Kennesaw State University.

**Mark D. Beck, DNP, MSN, BS, RN,** is Assistant Professor and Interim Program Director at Samuel Merritt University.

**Wanda J. Borges, PhD, RN, ANP-BC,** is Dean and Professor, and Associate Director of Graduate Programs in the School of Nursing at New Mexico State University.

**Sylvia T. Brown, EdD, RN, CNE, ANEF,** is Dean and Professor at the East Carolina University College of Nursing.

**Chantal Cara, PhD, RN, FAAN, FCAN,** is Professor at Université de Montréal and a Distinguished Caring Science Scholar at the Watson Caring Science Institute.

**Laura Caramanica, PhD, RN, CNE, CNEP, FACHE, FAAN,** is Graduate Program Director and Professor at the University of West Georgia.

**Gabrielle Dawn Childs, MA, MPH, RN,** is a PhD Candidate at the American Graduate School in Paris and a Program Manager for the Peace Corps' Advancing Health Professionals program.

**Peggy L. Chinn, PhD, DSc(Hon), RN, FAAN,** is the Editor of the journal *Advances in Nursing Science* and Professor Emerita at the University of Connecticut.

**Carey S. Clark, PhD, RN, AHN-BSC RYT, FAAN,** is Professor of Nursing at Pacific College of Health and Science.

**Jim D'Alfonso, DNP, PhD(h), RN, NEA-BC, FNAP, FAAN,** is Executive Director, Professional Excellence and the KP Scholars Academy, & Adjunct Faculty at the University of San Francisco.

**Erica DeKruyter, MSN, RN,** is Manager of Educational Resources at Sigma Theta Tau International Honor Society of Nursing (Sigma).

**Jennifer J. Doering, PhD, RN,** is Associate Dean for Academic Affairs and Associate Professor at the University of Wisconsin-Milwaukee College of Nursing.

**Diana Drake, DNP, APRN, WHNP, FAAN, FNAP,** is Clinical Professor and Director of the Women's Health Gender-Related Nurse Practitioner specialty at the University of Minnesota School of Nursing.

**Karen J. Foli, PhD, RN, FAAN,** is Associate Professor in the Purdue University School of Nursing.

**Lynn Gallagher-Ford, PhD, RN, NE-BC, DPFNAP, FAAN/Evidence-based Practice (CH),** is Chief Operating Officer and Director of the Helene Fuld National Trust Institute for Evidence-based Practice in Nursing and Healthcare at the Ohio State University College of Nursing.

**Stephanie D. Gingerich, DNP, RN, CPN,** is Clinical Assistant Professor at the University of Minnesota School of Nursing.

**Kaboni Whitney Gondwe, PhD, RN,** is Assistant Professor at the University of Wisconsin-Milwaukee College of Nursing.

**Ernest J. Grant, PhD, RN, FAAN,** is President of the American Nurses Association.

**Sarah E. Gray, DNP, RN, CEN, FAEN,** is Chief Nursing Officer at Sigma Theta Tau International Honor Society of Nursing (Sigma).

**Christine Griffin, PhD, RN, NPD-BC, CPN,** is a Caritas Coach and Professional Development Specialist at Children's Hospital Colorado.

**Senem Guney, PhD,** is Vice President of Language Analytics for Press Ganey.

**Sonya R. Hardin, PhD, CCRN, NP-C, FAAN,** is Dean and Professor at the University of Louisville.

**Grissel Hernandez, PhD, RN, MPH, HNB-BC, NPD-BC, SGAHN,** is Executive Director at Stanford Health Care's Center for Education and Professional Development.

**Marcia Hills, PhD, RN, FAAN, CFAN,** is Professor and Associate Director of Research and Scholarship at the University of Victoria's School of Nursing.

**Phyllis N. Horns, PhD, RN, FAAN,** is Professor of Nursing and Director of the East Carolina Consortium for Nursing Leadership at the East Carolina University College of Nursing.

**Matthew S. Howard, DNP, RN, CEN, TCRN, CPEN, CPN,** is Director of Scholarship and Leadership Resources at Sigma Theta Tau International Honor Society of Nursing (Sigma).

**Rachel Johnson-Koenke, PhD, LCSW,** is Assistant Professor at the University of Colorado College of Nursing.

**Christie Kerwan, MSN, RN,** is Director of Strategic Partnerships—Healthcare for PowerDMS .

**Judy Ngele Khanyola, MSc, BSN, RN,** is Chair for the Center for Nursing and Midwifery at the University of Global Health Equity in Rwanda.

**Carol Ann King, DNP, MSN, BSN, RN, FNP-BC, NHDP-BC,** is Clinical Professor in the Doctor of Nursing Practice–Family and Adult-Gerontology Nurse Practitioner programs at East Carolina University.

**Dame Donna Kinnair, MA, RGN, HV, LLB, PGCE,** is Chief Executive and General Secretary of the Royal College of Nursing in the UK.

**Wipada Kunaviktikul, PhD, RN, RM, FAAN,** is Professor Emerita and Assistant to the President of Health Science Academic Affairs at Panyapiwat Institute of Management in Thailand.

**Donna Lake, PhD, RN, NEA-BC, FAAN,** is Clinical Professor at the East Carolina University College of Nursing.

**Jeneile Luebke PhD, RN,** is a post-doctoral Nurse Research Fellow at the University of Wisconsin-Madison.

**Elizabeth A. Madigan, PhD, RN, FAAN,** is Chief Executive Officer of Sigma Theta Tau International Honor Society of Nursing (Sigma).

**Kathy Malloch, PhD, MBA, RN, FAAN,** is Clinical Professor at the Ohio State University College of Nursing.

**Lucy Mkandawire-Valhmu, PhD, RN,** is Associate Professor at the University of Wisconsin-Milwaukee College of Nursing.

**Chelsie Monroe, MSN, APRN, PMHNP-BC,** is a Psychiatric Mental Health Nurse Practitioner and Owner of Balanced Mental Wellness in Colorado.

**Melissa T. Ojemeni, PhD, RN,** is Director of Nursing Education, Research and Professional Development for Partners In Health in Boston.

**Crystal Oldman, EdD, MSc, MA, RN, RHV, QN, FRCN, CBE,** is Chief Executive at the Queen's Nursing Institute in the UK.

**Danielle EK Perkins, PhD, RN,** is the former Manager of the Center for Excellence in Nursing Education at Sigma Theta Tau International Honor Society of Nursing (Sigma).

**Daniel J. Pesut, PhD, RN, FAAN,** is Emeritus Professor at the University of Minnesota School of Nursing and Emeritus Katherine R. and C. Walton Lillehei Chair of Nursing Leadership at the University of Minnesota.

**Tim Porter-O'Grady, DM, EdD, ScD(h), APRN, FAAN, FACCWS,** is Senior Partner for Tim Porter-O'Grady Associates LLC & Clinical Professor at the Emory University School of Nursing.

**Teddie M. Potter, PhD, RN, FAAN, FNAP,** is Clinical Professor, Director of Planetary Health, and Coordinator of the Doctor of Nursing Practice in Health Innovation and Leadership program at the University of Minnesota School of Nursing.

**Katherine Reed, LPC,** is Program Manager of the Ponzio Creative Arts Therapy program at Children's Hospital Colorado.

**Jennifer Reese, MD,** is Associate Professor of Clinical Pediatrics at the University of Colorado School of Medicine and Section Head of the Pediatric Hospital Medicine.

**William E. Rosa, PhD, MBE, NP-BC, FAANP, FAAN,** is Chief Research Fellow at Memorial Sloan Kettering Cancer Center's Department of Psychiatry and Behavioral Sciences.

**Barbara Sattler, DrPH, RN, FAAN,** is Professor Emerita at the University of San Francisco School of Nursing and Health Professions.

**Gwen Sherwood, PhD, RN, FAAN, ANEF,** is Professor Emerita at the University of North Carolina at Chapel Hill School of Nursing.

**Michelle Taylor Skipper, DNP, FNP-BC, NHDP-BC, FAANP,** is Director of the Adult-Gerontology and Family Nurse Practitioner specialties of the DNP program at the East Carolina University College of Nursing.

**Chandra L. Speight, PhD, RN, NP-C, CNE,** is Assistant Professor in the Department of Advanced Nursing Practice and Education at the East Carolina University College of Nursing.

**Allison Squires, PhD, RN, FAAN,** is Associate Professor and Director of the PhD program at the New York University Rory Meyers College of Nursing.

**Dennis A. Taylor, DNP, PhD, ACNP-BC, NEA-BC, FCCM,** is a Trauma Acute Care Nurse Practitioner and teaches in the Department of Academic Nursing at Wake Forest Baptist Health.

**Todd E. Tussing, DNP, RN, CENP, NEA-BC,** is Assistant Professor of Clinical Nursing at the Ohio State University College of Nursing.

**Gisela H. van Rensburg,** is Professor at the University of South Africa.

**AnnMarie Lee Walton, PhD, MPH, RN, OCN, CHES, FAAN,** is Assistant Professor at the Duke University School of Nursing.

**Kefang Wang, PhD, RN, FAAN,** is Dean and Professor in the School of Nursing and Rehabilitation at Shandong University in China.

**Jean Watson, PhD, RN, AHN-BC, HSGAHN, FAAN, LL (AAN),** is Distinguished Professor and Founder/Director of the Watson Caring Science Institute in Colorado.

**Ena M. Williams, MBA/MSM, RN, CENP,** is Senior Vice President and Chief Nursing Officer at Yale New Haven Hospital.

**Kenichi Yamaguchi, PhD,** is Associate Professor at the Okinawa Prefectural College of Nursing in Japan.

# TABLE OF CONTENTS

## 11　PROMOTING EXCEPTIONAL PATIENT EXPERIENCE THROUGH COMPASSIONATE CONNECTED CARE . . .285

## 12　APPLYING COMPLEXITY SCIENCE IN PROMOTING COMMUNITY AND POPULATION HEALTH . . . . . . . . .311

# FOREWORD

Caring does not burn us out; not caring is actually what is most dangerous for our patients *and* for us as healthcare providers. I first learned this years ago in my research with 247 nurses who showed me that nurses with higher empathic concern were less burnt-out and more personally fulfilled than nurses with lower empathic concern. I was unable, however, to explain this phenomenon using the psychological theories of that time. Now I can. In the years that followed, I learned about Caring Science in nursing and discovered how nursing has led the way in its scientific insights about compassionate caring for over 40 years. Along with the additional supportive research from the neuroscience of compassion, we can now explain why it happens that caring is not only related to the best quality of care for our patients but that it is also essential for our own well-being as healthcare providers. And the most effective way to support that individual caring capacity at the bedside is to create caring-centered organizations that cultivate and protect that compassionate caring in every facet of the organization. *Visionary Leadership in Healthcare* provides us with a transformative resource to do this work.

We are in a critical transition time as we work our way through the COVID-19 pandemic. There are challenging upheavals occurring throughout our society and the world. Nursing, at the forefront of patient care, plays an indispensable role in this time of crisis. While nurses are heralded as heroes, there is also an acute awareness of the tremendous costs on nurses as individuals, on the nursing profession, and on everyone who works in healthcare. We are now wrestling with major questions of who we will be in light of the great and noble lineage of nursing facing new challenges. Things will not be as they once were, yet our caring foundations in nursing will enable us to guide who we will become and what our role will be in the incredible shifts that are occurring. Caring Science is what will help us go from where we are now to this better place in which we are grounded in our care and interconnectedness with each other in the global community.

The nurse leader is charged with caring for the nurses and the organization that takes care of the patients. We could focus only on the individual nurse-patient relationship as the focus of Caring Science. But it is only the first ring of concentric circles all focused on caring for patients. The nurse takes care of the patient, but who takes care of the nurses who take care of the patients? Who makes sure nurses have what they need to do their work well? Who takes care of the organization that takes care of nurses and all other healthcare team members who take care of the patients? And who takes care of the leaders who are charged with taking care of the organization, the staff, and the patient? *Visionary Leadership in Healthcare* is not only a sourcebook but also a touchstone for this work of taking care of the organization, the staff, and the nurses who care for our patients. Compassionate caring is the essence of effective leadership—for our patients, our staffs, our organization, our societies, and ourselves.

Nursing has been among the helping professions in its empirical study and understanding of compassionate caring. In my work researching the science of compassion and training healthcare professionals in many different disciplines and specialties, only nursing has fully developed a theoretical understanding of caring that helps practically guide us in everything we do in healthcare. Typically, helping professions are not systematic in their overall conceptions of the caring process. To use an analogy with atomic theory, it is one thing to catalog the properties of individual chemicals. It is a whole other thing to have the periodic table showing us how all the elements fit together. While the helping professions have, in various ways, deeply investigated and improved various specific aspects of healing work, this has been done at a more granular level of analysis. It is nursing that has been showing us that we have to understand how it all fits and works together. Nursing is now showing the other helping professions the importance of having this theoretical understanding, this "caring periodic table" that helps us understand how to most effectively respond to the suffering of our patients. I work with many helping professions, and nursing leads all of them in its ability to reflect deeply on itself. Perhaps it is the fact that nurses must engage those who are suffering at the levels of mind and spirit, as well as body, that has launched nursing into this leadership role. Nursing has a history of knowing that one must have a regular practice of reflecting on this continual encounter with patients in their wholeness to understand fully what our patients need in whatever circumstances emerge. This has been a gift that nursing has given to me and all the helping professions as we make our way through these times.

*Visionary Leadership in Healthcare* covers all the aspects of healthcare leadership. It is a sourcebook for whatever area you would need to review, a checklist to make sure you have covered all the bases in being an effective leader, and a source of inspiration to help you know this can be done and be done well. In every chapter, you are given the vision and theoretical background of that aspect of healthcare leadership. You will get a summary of the pertinent information and research related to that area as well as resources for it. Then the experts in those areas offer ways to apply this practically, along with exemplars and case examples. It is very current with ways these areas have been applied in the complexities that have emerged during the COVID-19 pandemic. Each chapter offers ways to reflect on its particular topic for both individual readers and workgroups. The vision, theory, and practical information embedded in every chapter make it not only a great resource to work on every aspect of healthcare leadership but also a book that invites readers to be creative and courageous in their leadership journey.

We are creating something new in the nursing profession and in healthcare, but we need a lot to get there from here. What will help us find our way through stormy seas? The road map provided by Caring Science and the principles that have always grounded nurses are our rudder helping us tack into the wind as we work to sail through turbulent times, finding our way through pandemic change and global transformation. May the wisdom and deep caring of each author in this book help you be the leader who will provide what we desperately need in these times.

–Dominic O. Vachon, PhD, MDiv
Director, Ruth M. Hillebrand Center for Compassionate Care in Medicine
Professor of the Practice, University of Notre Dame
Author, *How Doctors Care: The Science of Compassionate and Balanced Caring in Medicine,* and co-author, *The Power & Pain of Nursing: Self-Care Practices to Protect & Replenish Compassion*

# INTRODUCTION

*"A leader sees greatness in other people."*

*"People will forget what you said, people will forget what you did, but people will never forget how you made them feel."*

–Maya Angelou

*"We don't have to wait for some grand utopian future. The future is an infinite succession of presents, and to live now as we think human beings should live, in defiance of all that is bad around us, is itself a marvelous victory."*

–Howard Zinn

Why this leadership book? Why now? Healthcare is in dire need of a bold and courageous vision and sacred actions that move beyond an illness narrative toward one that focuses on health and healing, serving all of humanity. This book aims to inform, expand, and empower healthcare leaders to envision and transform the current system into one with an expansive vision for health. It will enlighten a visionary leadership journey and guide nurses' and health professions' leaders to see beyond the daily care practice toward an evolved worldview. While most of the contributors of this book are grounded and rooted in the discipline of nursing, this text is a call to all healthcare professionals who seek to recenter care in healthcare. It addresses the need to balance the empirical, practical, technical, and vocational aspects of education, practice, and research with the ontological, epistemological, and critical humanities. To balance medical science with Caring Science. As a theoretical and moral matter, it is time to commit ourselves to care and to sacred actions for humanity.

This book informs healthcare leaders to implement leadership theories at the micro and macro systems level. At a micro level, it explains how leaders build and maintain a healthy work environment at the individual or team levels. At the macro level, the book discusses leadership's role in facilitating change at the organizational, health system, national, global, and even planetary levels. It also expands leadership knowledge on how leaders can influence and transform practice, including policy change, disaster management, political and social determinants of health, diversity, equity, inclusion, and the Ethics of Belonging. Each chapter has a section to introduce how to integrate theories into practice.

This book is timely, especially during this challenging time of pandemic. The chapters address ways to nurture a healthy work environment, mitigate organizational trauma, foster resilience, improve interprofessional collaboration, and promote exceptional patient experiences. The book gathers great minds in healthcare to make it unique from others. Each chapter uses a collective voice to shape the future of healthcare. The authors provide practical strategies for healthcare leaders to face the challenges regarding innovation, complexity, systems, and partnership in healthcare.

The book comprises five parts, which support leadership development in clinical practice or academic settings. With an emphasis on collaboration and partnerships, it moves away from hierarchical forms of leadership to more engaged, open, equitable, inclusive, authentic, and caring styles. Following is a brief introduction of the five parts.

Part 1 presents leadership theories in organizations. There are four chapters in this part, which are closely connected. The first chapter introduces the evolution of leadership theories from ancient times to the present. It ends with contemporary theories, including transformational, complexity, and visionary leadership. Chapter 2 examines nursing as both discipline and profession shaped by the conditions and attributes of influential nurse leaders, historically relevant theoretical and philosophical perspectives, and the paradigm shifts in healthcare. Using the past, present, and future of leadership viewed in the context of Hindsight, Insight, and Foresight leadership, new leadership literacies are explored that are essential to navigate evolving systems of practice. Chapter 3 fosters thinking around leadership concepts. It emphasizes that a greater understanding of complex adaptive systems and the neuroscience of interactions provide the framework for healthcare leadership development and implications for practice. For example, the multiple leadership development programs and academies from Sigma Theta Tau International Honor Society of Nursing (Sigma) are discussed to express how our knowledge and use of leadership tools have evolved over the years. Chapter 4 presents approaches to help readers develop effective leadership skills and capacity. The chapter introduces strengths-based leadership, positive leadership, power, and politics and provides tips for readers to promote effective communication, conflict management, team-building, and leadership influences.

Part 2 addresses healthy work environments. The four chapters in this part support readers in establishing and promoting organizational culture and environments. Chapter 5 discusses ways to nurture a healthy and healing environment, followed by Chapter 6, which specifies leadership's roles in promoting a resilient workforce. Chapter 7 identifies leadership's opportunities in mitigating organizational trauma and offers supportive strategies from a Caring Science perspective. Chapter 8 discusses planetary and environmental health, which is instrumental in leading and enhancing human-universe relationships.

Part 3 introduces and explains ways to apply novice leadership theories to practice. Chapter 9 explains Quantum Leadership and ways to integrate it into nursing. Chapter 10 introduces caring leadership, using Caring Science to guide leadership practice. Chapter 11 exemplifies organizational strategies to promote exceptional patient experience through Compassionate Connected Care. Chapter 12 uses complexity theory to inform population and community health. The chapter uses global examples to illustrate how leaders promote population and community health globally.

Part 4 is about collaboration, leading change, and innovation. Chapter 13 enlightens a unifying workforce to improve interprofessional collaboration and healthcare, followed by Chapter 14, which reinforces leadership's roles in collaboration for disaster preparedness and response. Chapter 15 further enforces collaboration and leading change at a global level. Chapter 16 focuses on promoting research, quality, and evidence-informed practice.

Part 5 is about envisioning the future of healthcare leadership. Chapter 17 defines the nature of wisdom leaders to inform personal and professional leadership development. It describes the strategies and tools to develop wisdom leadership capacities to support career development and building wisdom in healthcare organizations. Chapter 18 addresses diversity, equity, and inclusion in academia and clinical settings and provides specific strategies and recommendations to support Black, Indigenous, and people of color scholars. The chapter calls nurse leaders to recognize racism in healthcare and lead forward. Chapter 19 calls for advocacy and policy change. Chapter 20 further discusses leadership in social and political determinants of health. The book's final chapter, Chapter 21, calls on leaders to create a more connected world through Ethics of Face and Belonging.

Finally, this book guides readers to explore leadership possibilities and prospects from different standpoints. Our interpretation of leadership continues to grow. Through this leadership book, we hope readers create a vision beyond our current systems toward a global, life-sustaining perspective, inspired and moved to actions that promote the transformation and revolution of healthcare by leading to sustainable health and humanity.

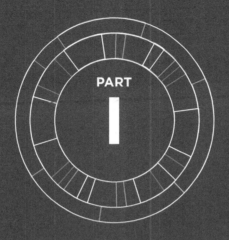

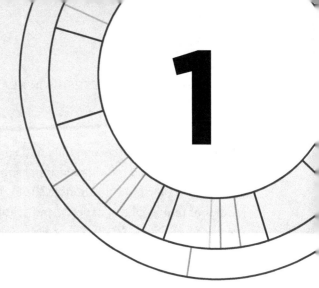

# THE EVOLUTION OF LEADERSHIP THEORIES

Holly Wei, PhD, RN, NEA-BC, FAAN
Sylvia T. Brown, EdD, RN, CNE, ANEF
Phyllis N. Horns, PhD, RN, FAAN

## LEARNING OBJECTIVES

After completing this chapter, you should be able to understand the:

- Evolution of leadership theories
- Definitions of leadership theories
- Strengths and weaknesses of the theories
- Implications of the theories in leadership practice

The world is constantly changing, and so is the development of leadership theories. Leadership is a multidimensional subject, and numerous factors determine successful leadership (Northouse, 2021). *Leadership theories* are the views and studies of philosophers, experts, and scholars describing the qualities making great leaders (Yukl, 2019). Diverse schools of thought express different beliefs on what makes a great leader, such as inborn traits, learned behaviors, and relationship based leadership.

The practice of leadership has changed significantly over time. Beginning with the Great Man Theory from the 19th century, the search for effective leaders and leadership styles continues. Throughout leadership's evolving history, the practice of leadership has gone through the following major leadership theories:

- Great Man Theory (the mid- to late-1800s)

- Trait Theory (the 1910s–1940s)

- Behavioral Theory (the 1950s–1970s)

- Contingency Theory (the 1960s–1990s)

- Contemporary Theory (the 1970s onwards)

# GREAT MAN THEORY

The Great Man Theory was mainly documented in the mid-late 1800s. The saying "Great leaders are born, not made" summarizes a fundamental belief of the Great Man Theory (Carlyle, 1888/2013). The theory believes that the ability of one's leadership is innate. According to the Great Man Theory, leaders' capabilities are naturally inborn and not acquired (Spector, 1874/2016). One is either born as a leader or not. The phrase "Great Man" was utilized because, in the 1800s, male superiority was largely unquestioned.

The Great Man Theory became prevalent in the 19th century, with an underlying assumption that leaders were heroes. The Great Man Theory was popularized by a Scottish historian and philosopher, Thomas Carlyle, in the 1840s and furthered by Francis Galton in his book *Hereditary Genius* (1892/2000). According to Carlyle, the world's history was mainly the biography of great men, and effective leaders exhibited exceptional inspirations and great characters (Carlyle, 1888/2013). Galton (1892/2000) described leadership as an inimitable property gifted to exceptional people whose leadership characteristics were immutable and could not be learned or developed. In addition, the mythology behind some great leaders, such as Plato, Lao Tzu, Aristotle, Julius Caesar, and Alexander the Great, led to the thought that great leaders were born and not made.

Some of the earliest leadership research studied those people who were already prominent leaders. Some of these people took leadership positions through their birthright, such as the aristocratic rulers. The notion was that people with higher social status were more able to achieve leadership positions and become successful figures than those with lower social status and fewer opportunities to attain leadership positions. This phenomenon led to the concept that leaders were born, and leadership was an innate ability. However, a noted philosopher and sociologist, Herbert Spencer (1874/2016), proposed a contrasting perspective on the theory. He contended that leaders are the creation of the society and social situations of their time. In his book *The Study of Sociology*, Spencer believed that before leaders changed society, society had changed them. Thus, society and social environments created leaders at the time.

The Great Man Theory is one of the earliest means to explore leadership. It ignited researchers' interest in studying the qualities of leadership. The major issues with the Great Man Theory were that it did not consider the complexity of leadership and that not all individuals owning the leadership characteristics were successful leaders. Therefore, research started to study the leadership traits of successful leaders in their time and history, leading to the Trait Theory of Leadership.

# TRAIT LEADERSHIP THEORY

Between the 1910s and 1940s, influenced by the Great Man Theory, Trait Leadership Theory intended to identify the personality characters and inheritable traits tied to great leaders. People assumed that leaders were born with certain personalities and superior traits, setting them apart from the mass society. Some personality traits included persistence, dominance, desire for control, intelligence, energy, self-confidence, self-discipline, self-motivation, responsibility, initiative, social interactions, moral force, aspiration for success, and insightfulness (Mann, 1959; Stogdill, 1948; Stogdill & Coons, 1957). Thus, the foci of leadership studies at the time were on leaders' inborn traits.

However, in 1948, after analyzing leadership works from 1907 to 1947, Ralph Melvin Stogdill, a professor and researcher on leadership and organizations, challenged the traditional trait-based leadership theory. Stogdill (1948) suggested that leaders' traits were not constant across different situations, the descriptions of leadership traits were in no way exclusive, and not all individuals who have leadership traits become leaders. This conclusion has been considered the end of Trait Theory as the mainstream leadership theory. It is believed that while certain leadership traits are great characteristics for leaders to have, leaders' behaviors and the ability to influence were essential to lead. Consequently, behavioral and situational leadership theories have emerged.

# BEHAVIORAL LEADERSHIP THEORY

The Behavioral Leadership Theory was studied mainly between the 1940s and 1970s, a paradigm shift from the Trait Theory. While the Great Man and Trait theories considered leaders to be born with certain personalities and traits, behavioral theories suggested that leadership behaviors can be trained in response to specific situations and that individuals can learn to lead. As a result, leadership research started to focus on the behaviors people could learn and develop to lead and leaders' and followers' behavioral characteristics. Noticeable behavioral leadership studies included Lewin's Behavioral Study, Ohio State University Studies, Michigan Leadership Studies, and Blake and Mouton's Leadership Grid.

# LEWIN'S BEHAVIORAL STUDY

In 1939, psychologist Kurt Lewin led a group of researchers to identify different leadership styles. The researchers assigned schoolchildren into three leadership-style groups, where children participated in an arts and crafts project with an authoritarian, a democratic, or a laissez-faire leader. Researchers monitored the children's behaviors in each group under the different leadership styles. They found that the children under the democratic leaders outperformed those in other leadership styles. In addition, democratic leadership was better in motivating the children to perform. This study was instrumental in establishing more defined leadership styles (Burnes, 2007; Lewin, 1951; Lewin et al., 1939).

## AUTHORITARIAN

The authoritarian leadership style is sometimes called the autocratic style. Leaders tell their subordinates their decisions, such as goals, deadlines, and ways to complete tasks. While making decisions, authoritarian or autocratic leaders tend to decide on their own, seeking little consultation with others. These leaders are usually not involved in group works, less likely to suggest creative choices, and are often seen as dictatorial by others. However, this leadership style is critical in situations requiring immediate actions to meet high-risk, short-timeline results.

## DEMOCRATIC

This leadership style is also called the participative style. Leaders express their priorities for goals, missions, and decisions to colleagues, participate in group works, and accept others' suggestions. Democratic leaders invite other's participation in decision-making processes, yet they make the final decision. This leadership style motivates followers' involvement in problem-solving and innovation more than the authoritarian leadership approach but may take longer to reach the final decision.

## LAISSEZ-FAIRE

The laissez-faire style is sometimes referred to as delegative leadership. These leaders use a more hands-off approach and pass the responsibilities to the group. Laissez-faire leaders allow team members to take charge in setting goals, delineating individuals' roles, and deciding approaches to working and achieving results. This leadership style may work well when leaders trust the team members to be highly motivated and share the same goals as leaders and organizations.

# OHIO STATE UNIVERSITY STUDIES

Conducted in the 1940s, the Ohio State Studies became one of the most significant research series in leadership and organizational behaviors. This study series has transformed how leadership can be studied, measured, and advanced. Researchers developed the Leader Behavior Description Questionnaire and the Supervisor Behavior Description Questionnaire to study leaders' and subordinates' behaviors and enable researchers to explore leadership behaviors systematically (Kerr et al., 1974; Schriesheim & Kerr, 1974). The studies focused on leaders' observable behaviors, found some similar behaviors in successful leaders, and established the two most widely known leadership behavior categories, *initiation of structure* and *consideration* (Fleishman, 1957, 1973, 1995):

- **Initiating Structure Behavior:** Initiating Structure Behavior is task oriented. Leaders' behaviors define the leader-subordinate relationship and subordinates' roles. Subordinates understand what is expected, establish formal lines of communication, and perform tasks as predetermined.

- **Consideration Behavior:** Consideration Behavior is people-oriented and aligns with interpersonal skills. Leaders are concerned for their subordinates and try to create a warm, compassionate, and supportive atmosphere.

Based on the scores in the two dimensions, leaders' behaviors can be categorized into four quadrants: High Consideration and Low Structure, Low Consideration and Low Structure, High Consideration and High Structure, and Low Consideration and High Structure (see Figure 1.1). The four quadrants indicate the leader-subordinate relationships that are associated with subordinates' performance and task outcomes. The Ohio State Leadership Studies suggest that successful leaders can balance work structure and relationships and build a highly functional and cohesive team to accomplish work and achieve team goals.

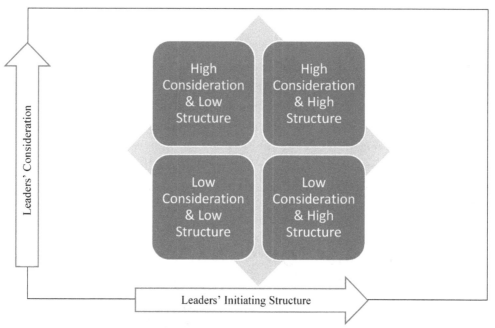

**FIGURE 1.1** Ohio State Model of Leadership (based on the sources by Fleishman, 1957, 1973, 1995).

# MICHIGAN LEADERSHIP STUDIES

The Michigan Leadership Studies were conducted in the 1950s, examining the relationships between supervisors' leadership styles and behaviors and workers' productivity and satisfaction. The studies recognized the leadership styles and principles leading to greater productivity and enhanced job satisfaction among workers. In addition, the behaviors were categorized into two leadership orientations, employee orientation and production orientation:

- *Employee orientation*: Leaders tend to have more relationship-oriented behaviors, care for employees' human factors, and establish effective workgroups with high implementation goals.

- *Production orientation*: Leaders have more task-oriented behaviors and pay more attention to the technical elements of employment and employee performance.

Rensis Likert (1961), a psychologist at the University of Michigan, expanded the studies to explore the differences between effective and ineffective managers. Likert's studies found that production or job-centered managers were less effective and productive than employee-centered managers. The more effective managers set clear goals and empowered employees with the freedom to achieve them. When coupled with general instead of close supervision, the employee-centered leaders could lead to better productivity and satisfaction. The Michigan Leadership Studies recognized the leadership styles that led to the highest employee satisfaction and productivity.

# BLAKE AND MOUTON'S LEADERSHIP GRID

In the 1960s, Blake and Mouton reevaluated the two dimensions (people and structure) of the Ohio State and Michigan studies. As a result, they developed the Blake and Mouton's Leadership Grid, formerly referred to as the Managerial

Grid (Blake & Mouton, 1969). The Leadership Grid helps managers assess their leadership styles and provides ways to become desired managers. The grid uses a two-dimensional grid to indicate leaders' behaviors.

The leadership grid has two axes; the *x*-axis shows leaders' emphasis on tasks, like the initiating structure or job-centered behaviors in the Ohio State Studies. The *y*-axis signifies leaders' concerns for people and aligns with consideration or employee-centered behaviors in Ohio State Studies. Both axes contain a 9-point scale, ranging from 1 (low concern) to 9 (high concern), suggesting leaders' task versus person orientation levels. Blake and Mouton's Leadership Grid suggests five major leadership styles (see Figure 1.2; Blake & Mouton, 1969):

- **Impoverished Management (1, 1):** Impoverished managers have low scores for both production and people. Leaders employ minimal efforts to have the required work completed or uphold interpersonal relationships. This leadership style is comparable to the laissez-faire style, avoiding responsibility and errors.

- **Country Club Management (1, 9):** These managers have a low concern for production and high regard for people. Managers with this style try to avoid conflict and create a safe work environment. The resulting work atmosphere is welcoming and easygoing yet may not be very productive. Highly task-focused individuals may feel frustrated.

- **Authoritarian Management (9, 1):** Authoritarian managers focus more on production than people. This style is consistent with McGregor's Theory X (McGregor, 1960). Authoritarian leaders tend to make decisions with little or no input from their followers.

- **Team Management (9, 9):** These managers show high concerns for both production and people. This management style is often considered the most effective style. It aligns with McGregor's Theory Y (McGregor, 1960), believing that employees are intrinsically motivated, like their job, and want to do a good job.

- **Middle-of-the-Road Management (5, 5):** These managers have moderate concerns for production and people. They try to balance organizations' and employees' needs.

Leadership is a complex concept encompassing a multitude of factors. Being an effective leader requires more than individual traits and behaviors. Successful leadership also needs to consider situations' effects on leadership, which leads to the Contingency Leadership Theories.

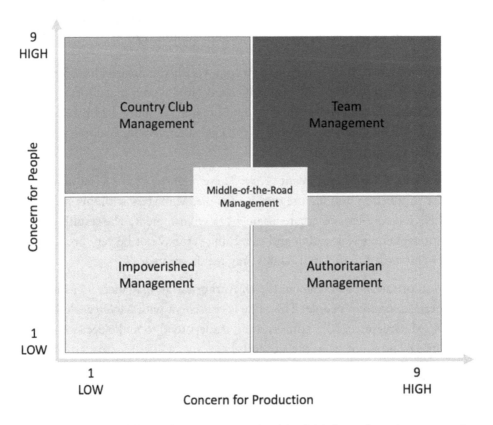

**FIGURE 1.2**   Blake and Mouton's Leadership Grid (based on the sources by Blake & Mouton, 1969).

# CONTINGENCY LEADERSHIP THEORIES

Contingency Leadership Theories were popular between the 1950s and 1990s. The theories suggested that effective leadership was contingent and depended on situations and how well leaders' leadership styles matched the situations involved. It was recognized that merely studying leadership based on individual traits and behaviors could not capture the complexity of situations' effects on leadership (Yukl, 2019). Contingency theories shifted the focus from individual factors to situational characteristics. Analyzing and matching contingent factors and leadership styles can facilitate individuals to lead effectively.

The development of the Contingency Theories was notably influenced by the two leadership studies mentioned in the Behavioral Theory of Leadership, the Ohio State University Studies in the 1940s and the Michigan Leadership Studies in the 1950s. The premise of the Contingency Theories is that the success of leadership is situational. The better the match between leaders' leadership styles and the situations, the more effective their leadership is. Factors determining the success or effectiveness of a leader or leadership style include the leader's personality, group characteristics, and the situation at hand.

Contingency Theories concluded that there could not be one best leadership approach for various organizations. The success and effectiveness of leadership depended on factors such as the tasks at hand, leaders' personalities, and organizational structure. There are four main sub-theories within the Contingency Theories—Fiedler's Contingency Theory, House's Path-Goal Theory, Vroom-Yetton-Jago Decision-Making Model of Leadership, and Hersey and Blanchard's Situational Leadership.

# FIEDLER'S CONTINGENCY THEORY

Fred Fiedler proposed Fiedler's Contingency Theory in the mid-1960s. He studied leaders' characteristics and personalities and believed that individuals had well-established and inflexible leadership characteristics (Fiedler, 1965, 1967, 1970). Leaders are either *task-oriented* (active, structuring, and controlling) or *relation-oriented* (passive, considerate, and permissive). This theory claims leadership success depends on two factors: leaders' leadership style and situational control. Leaders could only improve their leadership effectiveness by electing to be in situations matching their leadership styles.

Fiedler's Contingency Theory proposes that if a manager's style and the situational control are satisfactorily matched, the organization's efficiency can be achieved (Fiedler, 1967). The Least-Preferred Co-Worker (LPC) Scale delineates two factors: leadership styles and situational favorableness (Fiedler, 1972). First, it outlines leadership styles by gauging subordinates with whom leaders are least likely to work to define leaders' personality dispositions and the situations suitable for their style. The second factor of the theory is situational favorableness, a leader's control over a situation. The degree of situational favorableness is determined by the following three factors:

- **Leader-member relations:** The leader-member relations indicate the trust and influence of leaders with subordinates. Leaders who have more confidence and impact in their groups are in more favorable situations than those the group members do not trust.

- **Task structure:** Task structure affects leaders' ability to control situations. Clear goals and structured procedures are favorable situations for leaders.

- **Leaders' position power:** Leaders' position power represents the power they must have to regulate situations and implement rewards or punishments to the groups. The more power leaders have, the more favorable the leaders' situations are.

Once leaders have measured their leadership styles and identified their situational favorableness, effective leadership styles can be determined and fit in certain situations. However, Fiedler's Contingency Theory faces criticisms. One of the main criticisms is the lack of flexibility. The theory believes that leaders' leadership styles are fixed, and the most effective way to control situations is to change leaders.

# PATH-GOAL THEORY

The Path-Goal Theory was first presented by Martin Evans in 1970 and advanced by House in 1971. This theory integrated the Ohio State Studies (consideration and initiating structure) and Victor Vroom's Expectancy Theory of Motivation (1964). The Expectancy Theory claims that individuals are motivated to choose the behaviors that help them reach their goals. The Expectancy Theory posits that there is a direct relationship between individuals' efforts and performance. Excellent performance leads to anticipated rewards satisfying individuals' needs, and there is a strong desire to fulfill the requirement by trying.

House's Path-Goal Theory (1971) postulates that leaders have the responsibility and capability of clearing the path and providing guidance and support to help their subordinates achieve organizational goals. This theory focuses on ensuring that leaders' styles or behaviors fit their situations and subordinates' needs and help their subordinates reach their goals. The goal is to increase employees' motivation, engagement, and satisfaction to become productive members.

House's Path-Goal Leadership Theory comprises four separate but integrated components: Leadership Behaviors, Environmental Factors, Subordinate Factors, and Outcomes. The Leadership Behaviors identified four kinds of leaders:

- **Directive leadership:** Leaders tell subordinates what they should do. Leadership behaviors include setting performance goals and behavior standards, planning, making schedules, and emphasizing rules and regulations.

- **Supportive leadership:** Supportive leaders show concern for subordinates' personal needs and interests. These leaders are open, friendly, and approachable and create an equal and inclusive team environment.

- **Participative leadership:** Leaders consult followers, seek opinions and suggestions, and involve subordinates in decision-making.

- **Achievement-oriented leadership:** Leaders set high expectations for followers, expect them to perform at their best, and trust their ability to meet the expectations.

The combination of Leadership Style, Environmental Factors, and Subordinate Factors determines Outcomes, including subordinates' performance and satisfaction. House and Mitchell (1974) found that leaders could impact subordinates' perceptions and motivation toward organizations' desired outcomes. Managers could do the following to promote efficiency: coaching and guiding subordinates as needed, having clear expectations, eliminating frustrating barriers, and improving subordinates' satisfaction and, thus, performance.

# DECISION-MAKING THEORY

Decision-Making Theory is also known as the Vroom-Yetton-Jago Decision-Making Model of Leadership. The Decision-Making Theory helps leaders identify the best decision-making method and leadership style that leaders can apply to match their particular situations. Victor Vroom and Philip Yetton initially developed this theory in their book, *Leadership and Decision-Making* (1973). Similar to the Contingency Theories' principle that there is no one best way to lead in all situations, the Decision-Making Theory proposes that no single decision-making process can fit every scenario. Instead, the theory intends to guide leaders to select the most suitable decision-making approach for the situations.

Three factors affect decision-making processes. When using this theory to guide decision-making, leaders need to consider the following elements:

- **Decision quality**: Leaders need to utilize resources, such as people, time, and information, to ensure that their actions are well thought out and of high quality.

- **Team commitment**: Some decisions can significantly impact the team, and members need to participate. Team collaboration can promote the quality of the findings.

- **Time constraints**: When time is not the essence for decision-making, leaders can have more opportunities to conduct research and include others involved in the process. If time is limited, it may not be possible to include others or conduct thorough research.

## SITUATIONAL LEADERSHIP THEORY

Situational Leadership Theory believes that one cannot use a static method to lead. Instead, leaders need to modify their styles based on the situation, group composition, and organizational environments. The theory asserts that while organizational structure and settings cannot change, leaders can alter how they lead. Thus, the most successful leaders can adapt their leadership styles to particular situations and their subordinates' maturity and developmental state. These leaders observe the conditions—including tasks, group characteristics, and other factors—influencing job completion.

There are several sub-theories, one of which is Hersey and Blanchard's Situational Leadership Theory. The theory was first introduced as the "Life Cycle Theory of Leadership" (Hersey & Blanchard, 1969) and was further developed and named the Situational Leadership Theory in the mid-1970s (Hersey & Blanchard, 1977).

Hersey and Blanchard's Situational Leadership Theory proposes that the circumstances determine the most applicable leadership style. Leaders need to vary their leadership styles based on three factors:

- *Task behavior* is leaders' clear description of work roles and responsibilities.

- *Relationship behavior* is the personal relationship between leaders and subordinates.

- *Subordinates' maturity level* determines the task behavior and relationship behavior. Subordinates' maturity is characterized by the following criteria: subordinates' motivation level, willingness to take responsibilities, and experience and education.

Depending on employees' needs and abilities, leaders adjust their styles to have the following emphases:

- **Task emphasis**: more on guidance and direction

- **Socio-emotional emphasis**: focusing on relationship support

- **Readiness level** (maturity or development level): ability and willingness to work

As employees grow with knowledge, skills, and abilities, managers may change their leadership styles to increase expectations, fit employees' developmental needs, and modify the amount of directing, coaching, supporting, and delegating. Based on the varying extents of leaders' direction and support, four leadership styles are theorized: Telling, Selling, Participating, and Delegating. Leaders can adjust their styles to fit followers' developmental stages, needs, and abilities.

# CONTEMPORARY LEADERSHIP THEORY

Contemporary Leadership Theory emerged from the 1970s. The contemporary leadership styles acknowledge that leaders are more effective if they recognize the complexity of work and the changing environment. Major contemporary leadership styles include transactional, charismatic, servant, transformational, collaborative, complexity, and visionary.

# TRANSACTIONAL LEADERSHIP THEORY

Transactional leadership became trendy mainly in the 1970s to1990s. Transactional leadership was believed to have evolved from the rational-legal or bureaucratic leadership style proposed by Max Weber, a 20th-century German sociologist. Weber had studied leadership and divided it into three categories: traditional leadership, charismatic leadership, and rational-legal or bureaucratic leadership. The idea of the Transactional Leadership Theory is to exchange, meaning that managers give subordinates something they want, in exchange, to get something the managers want. The basic principle of the exchange is that subordinates require structure, direction, and supervision to complete tasks correctly and on time; in other words, subordinates depend on a reward-penalty system to stay motivated (Bass, 1985; Burns, 1978).

The Transactional Leadership Theory believes that subordinates can be motivated through reward and penalty systems; be managed and controlled by procedures and policies; and require supervision, direction, organization, and performance-watching to complete tasks on time (Bass, 1985; Burns, 1978). This leadership style keeps situations stable and predictable, with an overall goal to produce well-organized and routine procedures. When errors occur, transactional leadership focuses on finding fault and using punishments to solve problems.

Transactional leaders are more likely to lead organizations and programs that depend on rules and regulations to complete tasks and achieve goals on time. This type of leader usually has formal organizational leadership positions and authority to set criteria and evaluate subordinates based on organizations' formally established requirements. Performance reviews are a common way to judge subordinates' performance.

Transactional leadership tends to exhibit the following characteristics:

- **Contingent reward**: Leaders and followers exchange contracts of rewards for effort, ensure employees rewards for good performance, and acknowledge accomplishments.

- **Management by exception**: There are two approaches:
  - *Active leadership approach*: Leaders observe and look for nonconformities from rules and standards. Once finding deviations, they take corrective actions.
  - *Passive approach*: Leaders intervene when employees do not meet standards.

- **Laissez-faire**: Leaders renounce their obligations and avoid making decisions.

Transactional leaders can be a good fit to work with subordinates who like to work in a structured and guided environment and are motivated by the reward-penalty system but not for organizations that value their employees' creative or innovative thoughts. Their focus is to maintain the status quo of an organization—following the existing rules and regulations and maintaining job routines. These leaders are more of a "telling" leadership style, use positive and negative reinforcements, and emphasize self-interest.

# CHARISMATIC LEADERSHIP THEORY

Charismatic leadership primarily occurred in the 1970s–1990s. Leaders use their charm to inspire their followers to make changes. Charismatic leaders use their charming personalities and communication styles to attract and invite followers' admiration (Shamir et al., 1993). These leaders communicate effectively, show their compassion and sensitivity, emphasize social connections, and control their emotions in situations that provoke stress or disturb followers. Charismatic leadership influences others (individuals, groups, and organizations) to make them better entities.

The driving force of the Charismatic Leadership Theory was Max Weber's study on political obligation. Weber found that people followed a leader because they felt that its authority was a suitable form of power. According to Weber (1947, 1968), *charisma* was the characteristic that set leaders apart from ordinary people. It was thought to be the supernatural and superhuman powers or qualities attributed to leaders and regarded as divine. Charismatic leaders were those who had a personality that was attractive, appealing, and influential to followers. There were three types of authority depending on how leaders control others: charismatic authority, traditional authority, and legal and bureaucratic authority. Despite the influence of Weber's work, the charisma concept stayed latent until the 1970s, when scholars started to reexamine and explain this concept.

Robert House (1977) advanced the concept to a more testable theory. House proposed that the core of charismatic leadership was an attributional process in which followers attributed extraordinary abilities to leaders based on leaders' behaviors. House (1977) used four terms to define charismatic leadership: dominant, influential, confident, and a strong sense of personal morality. Based on House's Charismatic Leadership Theory, researchers started to study the characteristics of charismatic leaders.

Charismatic leaders have high self-confidence and high expectations and trust in subordinates (Shamir et al., 1993). The followers of charismatic leaders are loyal to the leaders, admire their actions, trust them, and have confidence in their vision and goals. Charismatic leaders' relationship and connectedness with their followers is profound, facilitating followers' performance and outcomes. The followers of charismatic leaders are willing to place team or organizational goals and interests above their own. Thus, charismatic leaders have a potent influence on followers.

# SERVANT LEADERSHIP THEORY

Robert K. Greenleaf initially presented Servant Leadership Theory in his essay, "The Servant as Leader," in 1970 (Greenleaf, 1977). Servant leadership focuses on meeting people's needs and helping them achieve their visions and goals. Servant leaders have a well-defined and compelling vision that enthuses followers' passion and commitment to achieving goals. This leadership type values followers' strengths and motivates them to use their talents to better their organizations. Greenleaf's writings delineated certain servant leaders' characteristics, such as listening, attending, being empathetic, healing, consciousness, encouragement, prudence, assurance, commitment, and caring for the community (Greenleaf, 1977).

Servant leadership stresses leaders' professional development, self-awareness, and knowledge for them to become better leaders. Servant leaders are committed to serving others, including individuals, organizations, and communities. They achieve desired organizational results and outcomes through serving, giving their whole-hearted attention to followers, and meeting their needs. Instead of using one's power to influence followers down the organizational hierarchy, servant leaders focus on collaborating with followers, building trust, and showing empathy toward them. The theory assumes that followers will reciprocate through an improved commitment to the organization, teamwork, engagement, and performance when leaders care about followers' needs and desires.

Servant leadership recognizes the values of mentorship in helping followers grow and develop personally and professionally. Researchers Blanchard and Hodges (2003) identified three factors servant leaders can use to improve mentorship:

- **Performance planning:** Leaders set goals and objectives to achieve.

- **Day-to-day coaching:** Servant leaders provide support and the environments to help followers achieve the established goals.

- **Performance evaluation:** Leaders evaluate individual performance and provide feedback and suggestions to aid followers' professional developmental needs.

Servant leaders have a giving mentality. They accept the responsibility to help others and invest in others' development and growth. They do not feel superior to their followers, and it is their hope and belief that followers can become leaders when time and occasions permit. This belief drives servant leaders to invest in, coach, and mentor followers to facilitate the process and followers' career advancement. However, there are concerns that servant leaders may be so focused on followers' needs that they fail to care for organizations' needs as a result.

## TRANSFORMATIONAL LEADERSHIP THEORY

Transformational Leadership Theory was started by James V. Downton in 1973, extended by James Burns in 1978, and further developed by Bernard M. Bass in 1985. This leadership style supports leaders to show authenticity and believes that employees are inspired to perform at their best capability. Because transformational leaders lead by aligning employees and organizational goals, employees work toward the organization's mission, goals, and well-being (Bass, 1985; Burns, 1978). Transformational leaders focus on renovation and transformation by inspiring, encouraging, and influencing others to transform and change.

Transformational leaders demonstrate consideration and bonding between leaders and followers. In addition, they exhibit the following characteristics, which can influence employees and promote commitment to meet organizations' goals:

- **Charisma**: Transformational leaders provide vision, instill pride, and inspire employees' confidence and commitment. Leaders with charisma tend to attract people and gain employees' respect and trust.

- **Inspirational motivation**: Leaders are inspirational, have motivational visions and expectations, focus on strengths, and communicate critical purposes in simple language.

- **Intellectual stimulation**: Leaders challenge the existing norms and status quo, encourage innovation, and stimulate intelligence and creative problem-solving.

- **Individualized consideration**: Leaders demonstrate personal care and compassion for followers' well-being, treat everyone as a valued individual, and coach and mentor others.

The transformational leadership style focuses on encouraging, inspiring, and motivating followers to challenge the status quo and make changes to shape organizations' future and success. Transformational leaders inspire followers' visions and insights about organizational outcomes. They foster employees' professional development and growth and mentor them to challenge their thinking and performance.

# COLLABORATIVE LEADERSHIP THEORY

While the previous leadership theories focused more on leader-follower relationships, collaborative leadership emphasizes leadership processes. Collaborative Leadership Theory delineates leaders' course of actions and capacity to engage individuals and groups with diverse backgrounds in cultural values, thoughts, and norms; inspire them to become a cohesive team; and work toward common goals

(Bolden, 2011). The underlying premise of collaborative leadership is that when people get together in constructive ways, they can cultivate visions, create strategies, share common concerns, and work together to achieve organizational goals. Thus, effective collaboration requires collaborative leadership.

Collaborative leadership requires leaders to achieve success by motivating individuals in different groups, bringing them together, creating commonalities, and aligning multiple stakeholders' goals and visions (Borkowski & Meese, 2020; Borkowski & Perez-Deppman, 2019). In complex healthcare settings, collaborative leadership needs to establish and maintain an interactive and synergistic work environment. A cooperative work environment can facilitate understanding, integrate diverse cultures, and unify visions and values. Thus, collaborative leadership can promote collaboration among multiple stakeholders, support interdisciplinary professionals to work together, and improve practices and outcomes.

Collaborative leaders demonstrate the following characteristics:

- Confidence in achieving organizational goals and objectives
- Effective communication skills (especially listening skills) with multiple stakeholders
- Excellent interpersonal skills in decision-making and collaboration

These collaborative skills can be learned and implemented through appropriate training. Collaborative leadership is an important leadership style to lead in diverse and complex settings. Improved collaboration is an essential strategy in facilitating team cohesion and collaboration.

## COMPLEXITY LEADERSHIP THEORY

Whereas collaborative leadership moves attention from leader-follower relationships to leadership processes, Complexity Leadership Theory has further broadened leadership to systems and universal levels and taken systems' complexity and non-linearity into consideration. It looks at systems and how humans and environments, including organizational environments, interact. As a result, Complexity Leadership Theory breaks traditional organizational structure (organized, linear, and predictable) and redefines leadership processes and successes.

Complexity Leadership Theory emerged from complexity science to fit the complexity systems. With ever-changing environments and complex adaptive systems, complexity leadership enables adaptability, facilitates members' performance and innovation, and promotes individuals' everyday interactions in response to the stresses and opportunities in their local contexts, systems, and environments (Plsek & Wilson, 2001; Snowden & Stanbridge, 2004; Uhl-Bien & Marion, 2009). The local systems' responses then interact with and influence one another to generate powerful emergent phenomena (Lichtenstein & Plowman, 2009). However, these interactions and emergences are challenging to produce because of the bureaucracy and silos that healthcare organizations practice and encounter, creating obstacles to interconnectivity.

Complexity leadership applies complexity theory in leadership practice and organizational behaviors (Marion & Uhl-Bien, 2001). An adaptive system comprises a collection of interacting or interrelated entities that are unified to react and respond to changes in the dynamic systems or environments. There is no hierarchy of power, command, or control in complex adaptive systems. Yet, organizations continuously re-organize based on constant feedback processes to find the best fit in the constantly changing environments.

This leadership theory helps leaders understand organizations as dynamic and complex systems of social interactions. Complexity leaders have complexity thinking (versus linear cause-effect thinking), look at the trends, constantly evaluate what is working and what is not, and create the conditions for emergence (Uhl-Bien, & Arena, 2018; Uhl-Bien & Marion, 2009). This adaptation helps systems get to the new order. Leaders can implement complexity leadership in an organization through (Marion & Uhl-Bien, 2001; Uhl-Bien & Arena, 2018; Uhl-Bien & Marion, 2009):

1.  Creating space for change and innovation

2.  Fostering natural interactions taking place in organizations

3.  Accepting and increasing organized complexity

4.  Enabling instead of dictating organizational change

5.  Fostering autonomy and self-responsibility

Complexity Leadership Theory emphasizes social interactions and networks as the driving force for autonomy, self-responsibility, and performance.

# VISIONARY LEADERSHIP THEORY

Emerging in the 1980s, *visionary leadership* refers to constructing and communicating a compelling sense of vision, direction, and purpose to work for an organization (Nanus, 1992; Sashkin, 1988). Visionary leaders use clear visions as the foundation of their work. The leaders create their vision, integrate it with their mission, and help team members build a shared vision. The shared vision bonds individuals to align their goals and create a coherent team. Visionary leadership is significantly associated with team creativity and innovation through personal and organizational goal alignment (Mascareño et al., 2020; Taylor et al., 2014; Wei et al., 2020). With visionary leaders, team members work together and are committed to promoting organizational effectiveness.

Visionary leaders apply transformational and charismatic behaviors and characteristics to gather followers' dedication and promote organizational effectiveness. Visionary leaders demonstrate the following prominent attributes:

- Merging personal beliefs with organizational principles

- Creating and attaining shared goals with high commitment

- Developing organizational culture to promote a clear vision

- Being a visionary and innovator to stimulate team creativity

- Painting a future image to motivate others' commitment

Visionary leaders have a clear vision about the goals that organizations can achieve and the directions they go. Teams' commitment and creativity are achieved when they align personal and organizational missions and goals. Visionary leaders have an image of their organizations in the future. Effective communication skills help team members see the picture they paint for the organizations in the future and encourage them to get on board and contribute.

# IMPLICATIONS FOR PRACTICE

Leadership and healthcare exist in complex organizations, which require both skill and knowledge by nurse leaders. The healthcare arena can be characterized as ever-changing and filled with uncertainty and unpredictability. It involves the use of various leadership theories to resolve multifaceted problems that occur in an organization. Leadership is not a one-size-fits-all approach. It is essential to understand the advantages and disadvantages of various leadership theories so nurses can utilize an appropriate approach and solution to resolve complicated issues. Effective leadership does take practice to ensure a culture of safety that results in positive patient outcomes and a positive work environment for staff. We have all heard the saying "practice makes perfect." While leadership practice is not that simple, as one encounters problems and uses various leadership theories in the clinical context, lessons can be valuable for future encounters and situations.

The development of leadership skills requires introspection into one's belief systems, abilities, and values. A deep reflection about oneself helps build self-awareness of strengths, weaknesses, and leadership qualities. A leader needs introspection time to contemplate the culture, vision, and goals one has for the organization. A deeper understanding of what leadership theories would be most effective to utilize can become more evident through self-analysis. Ethics play a vital role in the leadership process because it is imperative for leaders to treat followers and their ideas with respect and dignity.

Clinical leaders have a significant impact on their teams, which ultimately affects the quality of care and the effectiveness of the health system, directly impacting patient outcomes. Leaders with high emotional intelligence will invest in others and bring together a more motivated team that will focus on a shared vision. Productivity and performance are directly influenced by the leader's influence on the organizational culture. A set of shared values defined, developed, and inspired by the leader helps achieve a successful organization. When leaders make diversity, inclusion, and equality a priority, it can help nurse retention and staff engagement. In addition, it sets the climate for an environment that transcends to patients and their families. Staff empowerment through creating opportunities leads to the team's growth, enhanced self-confidence, and the ability to handle change and uncertainty in a complex environment. As leaders, coaching and mentoring nurses to identify their strengths will help them build confidence and competence.

Leaders must work collaboratively with others, including other health professionals. Healthcare is a team effort. As nurse leaders, it is critical to advocate for reform efforts to improve patient outcomes and needed reform in the healthcare system. Interprofessional collaboration can lead to improved patient outcomes, a better patient experience, and greater job satisfaction. Serving in roles from the bedside to the boardroom will improve and redesign the practice environment's healthcare system. As leaders, it is critical to bring a nursing perspective to influence health policy decision-making.

# SUMMARY

Leadership theories have developed over time from focusing on leaders' personality traits to considering a complex system with continuous interactions and interrelationships among leaders, followers, and situations. Many theories have emerged over time and will continue to evolve as change occurs. The advantages and disadvantages of each theory should be considered as leaders achieve the most effective outcome. Exploring the historical development of leadership theories provides a perspective on the complexity of the concept of leadership. No one theory has the solution to all leadership problems. Flexibility is essential in determining approaches to use in different encounters that one experiences daily. The challenge for leaders is to know which leadership theory is most relevant to achieve the organization's goals and apply the theory effectively in practice. Understanding various leadership theories can assist the leader in determining the right approach to use in a situation. Knowledge of leadership theories is a crucial tool to help leaders achieve success in the work environment.

# REFLECTIVE QUESTIONS

1.  How are Collaborative Leadership Theory and Complexity Leadership Theory similar? Different?

2.  What leadership style might be most effective in a situation where immediate action is required? Why?

3.  What are the four characteristics of transformational leaders?

4.  According to Situational Leadership Theory, what factors determine the appropriate leadership style?

5.  Explain how Behavioral Leadership Theory is different from Trait Leadership Theory.

# NARRATIVE

As a result of the COVID-19 pandemic, the healthcare industry has seen unprecedented disruption in its priorities, operations, and outcomes, challenging leadership and management to be much nimbler. Numerous changes in hospital patient population and services available have shifted to accommodate the influx of often seriously ill COVID-19 patients. At one hospital, all ancillary operations—outpatient surgery, hospice, wellness centers, community outreach, etc.—were closed and those staff either "rifted" or reassigned.

Your unit manager is preparing to move 25% of the nursing staff to help cover the growing COVID-19 units. At a staff meeting, the manager informs the group that this will be done by lottery, and anyone selected who refuses to go will be terminated.

Your friend who works on another unit informs you that his manager plans to poll all nurses to ascertain their thoughts and willingness to take on this new assignment and, if needed, confer individually with staff before making decisions.

Another colleague reported that her manager informed staff that it would be up to them to decide who would go to the COVID-19 units and that the group decision would be final.

What management styles are these three managers exhibiting?

# AUTHOR BIOGRAPHIES

**Holly Wei, PhD, RN, NEA-BC, FAAN,** is a Professor and Assistant Dean for the PhD program at the University of Louisville School of Nursing. Her overarching research focuses on healthcare organizational culture, leadership development, clinician well-being, stress genomic biomarkers, and patient care quality. She is known nationally and internationally for her nursing practice models and a Convergent Care Theory. Multiple healthcare systems have used Wei's nursing models to guide practice and promote organizational culture and patient care with significant improvements in nursing practice and patient care quality.

**Sylvia T. Brown, EdD, RN, CNE, ANEF,** Dean and Professor, East Carolina University College of Nursing, has spent most of her professional academic career at ECU, having served over 40 years in a variety of roles from faculty member, Associate Dean for Graduate Programs, to her current role as Dean of the ECU College of Nursing since 2009. As the dean of a college with over 1,400 students and over 130 faculty and staff, organizational culture and leadership is of high interest and importance. A widely published scholar, Brown's research interests include leadership development, organizational culture, contemporary pedagogical strategies for nursing education, and pain management.

**Phyllis N. Horns, PhD, RN, FAAN,** Professor, Director of the East Carolina Consortium for Nursing Leadership, former Vice Chancellor for Health Sciences, East Carolina University College of Nursing, has unique leadership status as one of East Carolina University's most outstanding graduates and distinguished administrators. She has successfully pioneered leadership roles in healthcare and academia time and again, serving 19 years as Dean of the ECU School of Nursing and 10 years as Vice Chancellor for Health Sciences, where she led programs in Medicine, Dental Medicine, Allied Health Sciences and Nursing. Under her leadership, Health Sciences grew markedly in program offerings, enrollment, faculty, and staff; expanded facilities for state-of-the-art disciplinary and interprofessional teaching, research, and clinical care; launched doctoral programs in Nursing, PT, OT, CSDI, Public Health, and Dentistry. She has held major leadership roles in state, national, and international professional organizations. Leadership is her life's work. Horns holds a BSN from ECU, MPH from UNC-Chapel Hill, and PhD from UAB.

# REFERENCES

Bass, B. M. (1985). *Leadership and performance beyond expectations*. Free Press.

Blake, R. R., & Mouton, J. S. (1969). *Building a dynamic corporation through grid organization development*. Addison-Wesley Pub. Co.

Blanchard, K. H., & Hodges, P. (2003). *The servant leader: Transforming your heart, head, hands, & habits*. Thomas Nelson.

Bolden, R. (2011). Distributed leadership in organizations: A review of theory and research. *International Journal of Management Reviews, 13*(3), 251–269. https://doi.org/10.1111/j.1468-2370.2011.00306.x

Borkowski, N., & Meese, K. (2020). *Organizational behavior in health care* (4th ed.). Jones and Bartlett Publishers.

Borkowski, N., & Perez-Deppman, B. (2019). Collaborative leadership. In L. Rubino, S. Esparza, and Y. S. Reid Chassiakos (Eds.), *New leadership for today's health professionals: Concepts and cases* (2nd ed., pp. 175–189). Jones and Bartlett Publishers.

Burnes, B. (2007). Kurt Lewin and the Harwood studies: The foundations of OD. *The Journal of Applied Behavioral Science, 43*(2), 213–231. https://doi.org/10.1177/0021886306297004

Burns, J. M. (1978). *Leadership*. Harper & Row.

Carlyle, T. (1841/2013). *On heroes, hero worship, and the heroic in history*. D. R. Sorensen & B. E. Kinser (Eds.). Yale University Press.

Downton, J. V. (1973). *Rebel leadership: Commitment and charisma in the revolutionary process*. Free Press.

Evans, M. G. (1970). The effects of supervisory behavior on the path-goal relationship. *Organizational Behavior and Human Performance, 5*, 277–298.

Fiedler, F. E. (1965). Engineer the job to fit the manager. *Harvard Business Review, 43*, 115–122.

Fiedler, F. E. (1967). *A theory of leadership effectiveness.* McGraw-Hill Book Company.

Fiedler, F. E. (1970). The contingency model: A theory of leadership effectiveness. In C. W. Backman & P. F. Secord (Eds.), *Problems in social psychology* (pp. 279–289). McGraw-Hill Book Company.

Fiedler, F. E. (1972). Personality, motivational systems, and behavior of high and low LPC persons. *Human Relations, 25*(5), 391–412. https://doi.org/10.1177/001872677202500502

Fleishman, E. A. (1957). A leader behavior description for industry. In R. M. Stogdill, & A. E. Coons (Eds.), *Leadership behavior: Its description and measurement.* Ohio State University, Bureau of Business Research.

Fleishman, E. A. (1973). Twenty years of consideration and structure. In E. A. Fleishman, & J. G. Hunt (Eds.), *Current developments in the study of leadership* (pp. 1–40). Southern Illinois University Press.

Fleishman, E. A. (1995). Consideration and structure: Another look at their role in leadership research. In F. Dansereau, & F. J. Yammarino (Eds.), *Leadership: The multiple-level approaches* (pp. 51–60). JAI Press.

Galton, F. (1869/1892/2000). *Hereditary genius: An inquiry into its laws and consequences.* Third corrected proof of the first electronic edition based on the text of the second edition 1892. Macmillan and Co. https://galton.org/books/hereditary-genius/text/pdf/galton-1869-genius-v3.pdf

Greenleaf, R. K. (1977). *Servant leadership: A journey into the nature of legitimate power and greatness.* Paulist Press.

Hersey, P., & Blanchard, K. H. (1969). Life cycle theory of leadership. *Training and Development Journal, 23*(5), 26–34.

Hersey, P., & Blanchard, K. H. (1977). *Management of organizational behavior: Utilizing human resources* (3rd ed.). Prentice Hall.

House, R. J. (1971). A path-goal theory of leader effectiveness. *Administrative Science Quarterly, 16*, 321–328.

House, R. J. (1977). A 1976 theory of charismatic leadership. In J. G. Hunt & L. L. Larson (Eds.), *Leadership: The cutting edge* (pp. 189–207). Southern Illinois University Press.

House, R, J., & Mitchell, T. R. (1974). Path-goal theory of leadership. *Contemporary Business, 3*, 81–98.

Kerr, S., Schriesheim, C. A., Murphy, C. J., & Stogdill, R. M. (1974). Toward a contingency theory of leadership based upon the consideration and initiating structure literature. *Organizational Behavior and Human Performance, 12*(1), 62–82. https://doi.org/10.1016/0030-5073(74)90037-3

Lewin, K. (1951). *Field theory in the social sciences.* Harper & Row.

Lewin, K., Lippitt, R., & White, R. K. (1939). Patterns of aggressive behavior in experimentally created "social climates." *The Journal of Social Psychology, 10*, 271–299. https://doi.org/10.1080/00224545.1939.9713366

Lichtenstein, B. B., & Plowman, D. A. (2009). The leadership of emergence: A complex systems leadership theory of emergence at successive organizational levels. *The Leadership Quarterly, 20*(4), 617–630. https://doi.org/10.1016/j.leaqua.2009.04.006

Likert, R. (1961). *New patterns of management.* Garland Science Publishing.

Mann, R. D. (1959). A review of the relationships between personality and performance in small groups. *Psychological Bulletin, 56*(4), 241–270. https://doi.org/10.1037/h0044587

Marion, R., & Uhl-Bien, M. (2001). Leadership in complex organizations. *The Leadership Quarterly, 12*(4), 389–418. https://doi.org/10.1016/S1048-9843(01)00092-3

Mascareño, J., Rietzschel, E., & Wisse, B. (2020). Envisioning innovation: Does visionary leadership engender team innovative performance through goal alignment? *Creativity and Innovation Management, 29*(1), 33–48. https://doi.org/10.1111/caim.12341

McGregor, D. M. (1960). *The human side of enterprise.* McGraw-Hill.

Nanus, B. (1992). *Visionary leadership: Creating a compelling sense of direction for your organisation.* Jossey-Bass.

Northouse, P. G. (2021). *Leadership: Theory and practice* (9th ed.). SAGE Publications, Inc.

Plsek, P. E., & Wilson, T. (2001). Complexity science: Complexity, leadership, and management in healthcare organisations. *BMJ: British Medical Journal, 323*(7315), 746–749. https://doi.org/10.1136/bmj.323.7315.746

Sashkin, M. (1988). The visionary leader: A new theory of organizational leadership. In J. A. Conger & R. N. Kanungo (Eds.), *Charismatic leadership: The elusive factor in organizational effectiveness* (pp. 122–160). Jossey-Bass.

Schriesheim, C., & Kerr, S. (1974). Psychometric properties of the Ohio State leadership scales. *Psychological Bulletin, 81*(11), 756–765. https://doi.org/10.1037/h0037277

Shamir, B., House, R. J., & Arthur, M. B. (1993). The motivational effects of charismatic leadership: A self-concept based theory. *Organization Science, 4,* 577–594.

Snowden, D. J., & Stanbridge, P. (2004). The landscape of management: Creating the context for understanding social complexity. *E:CO, 6*(1–2), 140–148. https://citeseerx.ist.psu.edu/viewdoc/download?doi=10.1.1.452.1904&rep=rep1&type=pdf

Spencer, H. (1874/2016). *The study of sociology.* Palala Press.

Stogdill, R. M. (1948). Personal factors associated with leadership: A survey of the literature. *Journal of Psychology, 25,* 35–71.

Stogdill, R. M., & Coons, A. E. (Eds.). (1957). *Leader behavior: Its description and measurement.* Ohio State University, Bureau of Busin.

Taylor, C. M., Cornelius, C. J., & Colvin, K. (2014). Visionary leadership and its relationship to organizational effectiveness. *Leadership & Organization Development Journal, 35*(6), 566–583. https://doi.org/10.1108/LODJ-10-2012-0130

Uhl-Bien, M., & Arena, M. (2018). Leadership for organizational adaptability: A theoretical synthesis and integrative framework. *The Leadership Quarterly, 29*(1), 89–104. https://doi.org/10.1016/j.leaqua.2017.12.009

Uhl-Bien, M., & Marion, R. (2009). Complexity leadership in bureaucratic forms of organizing: A meso model. *The Leadership Quarterly, 20*(4), 631–650. https://doi.org/10.1016/j.leaqua.2009.04.007

Vroom, V. H. (1964). *Work and motivation.* Wiley.

Vroom, V. H., & Yetton, P. W. (1973). *Leadership and decision-making.* University of Pittsburgh Press.

Weber, M. (1947). *The theory of social and economic organization* (T. Parsons, Trans.). Free Press.

Weber, M. (1968). *Max Weber on charisma and institutional building* (S. N. Eisenstadt, Ed.). The University of Chicago Press.

Wei, H., Corbett, R. W., Ray, J., & Wei, T. L. (2020). A culture of caring: The essence of healthcare interprofessional collaboration. *Journal of Interprofessional Care, 34*(3), 321–334. https://doi.org/10.1080/13561820.2019.1641476

Yukl, G. A. (2019). *Leadership in organizations* (9th ed.). Pearson-Prentice Hall.

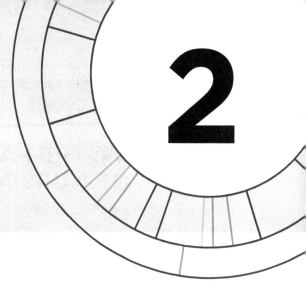

# 2

# GLOBAL PERSPECTIVES ON THE EVOLUTION OF NURSING LEADERSHIP

Gwen Sherwood, PhD, RN, FAAN, ANEF
Wipada Kunaviktikul, PhD, RN, RM, FAAN
Sara Horton-Deutsch, PhD, RN, PMHCNS, FAAN, ANEF

---

## LEARNING OBJECTIVES

After completing this chapter, the learner will be able to:

- Examine the distinction between the profession and the discipline of nursing

- Describe key attributes and expectations of nursing leaders from past, present, and future perspectives

- Apply theoretical and philosophical knowledge to nursing leadership

- Catalyze conversations and actions for global leadership development

---

## OVERVIEW: THE PAST, PRESENT, AND FUTURE OF NURSING LEADERSHIP

Nursing leadership is integrally linked to the history of the discipline and profession of nursing. The journey has been driven by a number of leading nurses during the 20th century who advanced the foundations, science, and practice of nursing. For nursing to continue to advance as a scholarly discipline and practice profession requires examining historical perspectives, contemporary influences, and confounding models and theories to reimagine a contemporary leadership vision to guide nurses.

This chapter examines nursing as both discipline and profession shaped by the conditions and attributes of influential nurse leaders, historically relevant theoretical and philosophical perspectives, and the paradigm shifts that illustrate the ever-changing healthcare environment. Using the past, present, and future of nursing leadership viewed in the context of Hindsight, Insight, and Foresight leadership informs the foundations of new leadership literacies essential to navigate evolving systems of practice (Pesut, 2019). Hindsight leadership builds from reflection on where we have been and helps visualize where we are now through current Insight. Insight leadership is experienced in the present, reflecting in action as a habit of the mind for situational awareness to adapt and evolve according to context. Foresight leadership stems from situation monitoring to anticipate likely scenarios emerging from current trends to be prepared for whatever may happen. Principles from these perspectives undergird explorations in this chapter of how leadership has been described, utilized, researched, and adapted in nursing to move to reimagining leadership futures.

# HINDSIGHT: EVOLUTION OF THE DISCIPLINE AND PROFESSION OF NURSING

Nursing has been variously described as a profession, a discipline, and/or an occupation (Northrup et al., 2004). Over the past few decades, the debate has examined nursing as embedded in its own distinctive knowledge base, experiences, purposes, and values versus its disciplinary status. Yet, learning from Hindsight, for nursing to advance as a scholarly academic discipline and practice profession, relationships among historical events, contemporary influences, and confounding definitions must be examined to guide and shape the evolution and leadership of nursing scholarship, practice, and education.

Now more than ever, it is important to understand and appreciate how the discipline informs the profession of nursing and serves as a guide to impact health and humanity globally. Disciplinary knowledge, grounded in nursing theories, informs professional identity and leadership paradigms. Therefore, understanding and valuing the discipline prepares and guides the profession of nursing and serves as a moral compass to meet nursing's covenant to humankind.

The discipline holds the timeless values, heritage, and traditions of the profession of nursing. The discipline adheres to nursing's philosophical orientation toward humanity and the global ethical covenant with humanity to sustain human caring-healing-health (Watson, 2017). The discipline holds nursing theories and orientation toward knowledge development and encourages critical discourse on what counts as knowledge for a more expansive view than utilitarian, conventional, medicalized ways of knowing alone. Diverse and innovative methodologies and orientations align with caring, healing, and person-centered health-illness experiences for which nursing is known. In essence, the discipline decides what counts as knowledge while the profession is associated with the unique knowledge it holds.

It is this convergence of knowledge, values, ethics, and caring that shapes nursing leadership. However, Watson (2017) has noted that nursing as a profession has detoured from its disciplinary foundation. The rise of external crises from new economics, management science, information overload, and technology contribute to medicalized, hospital-based practices and policies.

Yet, all members of the profession are expected to demonstrate their expression of nursing's unique knowledge and apply it in the work they do every day. Membership into the profession is earned, requiring members to express their leadership by demonstrating the ability to utilize their unique knowledge to advance the profession's roles and contributions to benefit the patient experience, co-create the work environment, and help shape healthcare. Nurses have the capacity to influence, drive change, and call for action through collective impact, the very definition of leadership.

> **THE DISCIPLINE OF NURSING IS CONCERNED WITH HOW NURSES INTERACT WITH PEOPLE IN RELATION TO THEIR HEALTH AND WITHIN THEIR TOTAL ENVIRONMENT.**
>
> A profession is **a recognized, disciplined group of individuals who adhere to common ethical standards, driven by** unique knowledge and skills built from a high level of research, education, and training.

# INSIGHT: THEORIES AND PHILOSOPHICAL KNOWLEDGE DRIVING NURSING LEADERSHIP

Leadership happens at the intersection of knowledge, values, and service. Inquiry guides knowledge work and evidence-based caregiving. Chapter 1 demonstrates the array of leadership theories and models that nurses have employed in both practice and academe. Through reflection and developing emotional intelligence, nurses become more conscious and intentional in professional being, thinking, feeling, doing, and acting. Reflection is inner work, mindful inquiry of self, and it results in engaging in outer service. Reflection in-and-on action supports meaning making and managing purpose in one's professional life (Horton-Deutsch & Sherwood, 2008).

# NURSING: A VALUES-BASED PROFESSION

Leadership is at the heart and foundation of nursing. In addition to a knowledge base, nursing as a profession is guided by values and ethics led by a consistent moral compass (Salvage & White, 2019). Values are the cornerstone for effective leadership and guide nursing leadership theory development. Values-based leadership helps build professional collaboration, enhances trust, provides a voice for nurses, and supports staff well-being, empowerment, job satisfaction, patient-focused outcomes, and quality care (James et al., 2021). Values-based leadership is often viewed as synonymous with authentic leadership (Alilyyani et al., 2018). A systematic review exploring values-based leadership in nursing identified three dominant leadership approaches as authentic, servant, and congruent leadership:

- **Authentic leadership** (James et al., 2021) is built on honest and ethical relationships that value the input of others, lead with truthfulness and openness, develop trust, and improve individual and team performance; Triola (2007) linked emotional intelligence with developing authentic leadership.

- **Servant leadership** (Honkavuo et al., 2018) is characterized by putting others first in an inverted pyramid; rather than the workers serving the leader, the leader shares power and works to enable others to improve and foster a positive work environment.

- **Congruent leadership** is recognized by the match of clinical leaders' actions with their values and beliefs and how they influence and unify a group around a common purpose or mission.

# CORE CONCEPTS FOR NURSING LEADERSHIP

Leadership is both art and science; effective leaders gain a knowledge base of leadership models built on evidence combined with the art of working with others effectively. Adopting a model of leadership can provide consistent approaches and interactions with others that help develop trusting relationships. Nurses are taught that all nurses are leaders. Leadership is influencing others to follow a chosen direction or vision. Leadership is knowing and following one's mission and values while inspiring or influencing others to journey together. All nurses have opportunities to lead through patient care, fulfilling positional leadership through formal appointment, or implementing a change in standards or guidelines. Leadership is about change—influencing patients to change health behaviors, faculty to approve curriculum updates, and governing bodies to adopt new policies.

> ## LEADERS MUST HAVE A CONSISTENT FOCUS ON THE MEANING AND PURPOSE, STAYING TRUE TO THEIR MISSION AND CORE VALUES YET ALIGNING WITH THE BIG PICTURE, HENCE MICRO AND MACRO.
>
> Leadership is not random but is purposeful in leading toward a preferred future. Leadership is guided by a common vision and passion. As such, leaders operate as social architects or generators; leaders provide a reason to care by inspiring others to follow the same vision and mission. Leaders are long-term thinkers, owning their role and responsibilities, and thus do not sacrifice long-term value for short-term results.

Leaders represent a group, whether individually or collectively. Therefore, leadership is often viewed in relational terms. Leaders act on behalf of the entire group, organization, or cohort more than for themselves or their own team. Leaders lead whatever the circumstances. Leaders can't opt out, saying, "That's not my job," but must consider overall goals, what others need and how to improve their experience, and advance each person's journey. Effective nurse leaders keep sight of the big picture while simultaneously being mindful of consequences at the micro or human level; that is, they connect the macro and the micro.

# CARING AND COMPASSION DEFINE NURSING LEADERSHIP

Caring is both a value and the core defining attribute for nursing. Solbakken et al. (2018) reported caring from the perspective of nurse leaders as nurturing and growing relationships to ensure best practices. Caring in nursing leadership consciously works among five domains, trying to connect actions that are best for each: 1) the patient, 2) staff, 3) one's superior, 4) oneself, and 5) the organization. As explored throughout this book, caring leaders develop conscious awareness of the various domains to balance equal attention and priorities among each to pursue patient outcomes, organizational mission, and self-care. Caring is a counterbalance with competence in managing multiple organizational demands without losing sight of the priority of the patient's needs with compassion.

As such, **compassion is the essence of effective leadership.** Caring leaders promote healthy relationships and positivity in the organization through empathy, cognitive knowing, and motivation (Johns, 2015). Leadership is about relationships and building connections with others; through empathy, one may need to walk in others' shoes to understand new perspectives.

Compassionate leadership is a mindful call to lead from head, heart, and hands that demonstrates **concern for others and their well-being.** Compassion opens the heart to nurture and bring out the best in others (Johns, 2015). Compassionate leaders have similar characteristics as authentic, servant, and congruent leaders described earlier. As such, they are more engaging, create higher levels of staff engagement, develop trusting relationships, inspire collaboration, and build connections among people (Papadopoulos et al., 2021). Compassionate leaders create environments where employees feel a greater sense of commitment to their organizations through three core domains, as shown in Figure 2.1.

| Empathy: | • Feeling the way another feels even if uncomfortable |
| Cognition: | • Understanding what somebody else is thinking and why through mindful listening |
| Motivation: | • Caring for the concerns of others to reduce suffering |

**FIGURE 2.1** Core domains of compassionate leadership.

Compassionate leadership starts from the inside out. Novice leaders often feel the need to make an impact on followers by acting tough or being abrasive. Compassionate leaders aim to make a difference by leading with inspiration, hope, and resilience. By modeling these attributes for others, compassionate leaders help others *become*, creating a bridge for belonging, which in turn reduces nurse turnover and burnout and enhances patient satisfaction (Saab et al., 2019). Compassionate leaders develop from the intertwining of horizontal and vertical perspectives (Pesut & Thompson, 2018). *Horizontal development* is cognitive learning focusing on the skills of leading and managing. *Vertical development* is reflective and mindful, focusing on lessons from the heart to see people as they are, helping them become and belong.

Watson's Theory of Human Caring is the basis of sustained, high-performance nursing leadership (Pipe, 2008). Like compassionate leadership described above, caring-based leadership is demonstrated through external behaviors grounded from the internal work of self-reflection and growth. A deeper discussion of Caring Science–informed leadership with exemplars is explored in Chapter 10.

> Caring leadership is one way to manage the urgent, high-stakes challenges of the evolving current healthcare environment that can easily bury the personal domains. Self-nurturance and caring-healing leadership of others undergird effective leadership.

Caring and compassionate leaders enhance patient satisfaction and quality of life while also reducing nurse burnout. Saab et al. (2019) measured the perceptions of nursing and midwifery leaders regarding the impact of the "Leaders for Compassionate Care Programme" using the Leaders for Compassionate Care Outcomes Evaluation Questionnaire. Participants reported an increase in their ability and motivation to support peer learning, manage conflict, and build trust with patients by applying what they learned in their practice.

Going further, Cardiff, McCormack, and McCance (2018) applied many of these same principles to develop a model of person-centered leadership. A combination of caring and compassion, person-centered leadership is a groundbreaking, complex, dynamic, relational, and contextualized way of leading that fosters self-actualization, empowerment, and well-being of the entire team, and thus applies in interprofessional practice as well.

Similarly, Leclerc et al. (2020) proposed a human-centered leadership theory to address the chaos of contemporary healthcare. Leadership embedded in complexity science reflects the challenges of modern healthcare delivery with three major constructs: 1) Awakening to cultivate people in a culture of excellence, 2) Connector for building a community of trust, and 3) Upholder to recognize humanity in others through a culture of caring. Further, these constructs help create an environment of excellence, caring, and trust.

The leadership models in this section—caring, compassionate, person-centered, human-centered—share similar characteristics. They are descendants of value-based leadership discussed earlier, illustrating the evolution of nursing leadership over these past decades, and all have common themes of values, authenticity, respect, knowledge, and caring and compassion (O'Conner, 2008). The embodiment of caring competencies by nurse leaders is summed up as communication, relationship management, and building and sustaining trust. These three attributes of caring and compassionate leadership through person-centered and human-centered leadership are the building blocks for healthy work environments and are summarized in Figure 2.2

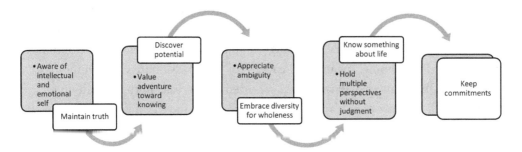

**Figure 2.2**   Nine dimensions of leadership that embody caring.
*Adapted from O'Conner, 2008.*

# FORESIGHT: THEORY-GUIDED LEADERSHIP TO NAVIGATE SYSTEMS TO INFORM PRACTICE

Much of healthcare has experienced mergers, acquisitions, and new payment models in response to healthcare's growing complexity and economics. Traditional bureaucratic leadership responses to "do more with less" have contributed to the increasing frustration with the work environment leading to provider burnout. Uhl-Bien et al. (2020) propose concepts from complexity leadership as a networked approach to enable people and organizations to adapt by "doing things better." Leaders work as collaborators to enhance the adaptability and fitness of the system (rather than working as managers following top-down directives), consistent with the previous discussion of congruent and authentic leadership.

# TRANSFORMATIONAL LEADERSHIP: APPLYING SYSTEMS THINKING

Transformational leadership has become a predominant leadership style practiced by leaders across many industries and disciplines (Giddens, 2018). Characterized by stimulating, inspiring, and motivating followers, transformational leaders focus on building relationships with people and creating change by emphasizing values (Albert et al., 2022). Giddens expands the more prevalent description of transformational leadership within the clinical arena to include the academic context.

Transformational leaders reflect to consider what is needed to match people and circumstances to accomplish goals. Reflective practice provides a guide for the process of learning from experience. Self-awareness is developed through *reflective practice*, the systematic examination of experiences to learn better ways to respond, develop the mental model to continually question how work is performed, monitor processes for reliability, and consciously examine consequences—outcomes—of actions. Reflective practice helps analyze contradictions in practice—how values align with actions—and make sense of challenging situations. Frontline leaders are key to sharing organizational culture and the subset of safety culture. Nurse leaders in both academic and clinical settings are in positions to facilitate and/or support continuing education that focuses on ongoing development in reflective practice and self-awareness and, as such, promotes learning organizations in the quest for continuous improvement.

Transformational leaders are also mindful leaders who use communication, relationship-building, and situational awareness to monitor context (Roussel, 2019). Three key actions of transformational leaders are paying attention, increasing awareness, and being sensitive to others to help build a positive work environment that mitigates risk for preventable harm. Mindful leaders help develop value-based outcomes related to both workers and patients, model clear communication and collaboration, and maintain a spirit of inquiry. These leaders coach team members to openly share ideas, think innovatively, and engage in creative design thinking—playing "what if" and plus thinking that provides alternatives—critical behaviors for leading in complex dynamic healthcare settings (Roussel, 2019).

Systems thinking is a core component of reflective learning organizations, those that want to improve and learn from events, including near misses and preventable harm. To help lead these improvements, nurse leaders must also ground themselves in all forms of knowledge and have skills for translating evidence to practice, promoting best practices. Transformational leaders likewise monitor individual and system responses to maintain situational monitoring and contextual awareness. Mindful leaders embrace transparency across all micro-systems, whether inpatient or outpatient primary care, to improve outcomes across all measurable dimensions.

An early systematic review by Pearson et al. (2007) holds true today in defining nursing leadership attributes that contribute to the development and sustainability of a healthy work environment. Staff and patients helped identify key themes that included developing collaboration, education, emotional intelligence, organizational climate, professional development, and positive behaviors and qualities to sustain a supportive environment. While these characteristics are consistent with the leadership styles mentioned in this chapter (authentic, servant, person-centered, caring, compassionate, and transformational), a combination of leadership styles and characteristics is likely to be more effective in developing and sustaining a healthy work environment than one single style.

## NURSES AS INTERPROFESSIONAL LEADERS

Healthcare occurs in teams. Strong and effective teams include multiple disciplines who collaborate, communicate, and coordinate patient-centered care. Leading teams from multiple professions to function interprofessionally rather than interdisciplinarily calls for unique competencies that have not been a part of nurse leadership development. Typically, each healthcare discipline has treated each patient independently; multidisciplinary teams are not focused on collectively working or seeking input from other team members. Nurses have traditionally accepted the physician as the person responsible for overall patient care. In contemporary healthcare, no one discipline can adequately provide total care. By contrast, the term *interprofessional* is a team-based approach of collective effort in which some responsibilities are shared, including leadership.

Smith et al. (2018) identified a set of core competencies that comprise the Interprofessional Team Leadership framework, enabling diverse members of the team to coordinate their efforts to improve performance and better patient outcomes, shown in Figure 2.3.

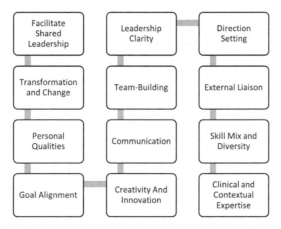

**Figure 2.3**  Leadership competencies for interprofessional healthcare providers.

While most attention is given to leadership characteristics and frameworks, the impact on the workgroup is important. Relational coordination as a leadership framework is similar to the previously discussed authentic, servant, and congruent leadership paradigms. Gittell's (2016) Relational Coordination Theory describes how leaders empower workers through a mutually reinforcing process of communicating and relating to achieve a common purpose.

Smith et al. (2018) described interprofessional leadership as similar to Relational Coordination, which is characterized by shared goals, shared knowledge, and mutual respect for what each brings to the team. Relational Coordination promotes bidirectional, frequent, timely, accurate, problem-solving communication and promotes respect for the unique knowledge of each team member. Relational Coordination is especially relevant when work is interdependent, uncertain, and time-constrained, such as nurses' daily work caring for patients and advanced practice nurses collaborating daily with multiple staff. As such, leaders always need skills in networking, team-building, and providing meaningful recognition. Chapter 13 will further explore how nurse leaders assemble and unify healthcare professions through interprofessional education and collaborative best practices.

## NURSING LEADERSHIP IN THE GLOBAL ARENA

Global nursing leadership has never been more important nor more in the public's eye due to four overlapping signature events. First, the COVID-19 global pandemic reinforced the universality of the nursing profession and highlighted the role of nursing leadership (Losty & Bailey, 2021). Around the world, nurses were hailed for their moral courage as frontline caregivers for a largely unknown and deadly disease. Yet, nurses demonstrated leadership in innovating the virtual connection between isolated patients with COVID-19 and family members unable to visit, redesigned procedures to maintain a safe environment, and joined in an analysis of the constant stream of new information for just-in-time application. COVID-19 was a real lesson in the global benefit of nursing leadership as nurses shared across borders and institutions (Lacy et al., 2020).

Secondly and ironically, 2020 was declared the first-ever Year of the Nurse and Midwife, and nurses demonstrated their leadership across the spectrum of healthcare as the COVID-19 pandemic became the dominant story of nursing (https://www.who.int/campaigns/annual-theme/year-of-the-nurse-and-the-midwife-2020). Thirdly and simultaneously, the World Health Organization released the first *State of the World's Nursing* (2020). Increasing nurse leaders' capacity both educationally and in service is a chief strategy of the report. Fourthly, Nursing Now launched as a global campaign to tie global policy action with local action to create a social movement to advance the image and impact of nurses in policy and decision-making. Nursing Now seeks to create and strengthen strategic nursing leadership in all countries to help nursing deliver its potential. Nursing Now also developed the Nightingale Challenge, focusing on leadership development of a younger generation of nurses (https://www.nursingnow.org).

Globally, nursing leadership has helped shape healthcare with increasing public recognition and in the professional literature. For example, a special topic issue of the *Journal of Nursing Management* in 2014 (Thompson & Hyrkas, 2014) shared the dynamics of global nursing leadership. A sample of recent articles have highlighted building leadership capacity in DNP graduate nursing programs within a global context (Chavez et al., 2019); applying a code of ethics for global leadership (Schick-Makaroff & Storch, 2019); and the role of professional organizations in developing global leaders (Rosser et al., 2017; Shin et al., 2016). Further exploration of attending to global health through nursing leadership can be found in Chapter 15.

Locally and globally, nurses influence policy through empowerment, competency development, and effective leadership, making a difference in the workforce and patient care safety issues (Disch, 2019). Global nurse leaders have been described as bringing a unique ethos akin to servant leadership that shapes the inner core of a caring culture and ethical value base (Kunaviktikul, 2014). Honkavuo et al. (2018) describe this through three patterns of heart, hand, and head found in early 20th century Nordic nurse leaders: 1) serving from the innermost room of the heart, 2) acting through the hands as acts of love, and 3) cultivating the head as knowledge development.

Villarruel (2017) posed an emerging theory of Latina Nurse Leadership. The framework considers leadership as discrete traits or qualities (integrity, vision, professional knowledge, skills and expertise, and emotional intelligence) and as a process in which skills and insights are derived from both professional and personal experiences: Latina cultural knowledge awareness skills, connection to communities, and relational knowledge and skills.

Im et al. (2018) proposed an integrated middle range theory on Asian women's leadership in nursing. The theory included two main domains: leadership frames and leadership contexts. The leadership frame includes human resources/networks, structure/organization, national or international policies, and symbols. Leadership contexts include cultural, sociopolitical, and gender contexts. Later, the researchers refined the middle-range theory on women's leadership in Asian culture by adding two additional main concepts to the domain of leadership context: demographic context and health workforce or system contexts (Im et al., 2020).

# THEORY-GUIDED LEADERSHIP TO INFORM PRACTICE

Leadership is critical in building quality work environments, implementing new models of care, and bringing health and well-being to an overextended nursing workforce. Complex, stressful, and ever-changing work environments, an aging nursing workforce, the continuing impact of the COVID-19 pandemic, and new graduate job changes impact patient outcomes and challenge nurse leaders.

## LEADERSHIP AND THE WORK ENVIRONMENT

Wong, Cummings, and Ducharme (2013) examined the relationship between nursing leadership practices and patient outcomes in a systematic literature review of 20 studies. Results indicate that positive relational leadership styles correlate with higher patient satisfaction and with lower patient mortality, medication errors, restraint use, and hospital-acquired infections. However, the nature of leadership style, how leadership should be enacted, and its associated outcomes require further research and understanding.

Leadership and management are related terms with different foci. Nurses have a more solid foundation in "management" than in "leadership." Laurent (2000) posits that early nursing theorists such as Orem, Roy, Neuman, Henderson, Rogers, and others whose work often formed the theoretical framework for academic curricula focused more on patient management than on leadership. Only Orlando's nursing model includes both patient care management and leadership. More recently, nurse educators in both clinical and academic settings have moved from theory-based curricula to include a wider range of non-nursing leadership models.

Nursing leadership and management are overlapping but unique roles. Jennings et al. (2007) compared leadership and management competencies in a literature review of 140 articles. Many competencies are fused between the roles, leaving considerable ambiguity, particularly for nurse educators in aligning course content to reflect practice realities. Managers are concerned with systems and processes, their position, and operations. Leaders are intentional, capable of turning vision into reality by focusing on people, expanding their thinking, motivating others to be a part, and serving as change agents, innovators, and even disruptors who challenge the process. Leaders seek to remain relevant in an ever-changing world through continuous learning and growth, hallmarks of a professional.

Stanley and Stanley (2018) explored clinical leadership through a comprehensive literature review of 27 studies, noting the dearth of clinical nurse leaders in upper administration. The data synthesis identified four categories: definitions of clinical leadership, characteristics most or least associated with clinical leadership, models applied to clinical leadership, and limits to clinical leadership development. Effective clinical leaders match values and beliefs with actions and interventions to impact innovation, change, and care improvements.

Cummings et al. (2018) examined relationships between various styles of leadership and outcomes on the nursing workforce and their work environments. Six outcome categories were: 1) staff satisfaction with job factors, 2) staff relationships with work, 3) staff health and well-being, 4) relations among staff, 5) organizational environment factors, and 6) productivity and effectiveness. The results revealed definite patterns between relational and task-focused leadership styles and how they impacted nurses and their work environments. Relational leadership styles were associated with higher nurse job satisfaction, whereas task-focused leadership styles were associated with lower nurse job satisfaction. Leadership focused solely on task completion is a barrier to optimal workforce outcomes. Similar to Gittell's Relational Coordination, relational leadership enhances nursing job satisfaction, retention, work environment factors, and individual productivity within healthcare settings.

# LEADERSHIP TO INFLUENCE POLICY

The development of strategic and policy leadership is inadequate in most nursing leadership programs. Nurses are the largest global health discipline and are often the interface between the health system and the community. This connection allows nurses to observe the impact of policy and politics on patients and communities. Nurses have inadequate representation on the boards and higher administration of healthcare organizations. A new paradigm of nursing leadership development can help nurses equalize the balance to ensure influence in decision-making. Furthermore, not only are there too few nurses on boards and in C-suites, but also there remain inequalities among gender, race, and social class representatives.

While policy and politics determine health and nursing practice, few nurses get involved in decisions. They merely carry out decisions made by others (Salvage & White, 2019). Advocacy is an essential leadership skill. *Advocacy* is getting people to listen, care, and act. Learning to use one's voice to speak to the issue to get attention and inform solutions can become a call to action. Learning to advocate and influence policy increases nurses' influence and status while taking advantage of the increasing knowledge base that characterizes professional nursing.

Nurse leaders must be informed, remaining active within the national and multinational arena, applying cross-disciplinary decision processes that drive healthcare practices and policies at home and abroad. Nurse leaders need new tools and knowledge to advocate for policies to benefit nursing. Global nurse leaders must have good knowledge to understand the healthcare system, combined with a vision for developing health and nursing services in their countries. With an understanding of the social and political context, the ability to plan strategically for and manage change, nurse leadership will have the competencies and confidence to be proactive in a challenging change environment. Additional considerations for how nurse leaders transform health policy are explored in Chapter 19.

## INCLUSIVE LEADERSHIP

Nurse leaders underrepresent racial and ethnic diversity. For example, Villarruel (2017) reports Latina and other ethnic and racial minorities deal with overt and covert discrimination and microaggressions in education and the workplace. Microaggressions include comments about language and accents, assumptions about social class, and perceptions of perceived advantages. Villarruel further reported that Latinos in leadership positions are sometimes told that they achieved their position because of their Latino status and because the organization needed diversity in leadership roles. Microaggressions and systemic racism diminish the leadership qualities that a person brings to their position and contribute to dissatisfaction and disillusionment. Chapter 18 expands this discussion.

## LEADERSHIP EDUCATION: TRANSFORMING CURRICULA

Graduate nursing programs need more focus on leadership development to position academic nurses, advanced practice nurses, and clinical nurse leaders to lead change and improvements (Chavez et al., 2019). To achieve systems leadership, Jenkins (2020) described curricular strands to address graduate-level competencies, including organizational and systems thinking to improve quality and safety, advocacy for policy development, and interprofessional collaboration to achieve population health outcomes.

Academic leaders have the opportunity and responsibility to support and encourage faculty to serve as role models and mentors as well as embed leadership theory and practice across nursing curricula. Regardless of the setting, all nurses benefit from mentors and role models. To fully develop leadership capacity, nurses benefit from clinical placements or internships that help them observe leaders in their daily work and see examples of problem-solving, leading change, and building broad networks and relationships. Leadership development is so critical that many institutions offer leadership academies, mentorships, and other coaching opportunities to provide feedback as novice leaders begin to engage in curriculum development, advocate for their patients, participate in shared governance, or lead quality improvement initiatives.

Curricular strands need to blend concepts of patient-centered care, evidence-based practice improvement, systems management, leadership, healthcare technology, quality and safety, integrative therapies, global health, and nursing practices focusing on health promotion and healing. To influence optimal health outcomes, nurses need to be able to lead and deliver comprehensive, coordinated, and compassionate patient-centered care, emphasize patient advocacy through systems leadership in a variety of practice environments, and influence the delivery of complex healthcare to patients across the trajectory of illness (Jenkins, 2020).

Formal learning is important, but informal learning by observing leadership in action is yet another way nurses learn and adopt theory-based leadership. The upcoming sidebar summarizes key points from an interview with Wipada Kunaviktikul, a well-known global leader who reflects on her own journey in leadership development. Her key point is that true leaders never stop learning and growing (Kunaviktikul et al., 2018).

# IMPLICATIONS FOR PRACTICE: INSPIRING ACTION

Nurse leadership has a key role as operator of social systems with human resources in the center. Leadership training is vital to positively affect nurses' job satisfaction and patient care quality indicators. Specchia et al. (2021) reported a significant correlation between leadership style and nurses' job satisfaction. Transformational leadership was associated with the highest number of positive correlations with nurses' job satisfaction, followed by authentic, resonant, and servant styles. A negative correlation was associated with passive-avoidant and laissez-faire styles. The transactional style showed both positive and negative correlations.

Leadership skills are critical during crises; the leader guides the response of the follower. Losty and Bailey (2021) explored the system challenges presented by the COVID-19 crisis and the changes in how healthcare professionals delivered care. Three themes characterized nurse executive leadership and innovation during the COVID-19 crisis: the importance of communication, the need for leadership presence, and mental toughness. Visibility in offering frontline support; maintaining clear, transparent communication; and remaining engaged were strategic leadership approaches that helped sustain the workforce (Rosser et al., 2020). The COVID-19 pandemic also demonstrated the importance of nurses' skills in research and evidence-based practice. As new data constantly evolved, knowing how to access, review, discern, and apply the outpouring of new information to develop new standards to guide practice, keep nurses safe, and maintain communication with patients and families was reflected in nurses' leadership across the pandemic.

**EXEMPLAR: GLOBAL LEADERSHIP IN ACTION**

Because many learn from the examples of others, this interview on developing global leadership for *Nursing and Health Sciences* shares the journey of a noted global leader. Wipada Kunaviktikul, former dean at Chiang Mai University in Thailand, reflected on many of the themes in this chapter. Foremost, leaders must be unafraid of hard work or stretching their comfort zone; both are part of strong leadership. Seeking mentors at strategic times or when approaching new opportunities is a sign of strength, of recognizing the role of continuous learning and improvement. However, more important is the willingness to listen to mentor feedback and coaching. Kunaviktikul named critical leaders' attributes consistent with transformational leadership style: listening, honesty, transparency, emotional intelligence, kindness, and an open mind. Treating others with respect helps build trust; recognizing the need to always be learning helps develop new skills and builds confidence. Leaders provide inspiration, set vision, and lead with purpose. Leaders must be visible and available and reach out to build networks and relationships locally and globally. Kunaviktikul explained that while she primarily subscribes to transformational leadership principles, she also finds it necessary to employ some aspects of transactional leadership to accomplish organizational tasks and human resource responsibilities (Kunaviktikul et al., 2018).

# SUMMARY

Various leadership models were described in this chapter encompassing authentic, servant, congruent, caring, compassionate, relational, and human/person-centered leadership. Using a framework of Hindsight (past), Insight (present), and Foresight (future) Leadership revealed common threads across these progressive models: the feeling of being valued, respected, and understood; working together for shared values, common visions, and purpose; knowing clear roles and responsibilities across the team; and supporting bidirectional team processes and communication. Foresight Leadership helps develop the capacity to anticipate disruptive innovations, manage consequences of challenging trends, and pivot to align with changing paradigms and circumstances. Using systematic reflections in hindsight to interpret lessons from past events and examine insights of current events, and in foresight to envision what can be, leaders use these lessons to reimagine the future.

Caring and compassionate leadership principles prioritize equity and inclusion of all community members and cultivate leaders with unique system leadership skills. Interprofessional leaders co-create with cross-sector partners, measuring and using the information to learn, adapt, and continuously improve. The domains of leadership described in this chapter build on individual and system strengths to improve workplace cultures by fostering relationships, creating trust, and respecting all participants. Global nurse leaders can be a force by influencing policy locally and globally, setting practice standards, and advocating guidelines for compassionate leadership—all help dispel distorted organizational cultures and system obstacles. In conclusion, nursing leadership must be visible, speak up to join decision-making, demonstrate to all nurses the importance of their well-being, maintain person-centered approaches, and harness strengths of active engagement to serve the well-being of patients and every member of the healthcare team.

# REFLECTIVE QUESTIONS

1. Identify a leader who influenced your own leadership journey. What stood out? What is an example of how this person has helped shape you as a nurse leader?

2. How did the global pandemic reveal your leadership capacity? What values and beliefs guided you?

3. What leadership lessons will you take from your experiences during the COVID-19 pandemic? How will you look back five years or even 10 years from now to reflect on this stage of your leadership journey?

4. How do leaders practice inclusive principles to help everyone feel they belong?

5. When is a time that you felt excluded or ignored by your leader? How did you respond? What have you learned from this chapter to guide a future response?

# NARRATIVE

Jennie notices that her post-operative patient has developed a urinary tract infection (UTI). She checks the chart and notes the number of days since the tubing had been changed, but no date is on the tubing. She sighs as she considers this lack of attentive nursing care. Jennie remembers that another nurse had also commented on the increase in UTIs. After confirming the standards of care for post-operative patients with an in-dwelling urinary catheter, Jennie found the other nurse and discussed her concern that the unit nurses may be slack in consistently following the evidence-based guidelines for catheter care. Should they speak up? Jennie has only been working on the unit for a year. She wonders if she has the leadership skills for bringing this to the unit council. Should she ask to lead a quality improvement project? She tries to recall leadership principles from her undergraduate program. While she feels inadequate, knowing that patients experienced unnecessary pain and suffering with a preventable UTI violates her values of quality patient-centered care.

- What steps should Jennie take next?

- What leadership principles can help guide her actions?

- What are ways novice leaders can become more confident in their leadership?

# AUTHOR BIOGRAPHIES

**Gwen Sherwood, PhD, RN, FAAN, ANEF,** Professor Emerita, University of North Carolina at Chapel Hill, is a global leader and mentor working in many countries. Her academic leadership includes Associate Dean for Academic Affairs and the founding Associate Dean for Global Initiatives. She is co-developer of QSEN, the award-winning Quality and Safety Education for Nurses competency model to improve quality and safety implemented nationally and internationally. She is senior faculty in the Academy for Emerging Leaders in Patient Safety and co-editor of four books; two received AJN Book of the Year awards: *Quality and Safety in Nursing: A Competency Approach* (translated into Swedish, Italian, Korean, and Chinese) and *Reflective Practice: Transforming Education and Improving Outcomes*. In recognition of her scholarship, awards, and professional and community leadership roles including Vice President of Sigma Theta Tau International Honor Society for Nursing, she received an Honorary Doctorate from Sweden's Jonkoping University in 2019.

**Wipada Kunaviktikul, PhD, RN, RM, FAAN,** is the Assistant to the President of Health Science Academic Affairs at the Panyapiwat Institute of Management in Thailand. She is a Professor Emerita and the former Dean of the Faculty of Nursing, Chiang Mai University, Thailand. She obtained her doctoral degree from the University of Alabama at Birmingham, USA, and was a research fellow at Harvard University School of Public Health USA in International Health and Policy. She served as the Director of Nursing Policy and Outcome Center, the Head of the WHOCC Center for Nursing and Midwifery Development, the Board of Directors of INDEN and the EAFONS. Kunaviktikul has conducted many research projects in nursing leadership and administration, policy, healthcare systems, and quality of care with more than 100 national and international publications and is invited to speak at national and international conferences. She has received several national and international awards including International Nurse Researcher Hall of Fame from Sigma, the UABSON's Visionary Leader and distinguished Srisa award in policy level of nurse leader, and others. She has also been a chair of many international conferences and more than 50 international trainings.

**Sara Horton-Deutsch, PhD, RN, PMHCNS, FAAN, ANEF,** is a Caritas Coach and a Professor and the Director of the Kaiser Permanente/USF Partnership at the University of San Francisco, where she mentors the next generation of nursing leaders through the lens of Caring Science and values-based leadership. She also serves as a Faculty Associate with the Watson Caring Science Institute. In 2021, she co-created and initiated the Caritas Leadership Program, a uniquely customized six-month program guiding participants through executive Caring Science leader dialogues, interactive circles, and participant transformation projects. She is also a founding partner of Better Together Healing, LLC, a holistic practice partnership specializing in an integrative approach to heal the self, build collaborations, and create healthy and bounded communities. As a therapeutic practitioner and Caritas leadership coach, she collaborates with healthcare professionals and organizations seeking balance and growth who are open to engaging in innovative approaches to healing. Her comprehensive approach includes certifications in professional coaching and training through the Leadership Circle and Working with Resilience, providing comprehensive profiles and assessments to raise the conscious practice of leadership and build regenerative success at work.

# REFERENCES

Albert, N., Pappas, S., Porter-O-Grady, T. & Malloch, K. (2022). *Quantum leadership: Creating sustainable value in healthcare* (6th ed.). Jones & Bartlett Learning.

Alilyyani, B., Wong, C. A., & Cummings, G. (2018). Antecedents, mediators, and outcomes of authentic leadership in healthcare: A systematic review. *International Journal of Nursing Studies, 83*, 34–64. https://doi.org/10.1016/j.ijnurstu.2018.04.001

Cardiff, S., McCormack, B., & McCance, T. (2018). Person-centred leadership: A relational approach to leadership derived through action research. *Journal of Clinical Nursing, 27*(15–16), 3056–3069. https://doi.org/10.1111/jocn.14492

Chavez, F., Kelly, T., Kunisch, J. R., & Kurth, A. (2019). Systems leadership doctor of nursing practice: Global relevance. *International Nursing Review, 66*(4), 482–489. https://doi.org/10.1111/inr.12527

Cummings, G. G., Tate, K., Lee, S., Wong, C. A., Paananen, T., Micaroni, S., & Chatterjee, G. E. (2018). Leadership styles and outcome patterns for the nursing workforce and work environment: A systematic review. *International Journal of Nursing Studies, 85*, 19–60. https://doi.org/10.1016/j.ijnurstu.2018.04.016

Disch, J. (2020). Nursing leadership in policy formation. *Nursing Forum, 55*(1), 4–10. https://doi.org/10.1111/nuf.12375

Giddens J. (2018). Transformational leadership: What every nursing dean should know. *Journal of Professional Nursing, 34*(2), 117–121. https://doi.org/10.1016/j.profnurs.2017.10.004

Gittell, J. H. (2016). *Transforming relationships for high performance: The power of relational coordination.* Stanford University Press.

Honkavuo, L., Eriksson, K., & Nåden, D. (2018). Discovering the ethos of serving in nursing leadership from the first half of the 20th century in three Nordic countries: An idea-historical research approach. *Scandinavian Journal of Caring Sciences, 32*(4), 1492–1501. https://doi.org/10.1111/scs.12590

Horton Deutsch, S., & Sherwood, G. (2008). Reflection: An educational strategy to develop emotionally competent nurse leaders. *Journal of Nursing Management, 16*(8), 946–954.

Im, E. O., Broome, M. E., Inouye, J., Kunaviktikul, W., Oh, E. G., Sakashita, R., Yi, M., Huang, L. H., Tsai, H. M., & Wang, H. H. (2018). An emerging integrated middle-range theory on Asian women's leadership in nursing. *Journal of Transcultural Nursing, 29*(4), 318–325. https://doi.org/10.1177/1043659618760397

Im, E. O., Wang, H. H., Tsai, H., Sakashita, R, Oh, E. G., Lin, C. C., Kunaviktikul, W., Inouye, J., Huang, L. H., & Broome, M. E. (2020). The refined middle-range theory on women's leadership in Asian countries. *Journal of Transcultural Nursing, 31*(6) 539–546.

James, A. H., Bennett, C. L., Blanchard, D., & Stanley, D. (2021). Nursing and values-based leadership: A literature review. *Journal of Nursing Management.* Advance online publication. https://doi.org/10.1111/jonm.13273

Jenkins, P. (2020). Effective leadership. In G. E. Armstrong & S. Sables-Baus (Eds.). *Leadership in DNP programs: A systems approach* (pp. 23–42). Springer Publishing.

Jennings, B. M., Scalzi, C. C., Rodgers, J. D., 3rd, & Keane, A. (2007). Differentiating nursing leadership and management competencies. *Nursing Outlook, 55*(4), 169–175. https://doi.org/10.1016/j.outlook.2006.10.002

Johns, C. (2015). *Mindful leadership: A guide for the health care professions.* Macmillan International Higher Education.

Kunaviktikul, W. (2014). Nursing towards the greater involvement of nurses in policy development. *International Nursing Review, 61*(1), 1–2.

Kunaviktikul, W., Turale, S., & Stone, T. E. (2018). Developing leadership and capacity building: Reflections of a nurse leader. *Nursing & Health Sciences, 20*(4), 411–414. https://doi.org/10.1111/nhs.12579

Lacy, S. R., Goodyear, C., & Hanson, M. D. (2020). An enduring crisis: Nurse leaders' perspectives. *Nursing Economic$*, *38*(5), 258–266.

Laurent, C. L. (2000). A nursing theory for nursing leadership. *Journal of Nursing Management*, *8*(2), 83–87. https://doi.org/10.1046/j.1365-2834.2000.00161.x

Leclerc, L., Kennedy, K., & Campis, S. (2020). Human-centered leadership in health care: An idea that's time has come. *Nursing Administration Quarterly*, *44*(2), 117–126. https://doi.org/10.1097/NAQ.0000000000000409

Losty, L. S., & Bailey, K. D. (2021). Leading through chaos: Perspectives from nurse executives. *Nursing Administration Quarterly*, *45*(2), 118–125. https://doi.org/10.1097/NAQ.0000000000000456

Northrup, D. T., Tschanz, C. L., Olynyk, V. G., Makaroff, K. L., Szabo, J., & Biasio, H. A. (2004). Nursing: Whose discipline is it anyway? *Nursing Science Quarterly*, *17*(1), 55–62. https://doi.org/10.1177/0894318403260471

O'Connor, M. (2008). The dimensions of leadership: A foundation for caring competency. *Nursing Administration Quarterly*, *32*(1), 21–26. https://doi.org/10.1097/01.NAQ.0000305944.23569.62

Papadopoulos, I., Lazzarino, R., Koulouglioti, C., Aagard, M., Akman, Ö., Alpers, L. M., Apostolara, P., Araneda-Bernal, J., Biglete-Pangilinan, S., Eldar-Regev, O., González-Gil, M. T., Kouta, C., Krepinska, R., Lesi ska-Sawicka, M., Liskova, M., Lopez-Diaz, A. L., Malliarou, M., Martín-García, Á., Muñoz-Solinas, M., Nagórska, M., ... Zorba, A. (2021). The importance of being a compassionate leader: The views of nursing and midwifery managers from around the world. *Journal of Transcultural Nursing*. Advance online publication. https://doi.org/10.1177/10436596211008214

Pearson, A., Laschinger, H., Porritt, K., Jordan, Z., Tucker, D., & Long, L. (2007). Comprehensive systematic review of evidence on developing and sustaining nursing leadership that fosters a healthy work environment in healthcare. *International Journal of Evidence-Based Healthcare*, *5*(2), 208–253. https://doi.org/10.1111/j.1479-6988.2007.00065x

Pesut, D. J. (2019). Anticipating disruptive innovations with foresight leadership. *Nursing Administration Quarterly*, *43*(3), 196–204. https://doi.org/10.1097/NAQ.0000000000000349

Pesut, D. J., & Thompson, S. A. (2018). Nursing leadership in academic nursing: The wisdom of development and the development of wisdom. *Journal of Professional Nursing*, *34*(2), 122–127. https://doi.org/10.1016/j.profnurs.2017.11.004

Pipe, T. B. (2008). Illuminating the inner leadership journey by engaging intention and mindfulness as guided by caring theory. *Nursing Administration Quarterly*, *32*(2), 117–125. https://doi.org/10.1097/01.NAQ.0000314540.21618.c1

Rosser, E. A., Scammell, J., Bevan, A., & Hundley, V. A. (2017). Strong leadership: The case for global connections. *Journal of Clinical Nursing*, *26*(7–8), 946–955. https://doi.org/10.1111/jocn.13562

Rosser, E., Westcott, L., Ali, P. A., Bosanquet, J., Castro-Sanchez, E., Dewing, J., McCormack, B., Merrell, J., & Witham, G. (2020). The need for visible nursing leadership during COVID-19. *Journal of Nursing Scholarship*, *52*(5), 459–461. https://doi.org/10.1111/jnu.12587

Roussel, L. (2019). Leadership's impact on quality, outcomes, and costs. *Critical Care Nursing Clinics of North America*, *31*(2), 153–163. https://doi.org/10.1016/j.cnc.2019.02.003

Saab, M. M., Drennan, J., Cornally, N., Landers, M., Hegarty, J., Savage, E., Lunn, C., & Coffey, A. (2019). Impact of a compassionate care leadership programme. *British Journal of Nursing*, *28*(11), 708–714. https://doi.org/10.12968/bjon.2019.28.11.708

Salvage, J., & White, J. (2019). Nursing leadership and health policy: Everybody's business. *International Nursing Review*, *66*(2), 147–150. https://doi.org/10.1111/inr.12523

Schick-Makaroff, K., & Storch, J. L. (2019). Guidance for ethical leadership in nursing codes of ethics: An integrative review. *Nursing Leadership*, *32*(1), 60–73. https://doi.org/10.12927/cjnl.2019.25848

Shin, S., Han, J., & Cha, C. (2016). Capacity building for global nursing leaders: Challenges and experiences. *International Nursing Review*, *63*(4), 580–587. https://doi.org/10.1111/inr.12323

Smith, T., Fowler-Davis, S., Nancarrow, S., Ariss, S. M. B., & Enderby, P. (2018). Leadership in interprofessional health and social care teams: A literature review. *Leadership in Health Services, 31*(4), 452–467. https://doi.org/10.1108/LHS-06-2016-0026

Solbakken, R., Bergdahl, E., Rudolfsson, G., & Bondas, T. (2018). International nursing: Caring in nursing leadership: A meta-ethnography from the nurse leader's perspective. *Nursing Administration Quarterly, 42*(4), E1–E19. https://doi.org/10.1097/NAQ.0000000000000314

Specchia, M. L., Cozzolino, M. R., Carini, E., Di Pilla, A., Galletti, C., Ricciardi, W., & Damiani, G. (2021). Leadership styles and nurses' job satisfaction. Results of a systematic review. *International Journal of Environmental Research and Public Health, 18*(4), 1552. https://doi.org/10.3390/ijerph18041552

Stanley, D., & Stanley, K, (2018). Clinical leadership and nursing explored: A literature search. *Journal of Clinical Nursing, 27*(9–10), 1730–1743. https://doi.org/10.1111/jocn.14145

Thompson, P., & Hyrkas, K. (2014). Global nursing leadership. *Journal of Nursing Management, 22*(1), 1–3. https://doi.org/10.1111/jonm.12215

Triola, N. (2007). Authentic leadership begins with emotional intelligence. *AACN Advanced Critical Care, 18*(3), 244–247. https://doi.org/10.4037/15597768-2007-3002

Uhl-Bien, M., Meyer, D., & Smith, J. (2020). Complexity leadership in the nursing context. *Nursing Administration Quarterly, 44*(2), 109–116. https://doi.org/10.1097/NAQ.0000000000000407

Villarruel, A. M. (2017). A framework for Latino nursing leadership. *Nursing Science Quarterly, 30*(4), 347–352. https://doi.org/10.1177/0894318417724476

Watson, J. (2017). *Discipline vs. profession of nursing.* Unpublished working manuscript as Watson portion of AAN Expert Panel Draft Paper, shared with Watson Caring Science Postdoctoral Scholars Seminar on July 7, 2017, in Boulder, Colorado.

Wong, C. A., Cummings, G. G., & Ducharme, L. (2013). The relationship between nursing leadership and patient outcomes: A systematic review update. *Journal of Nursing Management, 21*(5), 709–724. https://doi.org/10.1111/jonm.12116

World Health Organization. (2020). *State of the world's nursing 2020: Investing in education, jobs and leadership.* https://apps.who.int/iris/rest/bitstreams/1274201/retrieve

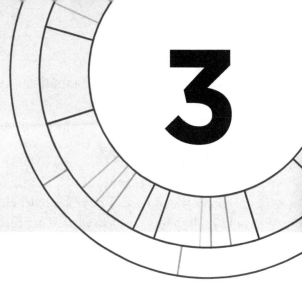

# 3

# TRANSCENDING LEADERSHIP AND REDEFINING SUCCESS

Matthew S. Howard, DNP, RN, CEN, TCRN, CPEN, CPN
Christie Kerwan, MSN, RN
Elizabeth A. Madigan, PhD, RN, FAAN
Danielle EK Perkins, PhD, RN
Erica DeKruyter, MSN, RN
Sarah E. Gray, DNP, RN, CEN, FAEN

## LEARNING OBJECTIVES

At the completion of the chapter, the reader will be able to:

- Explain new models of leadership development based on complex adaptive systems and neuroscience

- Describe Sigma's experience with leadership development and lessons learned

- Create the future of leadership development

# OVERVIEW

Leadership development has had an evolutionary path, starting with personal, anecdotal, and prescriptive approaches (e.g., Jim Collins, *From Good to Great* [2001]) to more evidence-based approaches that describe what good leaders have in common (Kouzes & Posner, 2017). This evolutionary journey for leadership is now ready for the next step by recognizing that leadership occurs in complex adaptive systems and is significantly impacted by the interpersonal aspects of neuroscience. We propose that new leadership development models will incorporate knowledge from both the personal/anecdotal and the evidence-based, recognizing the impact of complex adaptive systems on the organization and incorporating the neuroscience of interpersonal relationships among leaders and their followers.

# COMPLEX ADAPTIVE SYSTEMS

Complex adaptive systems (CAS) are familiar to us, even if we do not call them by this name. A flock of birds, a beehive, or any system including humans are complex adaptive systems. CAS and the related complexity theory are well established in basic science and organizational science (Anderson, 1999) and, subsequently, in healthcare (Plsek & Wilson, 2001). There is no one view of CAS nor one complexity theory but several perspectives. Like most other early theoretical approaches, there are ongoing debates and critiques (Greenhalgh et al., 2010; Paley, 2010). Most simply, CAS rejects a deterministic approach to understanding leadership, meaning that there is no prescription for what makes someone a good leader. Instead, a good leader recognizes the extent of their influence and how change occurs in a non-linear or unpredictable system. The principles underlying CAS can be found in Table 3.1, from Chaffee and McNeill (2007).

**TABLE 3.1**  Principles Underlying Complex Adaptive Systems (CAS)

| PROPERTY | DESCRIPTION OF PROPERTY |
| --- | --- |
| Adaptable elements | Elements in a CAS can evolve. |
| Attractors | Catalysts in a CAS that allow new behaviors to emerge. |
| Co-evolution | Progress in the CAS occurs with constant tension and balance. |
| Context and embeddedness | The CAS resides within and interacts with other systems that influence it. |
| Emergent behavior | New behavior is a feature of the CAS represented by constant innovation and creativity. |
| Inherent order | Order is maintained in a CAS even without central control. |
| Nonlinearity | Implies that in response to a stimulus a variety of behaviors are possible, and the cause and effect relationship is not directly evident or linear. |
| Porous boundaries | The boundaries of the elements in a CAS are blurry and porous, allowing exchange and movement between them. |
| Self-organization | Process where many local interactions create order without direction from above. |
| Simple rules | Local application of simple rules can result in broad, complex outcomes. |
| Unpredictability | Forecasting is inexact in a CAS because elements change, behavior is emerging, and activities are nonlinear; the trajectory of a system is unknowable. |

*Chaffee & McNeill (2007). Reprinted with permission.*

The key elements for leaders to understand are nonlinearity and unpredictability. Specifically, these concepts explain why a leader cannot predict the future. Co-evolution helps explain why there is often tension within the system; this is the only way that progress occurs. Leaders, therefore, should expect and manage the tension within their team and their organization and not expect consensus and smooth sailing.

For leadership, the implications are many (Clarke, 2013). Leaders first recognize that all influence is interpersonal, meaning that the traditional focus on leadership development at the individual and intrapersonal level is insufficient. The phrase "you cannot be a leader without followers" captures the essence of this implication; leaders must recognize the interpersonal nature of leadership versus the individual development approaches of the past.

Second, CAS for leadership requires less deterministic thinking: "If we do X, then Y will occur" no longer applies. This implication suggests that small tests of change (Berwick, 1998) are likely the better approach. The leader also emphasizes the importance of a learning environment where things are tried; some work and some do not. Expecting and welcoming failure leads to a learning environment.

Third, the optimal environments are those that are adaptable to change. Open environments, where the adaptable elements (i.e., staff members) interact broadly with the outside world and internally, are more likely to succeed. The theory of weak ties indicates that more distant relationships (i.e., colleagues, not friends) provide leaders with important information that leads to new ideas, innovation, and connections (Aral, 2016). Because the principles of CAS apply here, there is an unpredictable element in knowing which weak ties will eventually provide a payoff. The leader's role is to nurture their weak ties and the weak ties of their organization.

Fourth, leaders are less focused on being mentors and coaches and more on creating an environment that facilitates change and adaptability by promoting self-organization. For example, core teams representing various levels of staff who self-select to work on a common project are examples of creating an accommodating environment.

Finally, tension is recognized as a good thing because of the different perspectives that adaptable elements (e.g., staff) have and bring to any decision. This requires a leader who is adept at conflict identification, can call out the conflict if it is unseen, and can bring the group to conflict resolution, recognizing that a healthy level of conflict promotes progress.

In summary, "leadership arises through a pattern of interactions between team members in organizations and the structural conditions in which they act" (Clarke, 2013, p. 144). Thus, the leader is no longer viewed as the captain of the ship but as a gardener. The gardener selects the right plants, avoids a monoculture (all plants of the same type), recognizes what they can control (e.g., amount of compost) and what they cannot (e.g., the amount of natural rainfall, pests), and creates and nurtures an environment for growth. The skills needed by a ship's captain and a master gardener are very different: the gardener creates the best from the uncontrollable natural system.

Because the leader's influence is interpersonal, leaders need to understand how they are perceived and how they perceive others. Humans have evolved to be finely attuned to interactions with others. Many of these perceptions are nonverbal, and we process or understand them without necessarily being conscious of them, thus the need to understand neuroscience impacts.

# THE NEUROSCIENCE OF INTERACTIONS

Merriam Webster defines *neuroscience* as "a branch of the life sciences that deals with the anatomy, physiology, biochemistry, or molecular biology of nerves and nervous tissue, especially with their relation to behavior and learning" (Merriam-Webster, n.d.). This branch of science has provided great insight into how and why people act/react in given situations.

A variety of researchers, behavioralists, and neuroscientists have studied the effects neuroscience has on one's ability to lead effectively, coining the area of study *neuroleadership*. Specific neuroleadership theory development was published by David Rock in 2008. His team's fundamental finding was that leadership effectiveness was determined by how leaders address employee concerns—they either trigger a reward response or a stress response controlled by the limbic system (Greenberg & Nadler, 2008; Rock, 2008). Five social qualities were found to determine the leader and the employee's reactions (Freedman, 2019). These reactions were identified as the SCARF Model (Status, Certainty, Autonomy, Relatedness, and Fairness) as shown in Table 3.2 (Rock, 2008).

**TABLE 3.2**    SCARF Model: The Reward and Threat Response to Five Social Qualities

| SOCIAL QUALITY | BIOLOGICAL IMPACT | RESPONSE |
| --- | --- | --- |
| Status | Increased/decreased cortisol release | Reward: longevity, health, calm |
| | | Threat: anxiety, stress |
| Certainty | Enhanced/inhibited neural connections between basal ganglia and motor cortex; adrenaline and dopamine release | Reward: confidence, innovation, productivity |
| | | Threat: diminished memory, disengagement, feeling overwhelmed |
| Autonomy | Increased/decreased adrenaline and dopamine release | Reward: calm; better decision-making |
| | | Threat: stress, disruption, feeling disengaged |
| Relatedness | Oxytocin release; increased endorphins (exact response as physical pain response) | Reward: friendly, collaborative, generous |
| | | Threat: lonely, isolated, rejected |
| Fairness | Increased/decreased endorphins | Reward: loyal, engaged, trust |
| | | Threat: untrusting, disruptive |

*Source: Rock, 2008.*

Using one's ability to identify, understand, and react to these social qualities is paramount to successful leadership. This ability has been identified as the Theory of the Mind (ToM) and is unique to the human species (Dimitriadis & Psychogios, 2020). Dimitriadis and Psychogios (2020) explain the ToM work for leaders and suggest that successful leaders try to understand the intentions of those they work with as a way to "decode their intentions" for better decision-making (p. 174).

A brain is a problem-solving machine; thus, leaders may allow their mental shortcuts to jump to conclusions. Leaders in modern organizations cannot go on with a mental state of fierce competition or a feeling of isolation from their social surroundings; instead, "embracing collaboration and cooperation, alongside the necessary competition and unavoidable conflicts, will advance them to true brain adaptive leaders" (Dimitriadis & Psychogios, 2020, p. 172).

There is evidence that cooperation, not competition, is how human brains evolved. Thus, the legend of the sole and powerful leader (e.g., Steve Jobs) is more myth than reality. However, we do not have to throw out basic constructs of leadership. One such construct is to *walk the talk*—touted in *Harvard Business Review* as the most ubiquitous aphorism in business (Taylor, 2014). The concept aligns with the second aspect of neuroscience relevant for leaders: recognizing the influence of mirror neurons. While there is still scientific debate about the presence and function of mirror neurons, there is evidence from psychology and organizational behavior that a leader's mental and emotional state will be reflected by their followers (Goleman & Boyatzis, 2008).

McGilchrist (2012) noted that imitation is a powerful brain mechanism that contributes directly to development, learning, group assimilation, cultural homogeneity, cooperation, and innovation at various stages of our lives (Dimitriadis & Psychogios, 2020). Therefore, leaders need to positively model the behavior they wish to see to take advantage of the human brain's imitation functions.

Understanding brain structure and function provides leaders with the evidence that they need to model positive behavior and interact with their colleagues and followers in ways that decrease threat and increase reward. Throughout neuro-leadership research and development, leaders are fundamental to the success of a complex system that requires them to navigate an ever more complex environment. Navigating the human psyche requires leaders to "speak" to three main functions—thinking, feeling, and behaving—to achieve success (Dimitriadis & Psychogios, 2020, p. 213).

There is some literature to give us pause to the extrapolation of organizational neuroscience, specifically in the domain of leadership. Some authors caution using inferential ambiguities that do not adequately consider the challenges of or solutions to reductionism in leadership studies (Lindebaum & Zundel, 2013). Therefore, the reader is encouraged to consider these recommendations and incorporate them in ethical ways that address their followers' needs.

# SIGMA'S EXPERIENCE WITH LEADERSHIP DEVELOPMENT PROGRAMS AND LESSONS LEARNED

Sigma Theta Tau International Honor Society of Nursing (Sigma) was founded as an organization to advance nursing as a profession (Sensor, 2021). The founders recognized the value of scholarship and leadership and its vital role in advancing nursing excellence in practice. Sigma focuses on professional leadership and career development for all nurses. Through its leadership, Sigma began to advance the nursing profession by becoming the first organization in the United States to fund nursing research in 1936. Even in its early years, Sigma members recognized the need for nurses to obtain knowledge and skills in leadership, scholarship, and service.

Leadership academies were established in the early 2000s to provide formal leadership development to nurses within clinical and academic settings. Sigma created several programs to develop nurse leaders. In 2002, Sigma convened a group of experts that developed the Nursing Leadership Academy. Working with industry leaders such as Johnson & Johnson, Sigma created several academies focused on developing nurses' leadership skills and abilities.

In 2010, *The Future of Nursing: Leading Change, Advancing Health* report called for nurses to lead (Institute of Medicine, 2011). This continued Sigma's stance that all nurses are leaders. Regardless of title or position within an organization or society, nurses play a leadership role in patients, clients, healthcare, and the profession. The 2010 Institute of Medicine (IOM) report provided further directions and justifications for the progression of Sigma's leadership academies. Since that time, the World Health Organization (WHO) released the *State of the World's Nursing Report 2020: Investing in Education, Jobs and Leadership* (WHO, 2020). This document provided further evidence of the necessity of nurse leadership development at all levels. Recent additions to both include the *Future of Nursing 2020–2030* (National Academies of Sciences, Engineering, and Medicine, 2021) with a focus on health equity, and the *World Health Organization Global Strategic Directions for Nursing and Midwifery*, with a focus on the continued need for nursing leadership development (WHO, 2021).

Sigma took a multifaceted programming approach to deliver leadership development to nurses globally. The initial academy, Maternal-Child Health Nurse Leadership Academy (MCHNLA), was developed in 2002 with a pilot cohort in 2004. This 18-month mentored leadership experience was designed to improve maternal-child health outcomes by maximizing the contributions made by nurses (Morin et al., 2015). Several additional academies quickly followed this leadership program. Academies focused on increasing the leadership acumen of gerontology nurses and nurses in academia. See Table 3.3 for a listing of Sigma's leadership-focused academies.

**Table 3.3**  Sigma Leadership Academies

| SIGMA ACADEMY | NUMBER OF COHORTS | LEADERSHIP FOCUS |
|---|---|---|
| Maternal-Child Health Nurse Leadership Academy (MCHNLA) | Eight (2004–2019) | Develop leadership skills and abilities to produce learning experiences that prepare and position individual maternal-child nurses to influence patient and practice outcomes |
| Gerontological Nursing Leadership Academy (GNLA) | Six (2006–2017) | Develop leadership skills and abilities to produce learning experiences that prepare and position individual gerontological nurses to influence patient and practice outcomes |
| Nurse Faculty Leadership Academy (NFLA) | Four (2010–2017) | Develop leadership skills of early-career nursing faculty with less than seven years of experience |
| Maternal-Child Health Nurse Leadership Academy-Africa (MCHNLA-Africa) | Four (2011–2019) | Develop leadership skills and abilities to produce learning experiences that prepare and position individual maternal-child nurses within Africa to influence patient and practice outcomes |
| Experienced Faculty Leadership Academy (ENFLA) | Three (2014–2019) | Develop leadership abilities of mid-career nursing faculty with more than seven years of experience |
| Experienced Educational Administrator Institute (EEAI) | Three (2015–2019) | Develop leadership abilities of experienced nursing faculty to obtain a formal leadership role in an academic setting |
| Experienced Academic Leadership Academy (EALA) | Two (2020–present) | Develop leadership abilities of mid-career nursing faculty with more than six years of experience |
| New Academic Leadership Academy (NALA) | Two (2020–present) | Develop leadership skills of early-career nursing faculty with less than five years of experience |
| Nurse Leadership Academy for Practice (NLAP) | Two (2020–present) | Develop leadership skills and abilities to produce learning experiences that prepare and position nurses to influence patient and practice outcomes regardless of their nursing specialty |

Sigma also developed asynchronous educational programming to aid in the leadership development of nurses. The Nurse Manager Certificate Program (NMCP) and the Healthcare Leader Certificate Program (HLCP) were developed to enhance the knowledge and skills of nurse leaders at various stages of their professional development. The NMCP is a web-based asynchronous educational activity. The program was designed to develop nursing leadership abilities necessary to function in the rapidly changing healthcare environment nurses face daily. The initial 12 courses have been enhanced and revised four times since initial development. The now 16-course curriculum was developed by nurses using evidence to guide its development. Currently requiring 85.1 hours to complete, the NMCP was designed for entry-level nurse managers or those wishing to develop leadership skills to obtain a formal leadership position.

The HLCP was developed to support the professional development and leadership acumen of existing, formal nurse leaders and graduate nursing students. Sigma recognized that nurse leaders were expected to exhibit a broad range of leadership skills necessary to keep job satisfaction and productivity levels high and turnover rates low. The curriculum for the HLCP was based on the testing blueprints of four nursing leadership and management credentialing certifications. Consisting of seven courses and more than 50 contact hours, the HLCP includes a pre-and post-assessment to gauge leadership knowledge and skills.

First, developing nurse leaders requires intrinsically motivated professionals interested in building upon their strengths and, more importantly, willing to take risks that involve discovering and working to strengthen less robust areas. The belief that some people are born to lead while others are not is strongly refuted by evidence derived from decades of research by Kouzes and Posner (2017). In their book, *The Leadership Challenge*, James Kouzes and Barry Z. Posner (2017) propose a framework for leadership development based upon their findings and interactions with leaders all over the world. Their model, The Five Practices of Exemplary Leadership, is the culmination of having engaged with successful and diverse leaders about their behaviors and actions that they felt were enacted when they were at their "personal best" (Kouzes & Posner, 2017). As shown in Table 3.4, the five practices include Model the Way, Inspire a Shared Vision, Challenge the Process, Enable Others to Act, and Encourage the Heart (Kouzes & Posner, 2017). From the very beginning, Kouzes and Posner's model has served as the primary evidence-based framework for all of Sigma's leadership development academies and programs. While leadership development is at the top of the hierarchy for the professional development of nurses at Sigma, other important evidence-based specialty guidelines meet the individualized needs of nurses according to their primary or desired work role and environment.

**TABLE 3.4** Kouzes and Posner's Five Practices of Exemplary Leadership

| PILLAR | DESCRIPTION | EXAMPLES |
|---|---|---|
| Model the Way | Clarify values by setting an example by your actions | Acknowledge recent failures |
| | | Use inclusive language |
| | | Share professional philosophy of leadership with team members |
| Inspire a Shared Vision | Imagine exciting possibilities and engage the assistance of others to work toward the shared aspiration | Explain the desired future state of a performance improvement project with authenticity and enthusiasm to a colleague or team member |
| | | Involve a first follower in a project |
| | | Speak passionately and vividly about the goal(s) of a project |

| | | |
|---|---|---|
| Challenge the Process | Search for new ideas and opportunities by seeking innovative ways to upgrade or enhance processes | Take a risk |
| | | Encourage a teammate to try new ways to do their work |
| | | Find innovative ways to improve something for the workplace or team |
| Enable Others to Act | Promote an environment of collaboration through trusting relationships | Embrace collaborations |
| | | Assist team members to learn new skills |
| | | Allow team members to determine solutions to a project or task |
| | | Empower team members to decide |
| Encourage the Heart | Recognize people for participation to increase awareness of their value to the organization | Provide personalized encouragement to a team member |
| | | Praise a colleague for a job well done |
| | | Send handwritten thank you notes |
| | | Celebrate project milestones with the team |

(Kouzes & Posner, 2017)

The American Organization for Nursing Leadership (AONL) has explicitly focused on developing core competencies for nurse leaders and aspiring nurse leaders working in various healthcare settings and with varying degrees of responsibility in the US (AONL, 2021). The organization is dedicated to supporting nurse leaders in their self-discovery of leadership skills, knowledge, and abilities in manager and executive functioning healthcare-based roles. The Nurse Manager and Nurse Executive competencies have lent focused guidance on developing curricula for leadership development and enhancing practicing nurses in the Nurse Leadership Academy for Practice.

The WHO Nurse Educator Core Competencies (2016) were developed because of a collaborative effort of key international stakeholders including, but not limited to, the International Council of Nurses (ICN), Global Alliance for Nursing and Midwifery (GANM), and the American College of Nurse-Midwives (ACNM). The resulting eight core competencies for global nurse educators identify cognitive, affective, and psychomotor learning domains relative to each area. The eighth competency focuses on management, leadership, and advocacy and completes the listing of essential nurse educator expectations. These competencies have helped frame curricula for several more contemporary nurse educator leadership academies at Sigma.

Likewise, the National League for Nursing's Certified Nurse Educator (CNE) exam blueprint, which includes many of the primary areas of focus included in the WHO Nurse Educator Core Competencies, has served to structure all of the current nursing faculty academies (Nick et al., 2013; Poindexter et al., 2019). Shared focus areas include program assessment/monitoring and evaluation, facilitating learning, and engaging in scholarship/research (Nick et al., 2013).

Nursing education is constantly evolving, and regardless of their years of experience, academic and clinical nurse educators must remain current on the standards of excellence for nursing education and essential competencies that inform nursing education curricula. The National League for Nursing (NLN) Hallmarks of Excellence in Nursing Education Model (Headlines from the NLN, 2004; NLN, 2020) and Quality and Safety Education for Nurses (QSEN) Competencies (American Association of Colleges of Nursing QSEN Education Consortium, 2012; Cronenwett et al., 2009) provided an additional direction for curricular development of Sigma's nurse faculty development academies. When nurse educators understand and are equipped to ensure that nursing education curricula reflect the latest innovations in healthcare and teaching, patient care and health outcomes are improved. For example, the QSEN competencies support the preparation of a nursing workforce that can meet the challenges of a complex healthcare system by proposing specific targets for the knowledge, skills, and attitudes developed in pre-licensure and graduate programs (Cronenwett et al., 2009). Using the IOM competencies for patient safety and quality as a guide, nursing academic and practice experts identified six competencies to guide curricular development of pre-licensure and graduate nursing programs. Likewise, the NLN Hallmarks of Excellence in Nursing Education Model results from expert input on strategies that best support meeting the needs of 21st-century nursing education (NLN, 2020). Academic nurse leaders, aspiring leaders, and nursing faculty alike must be equipped with this knowledge so that the next generation of nursing professionals are prepared to address healthcare challenges with innovative strategies and pedagogically sound curricula.

Many past participants in Sigma's leadership development programming have accomplished short- and long-term professional goals. Carolyn Hart, PhD, RN, CNE, is a former nurse leadership scholar and alumna of three Sigma Academies, including the Nurse Faculty Leadership Academy (NFLA), Experienced Nurse Faculty Leadership Academy (ENFLA), and Emerging Educational Administrator Institute (EEAI). As a result of supportive mentorship and expert guidance, Dr. Hart presented an abstract based on the creation of a governance structure using the Commission for Nursing Education Accreditation (CNEA) standards as a framework at her institution (Hart et al., 2017). This outcome exemplifies leadership strength and the benefits of an intensive and individualized focus on developing aspiring nursing education administrators.

Michael Joseph Diño, PhD, MAN, RN, LPT, describes developing and implementing electronic web-based learning resources at Our Lady of Fatima University, Valenzuela City, Philippines (Diño, 2019). Dr. Diño focused his individual leadership goals on developing a team of stakeholders at his institution to bring about foundational technology enhancements to better support the future of nursing education and the inclusion of virtual and online learning.

Past NFLA scholars were able to achieve several education-related certifications because of their participation in the academy. Examples included the Certified Healthcare Simulation Educator (CHSE), CNE, and TeamSTEPPS Primary Care Master Trainer credentials (Cleeter et al., 2015). Scholar growth has been enhanced through the promotion of an Individual Leadership Development Plan

(ILDP). The ILDP provides a projected path for achieving career leadership outcomes and establishes varying short- and long-term goals. Scholars, working collaboratively with their mentor and faculty advisor, develop their ILDP using the Kouzes and Posner model for leadership development as an overarching framework (Cleeter et al., 2015).

Nurse leaders and experts that support aspiring and novice leaders in nursing education and practice also benefit personally and professionally through their participation. The experience of mentoring and providing expert guidance to Sigma nurse scholars opens up opportunities for publishing about Sigma programming, scholar outcomes, and individual personal growth. For example, Patterson et al. (2020), a group made up of experienced Sigma mentors, reported on the perceptions of faculty leadership scholars regarding their 20-month experiential Sigma leadership academy matriculation. The participants' interview data analysis yielded an overarching theme of "Finding Authentic Leadership Voice," the shared experience among the group (Patterson et al., 2020). "Identifying Inner Strengths and Areas for Improvement" was one way the scholars manifested finding their authentic leadership voice (Patterson et al., 2020). Using Kouzes and Posner's leadership framework, faculty scholars gained insight into what they were doing well and areas needing strengthening.

One scholar stated, "I learned that my strengths were in setting up clear standards and expecting the best" (Patterson et al., 2020, p. 12). Although this scholar found that she was strong in Modeling the Way for others, she identified herself as being "weak" in Encouraging the Heart (Patterson et al., 2020). The insights regarding leadership behavior strengths and weaknesses supported individual growth. It also increased their focus on others, increased self-confidence, self-awareness, and clarifying aspirations for their future leadership (Patterson et al., 2020).

In addition to leadership development academies, Sigma has developed a robust global leadership mentoring community. Previous findings among Sigma leaders in the European region supported this work (Rosser et al., 2017). Nurse leaders surveyed emphasized the value of networking and communication as a primary benefit of membership (Rosser et al., 2017). As a result, piloting a global leadership mentoring program was the first logical step in advancing this benefit (Rosser, 2017). A total of 11 nurse leaders agreed to mentor aspiring nurse leaders or early-career leaders from global regions different from their own for approximately 12 to 18 months. The pilot was well received and considered a success and provided support for ongoing global leadership mentorship. Sigma continued the important work of providing opportunities for global mentors and mentees to connect and develop supportive and mutually beneficial relationships (Rosser et al., 2020). While numerous challenges existed, such as time zone, cultural, and language differences, mentors reported benefitting from their interactions with their mentees. Mentors shared that they were able to develop trusting and valuable relationships with their mentees. Mentees also described the benefits of their mentoring relationships. For example, one mentee stated, "Mentorship has been an invaluable supportive mechanism that has enabled me to retain my dignity in challenging situations" (Rosser et al., 2020, p. 489).

CAS and neuroscience are reflected in the Kouzes and Posner five methods of leadership development (2017). Successful leaders and those who aspire to leadership positions would do well to integrate the understanding that the work environment is a CAS populated by humans with highly evolved reward and threat response systems. Understanding the implications of these aspects and how the Kouzes and Posner model incorporates these other areas of science will lead to more effective leadership.

Based on the previous work, the future of leadership development programs needs to include both personal/anecdotal and evidence-based approaches. The programs need to be grounded in recognizing how change occurs within a complex adaptive system and in response to neuroscience. As a result, leaders will need to be exquisitely aware of their state of being and be deeply authentic. To do so will require deep reflection, experiential learning, and coaching to consider how one comes across.

# IMPLICATIONS FOR PRACTICE

As healthcare grows in complexity to meet the population's needs, nurse leaders must apply higher system thinking strategies. Nursing leaders are needed to add their valuable insights into orchestrating CAS in clinical, academic, and non-nursing specific CAS such as community boards where health and safety need to be prioritized. Prescriptive, linear leadership models are now recognized as less relevant. Nursing leadership training must evolve to include experiential opportunities, building a body of evidence to support the role of nurses as change agents and leaders.

Sigma has paved the way for nurses to have experiential learning opportunities that build the scientific body of evidence and develop individuals to affect their organization positively. Utilizing evidence-based frameworks, standards, and competencies ensures that training supports foundational elements in leadership.

# SUMMARY

Whereas leadership has not evolved, our thinking and understanding of it does. Our interpretation of leadership continues to grow. In order to promote a culture of evolutionary thinking around leadership concepts, nurse leaders must continually propose new leadership development models to incorporate the knowledge and understanding of the interpersonal aspects of neuroscience. A greater understanding of complex adaptive systems and the neuroscience of interactions provides the framework for nursing leadership development and its implications on nursing practices. For example, the multiple leadership development programs and academies from Sigma are discussed to express how our knowledge and use of leadership tools have evolved over the years.

# NARRATIVE

Jan has been a nurse for nine months; she works in a 30-bed intensive care unit. Typically, there are 17 nurses and one charge nurse on the unit during each shift, and the night shift charge nurse has been there for eight years; however, this night looks different. Tonight, there are only 14 nurses, 22 patients with the potential for eight admissions, and Jan was pulled to the charge nurse position with the possibility of having her own patient(s) depending on the number of admissions and the acuity of the patients. Jan was shifted to the charge role because she has the most experience on nights compared to the other nursing staff. The other nursing staff consists of four nurses who have six months of experience, and the others are newly off orientation. Jan is nervous about being the charge nurse for the night because she fears her lack of experience is not enough to lead the team, and she has not had an orientation to the role. The night shift team senses her nervousness and anxiety.

# REFLECTIVE QUESTIONS

1.  What type of environment cultivates leadership, and which theory is applicable to this type of environment?

2.  A leader is no longer viewed as the captain of the ship but rather as a gardener. How does a gardener represent leadership?

3.  What are the five social qualities used to determine the leader and her employees' reactions? What is the biological impact and response of these qualities on the body?

4.  How does Kouzes and Posner's five methods of leadership development affect complex adaptive systems and neuroscience?

5.  What facets must be considered for leadership development?

# AUTHOR BIOGRAPHIES

**Matthew S. Howard, DNP, RN, CEN, TCRN, CPEN, CPN,** is currently the Director of Scholarship & Leadership Resources at Sigma. While also serving as graduate faculty at Northern Kentucky University, Howard works as a staff nurse in the emergency department at Eskenazi Health in Indianapolis, Indiana, USA. His nursing career has taken him from stretcher-side nursing to academia and back. His clinical background includes EMS, emergency department nursing, flight nursing, and trauma nursing with several leadership positions throughout. Working behind the scenes, Howard serves on several local, national, and international councils and nursing associations including the Emergency Nurses Association, the International Network for Doctoral Education in Nursing, Sigma, and as an advisory board member to the National Nursing Education Research Network.

**Christie Kerwan, MSN, RN,** Director of Strategic Partnerships—Healthcare for PowerDMS and former Manager, Sigma Marketplace, Sigma, has a passion for understanding why nursing leaders fail and how the profession can establish safe, fail-proof environments for these leaders. She is pursuing a doctorate, and her work toward it centers around the impact cognitive dissonance has on middle management retention and success. This work is inclusive of fundamental neuroleadership concepts, as there are significant physiological responses that align with fledging leaders' subjective statements. Kerwan's career spans 20 years, in which 17 of those have involved various leadership roles that span the responsibility spectrum from being a team leader in a busy cardiac catherization lab to being a for-profit healthcare corporate executive managing a $43 million dollar portfolio. Each role has provided her with opportunities to develop and promote leader success through mentoring, developing leadership programs, implementing data-driven strategies, and innovating delivery platforms that removed barriers to success.

**Elizabeth A. Madigan, PhD, RN, FAAN,** has been the Chief Executive Officer at Sigma since 2017. She leads the organization to support more than 135,000 members from more than 100 countries. Sigma provides programming, events, and leadership development focused on scholarship and research and leadership development. Prior to her role at Sigma, she was a tenured endowed professor at Case Western Reserve University. During her time there, she ran the World Health Organization/Pan American Health Organization Collaborating Center for Home Care Nursing and the global health programs. Her clinical and research background focused on home healthcare, and she has been funded by the US federal government and foundations for her research. She is widely published in home healthcare and global health. She is a Fellow in the American Academy of Nursing and Fellow Ad Eundem at the Royal College of Surgeons, Ireland.

**Danielle EK Perkins, PhD, RN,** is the former Manager of the Center for Excellence in Nursing Education for Sigma. There, she oversaw the administration and ongoing review of nurse faculty leadership enrichment institutes and academies and led the development of professional role education for international nursing faculty. For more than half of her career, she has taught undergraduate baccalaureate nursing students in the clinical, classroom, and online settings in the areas of nursing research, psychiatric, medical-surgical nursing, and community health nursing. She is a member of several nursing organizations including Sigma, Chi Eta Phi Sorority, Incorporated, and the American Psychiatric Nursing Association.

**Erica DeKruyter, MSN, RN,** is the Manager of Educational Resources at Sigma. She develops continuing education content and programs for the global nursing community. Prior to Sigma, DeKruyter had eight years of experience in emergency nursing as a staff nurse and a night shift patient care coordinator. As a patient care coordinator, she led the nursing staff on the unit and oversaw the patient flow within the department. DeKruyter was a missionary nurse in Haiti for 14 months. While in Haiti, she coordinated and oversaw all the short-term medical teams coming to the Thomazeau area while serving in the local clinic.

**Sarah E. Gray, DNP, RN, CEN, FAEN,** Chief Nursing Officer for Sigma, is a creative visionary whose mission is to equip and empower others. She discovered her passion for service and transformational leadership during her 15 years in leadership roles in emergency and occupational nursing. She develops continuing education programs, domestic and international events, opportunities for the global nursing community, and oversees Sigma's consultative status and programming with the United Nations (UN). She is a presenter, author, and coach on practical solutions, innovation, and inspirational topics, specializing in professional branding and leadership.

# REFERENCES

American Association of Colleges of Nursing QSEN Education Consortium. (2012). *Graduate-level QSEN competencies: Knowledge, skills, and attitudes.* https://www.aacnnursing.org/Portals/42/AcademicNursing/CurriculumGuidelines/Graduate-QSEN-Competencies.pdf

American Organization for Nursing Leadership. (2021). *AONL nurse leader competencies.* https://www.aonl.org/resources/nurse-leader-competencies

Anderson, P. (1999). Perspective: Complexity theory and organization science. *Organization Science, 10*(3), 215–376. https://doi.org/10.1287/orsc.10.3.216

Aral, S. (2016). The future of weak ties. *American Journal of Sociology, 121*(6), 1931–1939. https://doi.org/10.1086/686293

Berwick, D. M. (1998). Developing and testing changes in delivery of care. *Annals of Internal Medicine, 128*(8), 651–656. https://doi.org/10.7326/0003-4819-128-8-199804150-00009

Chaffee, M. W., & McNeill, M. M. (2007). A model of nursing as a complex adaptive system. *Nursing Outlook, 55*(5), 232–241. https://doi.org/10.1016/j.outlook.2007.04.003

Clarke, N. (2013). Model of complexity leadership development. *Human Resource Development International, 16*(2), 135–150. https://doi.org/10.1080/13678868.2012.756155

Cleeter, D. F., Dzurec, L. C., Horsley, T. L., Hardy, E. C., & Embree, J. L. (2015). *Developing nursing education leaders through intentional behavior change and expanded scope of influence.* https://sigma.nursingrepository.org/handle/10755/603369

Cronenwett, L., Sherwood, G., Pohl, J., Barnsteiner, J., Moore, S., Sullivan, D. T., Ward, D., & Warren, J. (2009). Quality and safety education for advanced nursing practice. *Nursing Outlook, 57*(6), 338–348. https://doi.org/10.1016/j.outlook.2009.07.009

Dimitriadis, N., & Psychogios, A. (2020). *Neuroscience for leaders: A brain adaptive leadership approach.* Kogan Page

Diño, M. J. S. (2019). *Experienced nurse faculty leadership academy project outcome: Developing and implementing electronic web-based learning resources.* https://sigma.nursingrepository.org/handle/10755/18736

Freedman, B. D. (2019). Risk factors and causes of interpersonal conflict in nursing workplaces: Understandings from neuroscience. *Collegian, 26*(5), 594–604. https://doi.org/10.1016/j.colegn.2019.02.001

Goleman, D., & Boyatzis, R. (2008). Social intelligence and the biology of leadership. *Harvard Business Review, 86*(9), 74–81.

Greenberg, C., & Nadler, R. (2008, March 31). Neuroleadership [Audio podcast episode]. In *Leadership Development News.* https://www.voiceamerica.com/episode/28583/neuroleadership

Greenhalgh, T., Plsek, P., Wilson, T., Fraser, S., & Holt, T. (2010). Response to "The appropriation of complexity theory in health care." *Journal of Health Services Research & Policy, 15*(2), 115–117. https://doi.org/10.1258/jhsrp.2010.009158

Hart, C., Bell, P., & Dzurec, L. C. (2017). *Creating a governance structure consistent with the Commission for Nursing Education Accreditation (CNEA) standards.* https://sigma.nursingrepository.org/handle/10755/623244

Headlines from the NLN. (2004). Hallmarks of excellence in nursing education. *Nursing Education Perspectives, 25*(2), 98–101.

Institute of Medicine. (2011). *The future of nursing: Leading change, advancing health.* Washington, DC: The National Academies Press. https://doi.org/10.17226/12956

Kouzes, J. M., & Posner, B. Z. (2017). *The leadership challenge: How to make extraordinary things happen in organizations* (6th ed.). John Wiley & Sons.

Lindebaum, D., & Zundel, M. (2013). Not quite a revolution: Scrutinizing organizational neuroscience in leadership studies. *Human Relations, 66*(6), 857–877. https://doi.org/10.1177/0018726713482151

McGilchrist, I. (2012). *The master and his emissary. The divided brain and the making of the Western world.* Yale University Press.

Merriam-Webster. (n.d.). *Neuroscience.* In Merriam-Webster.com dictionary. https://www.merriam-webster.com/dictionary/neuroscience

Morin, K., Small, L., Spatz, D. L., Solomon, J., Lessard, L., & Leng, S. W. (2015). Preparing leaders in maternal-child health nursing. *Journal of Obstetric, Gynecologic & Neonatal Nursing, 44*(5), 633–643. https://doi.org/10.1111/1552-6909.12730

National Academies of Sciences, Engineering, and Medicine. (2021). *The future of nursing 2020–2030: Charting a path to achieve health equity.* The National Academies Press. https://doi.org/10.17226/25982

National League for Nursing. (2020). *Hallmarks of excellence.* http://www.nln.org/professional-development-programs/teaching-resources/hallmarks-of-excellence

Nick, J. M., Sharts-Hopko, N. C., & Leners, D. W. (2013). From committee to commission: The history of the NLN's Academic Certified Nurse Educator program. *Nursing Education Perspectives, 34*(5), 298–302.

Paley, J. (2010). The appropriation of complexity theory in health care. *Journal of Health Services Research & Policy, 15*(1), 59–61. https://doi.org/10.1258/jhsrp.2009.009072

Patterson, B. J., Dzurec, L., Sherwood, G., & Forrester, D. A. (2020). Developing authentic leadership voice: Novice faculty experience. *Nursing Education Perspectives, 41*(1), 10–15. https://doi.org/10.1097/01.NEP.0000000000000494

Plsek, P. E., & Wilson, T. (2001). Complexity, leadership, and management in healthcare organisations. *BMJ, 323*(7315), 746–749. https://doi.org/10.1136/bmj.323.7315.746

Poindexter, K., Lindell, D., & Hagler, D. (2019). Measuring the value of Academic Nurse Educator Certification: Perceptions of administrators and educators. *Journal of Nursing Education, 58*(9), 502–509. https://doi.org/10.3928/01484834-20190819-02

Rock, D. (2008). SCARF: A brain-based model for collaborating with and influencing others. *NeuroLeadership Journal, 1*(1), 1–9. http://web.archive.org/web/20100705024057/http://www.your-brain-at-work.com/files/NLJ_SCARFUS.pdf

Rosser, E. (2017). Developing our future leaders: The role of a global mentoring programme. *British Journal of Nursing, 26*(18), 1045. https://doi.org/10.12968/bjon.2017.26.18.1045

Rosser, E., Buckner, E., Avedissian, T., Cheung, D. S. K., Eviza, K., Hafsteinsdóttir, T. B., Hsu, M. Y., Kirshbaum, M. N., Lai, C., Ng, Y. C., Ramsbotham, J., & Waweru, S. (2020). The global leadership mentoring community: Building capacity across seven global regions. *International Nursing Review, 67*(4), 484–494. https://doi.org/10.1111/inr.12617

Rosser, E. A., Scammell, J., Bevan, A., & Hundley, V. A. (2017). Strong leadership: The case for global connections. *Journal of Clinical Nursing, 26*(7–8), 946–955. https://doi.org/10.1111/jocn.13562

Sensor, C. S., Sessler Branden, P., Clary-Muronda, V., Hawkins, J. E., Fitzgerald, D., Shimek, A. M., Al-Itani, D., Madigan, E. A., & Rosa, W. E. (2021). Nurses achieving the Sustainable Development Goals: The United Nations and Sigma. *American Journal of Nursing, 121*(4), 65–68. https://doi.org/10.1097/01.naj.0000742544.07615.db

Taylor, B. (2014, August 7). The best leaders "talk the walk." *Harvard Business Review*. https://hbr.org/2014/08/the-best-leaders-talk-the-walk#:~:text=Why%20words%20matter.&text=One%20of%20the%20most%20ubiquitous,for%20their%20colleagues%20and%20organization

World Health Organization. (2016). *Nurse educator core competencies*. https://www.who.int/hrh/nursing_midwifery/nurse_educator050416.pdf

World Health Organization. (2020). *State of the world's nursing report 2020: Investing in education, jobs and leadership*. https://apps.who.int/iris/rest/bitstreams/1274201/retrieve

World Health Organization. (2021). *The WHO global strategic directions for nursing and midwifery (2021–2025)*. https://www.who.int/publications/m/item/global-strategic-directions-for-nursing-and-midwifery-2021-2025

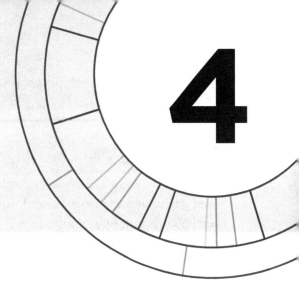

# 4

# DEVELOPING EFFECTIVE LEADERSHIP SKILLS AND CAPACITY

Nancy M. Ballard, PhD, RN, NEA-BC
Todd E. Tussing, DNP, RN, CENP, NEA-BC
Holly Wei, PhD, RN, NEA-BC, FAAN

## LEARNING OBJECTIVES

After completing this chapter, the learner will be able to:

- Identify principles and strategies to support strengths-based leadership.

- Define the role of politics and power in leadership.

- List strategies for dealing with politics and power in the leadership role.

- Identify components of effective communication.

- Describe the role conflict plays within work teams.

- Explain the role emotional intelligence and authenticity play in effective leadership.

- Develop positive leadership skills

# OVERVIEW

Leadership in organizations is a complex process dependent upon clear values based on maximizing personal and team strengths and understanding organizational politics and power. Leaders are expected to create a vision and actions that support the mission and outcomes for quality care while maintaining fiscal solvency. Paramount to accomplishing these objectives is the requirement of strong leadership, the use of evidence and information to acquire resources, and the inspiration of teams to collaborate and meet expected outcomes. Engagement with both executive leaders and teams is essential. Leadership skills—such as strengths-based leadership, power and politics, communication, conflict management, and team-building—will equip leaders with better tools for success.

# STRENGTHS-BASED LEADERSHIP

Performance improvement resulting from streamlining processes and cutting wastes to achieve improved outcomes requires leaders to build on personal and team strengths. During the 1990s, interest in leadership development changed its focus from identifying weaknesses to maximizing strengths. This change was rooted in a shift in the science of leadership toward a positive psychology approach (Welch et al., 2014). Collaboration by the Gallop Organization resulted in an assessment tool, *Clifton Strength Finder*, to measure leadership strengths in the belief that combining improvements in strengths with knowledge and skills would result in better outcomes. Other tools were subsequently developed, such as the *Values in Action* Inventory of Strengths (Peterson & Seligman, 2004), *Realize2* (Linley et al., 2010), and the *Reflected Best Self* (Roberts et al., 2005). While there is some disagreement on the substance of this approach (Warren, 2017), Ding and Yu (2020) found that strengths-based leadership mediated by work-related well-being was positively associated with enhanced task performance.

# DEVELOPING LEADER STRENGTHS

The development of strengths is an important area for leaders to explore. Welch et al. (2014) conducted interviews with executive coaches and determined areas contributing to developing strengths-based leadership for executives. From their research, four themes were identified.

The first theme is that strengths were intrinsically motivating and energizing. Leaders who incorporate motivators into their daily practice experience positive energy. They can discover "purpose" (i.e., what personally energizes them) and focus on building that same energy within the team they lead. Welch et al. (2014) point out that it is difficult to be passionate around a skill deficit. This does not mean that one can ignore the areas that aren't energizing, but if all the focus is on the weaknesses, the work suffers as those areas are energy-depleting. Leaders' attitudes and enthusiasm are contagious and encourage more energy in the team.

A second theme identified was the value of strength from building relationships. Identifying and incorporating strengths for the best outcome were energizing. For example, two parties with different strengths collaborate to achieve optimal results. One participant may have as a strength the ability to view the logistical steps of a project, and subsequently works with a partner with the talent to paint an inspirational vision. Together, the outcomes energize both parties and build on their strengths for a well-developed and inspiring plan. The resulting positive energy keeps everyone motivated. As indicated by Welch et al. (2014), leaders who work with their strengths subsequently encourage their team members to identify their own strengths as well. Combined with coaching, the result was that team members would work with more enthusiasm toward a goal.

The third theme involved leaders' awareness of personal blind spots while working on building strengths. Understanding one's blind spots and identifying corrective actions help leaders develop a good leadership balance. One example of a blind spot may be overusing one's strengths when working with a team. Such overuse can lead to unexpected results or irritation within the team. For example, if you are a good communicator and like to talk, you may not give ample time to others and thus deprive yourself of the team-related information needed for leadership. The practice of self-reflection on leadership strengths is an excellent exercise to identify blind spots. Additionally, working with an executive coach can be beneficial if you have difficulty discerning strengths, blind spots, or weaknesses and want to develop leadership strategies. Working with a peer and obtaining feedback is also helpful.

The fourth theme identified by Welch et al. (2014) was the need for self-awareness and taking time to reflect on what one is doing well, whether you are a leader or a coach for your team. One helpful exercise to assess self-awareness is to partner with another leader, list each other's strengths, and share perceptions of performance. While it may initially feel uncomfortable to spend time focusing on oneself, it has been shown to benefit a personal sense of well-being (Welch et al., 2014). In addition to self-reflection, lifelong self-development should be a continuous pursuit.

## STRENGTHS-BASED NURSING LEADERSHIP

Gottlieb et al. (2012) identified the principles for strengths-based nursing leadership, which leads to strengths-based nursing care. For a healthcare team to deliver the best care, leaders need to foster a culture that empowers staff to identify solutions and incorporate best practices. Recognition and cultivation of strengths support the development of a high-performing team, resulting in better patient outcomes. According to Gottlieb et al. (2012), strengths-based nursing care recognizes what works best and has potential. Factors critical to the development of strengths-based nursing care by leaders are (Gottlieb et al., 2012):

1.  Valuing the whole while recognizing the inter-relationship of the parts

2.   Recognizing the uniqueness of all team roles as well as the organization's role

3.   Creating a healthy work environment that promotes development

4.   Understanding subjective reality and the need for meaning

5.   Recognizing that the person and the environment should complement the work done and capitalize on the strengths that are associated with a good fit

6.   Promoting learning and recognize that readiness and timing are essential to success

Creating a culture that feeds on success incorporates role modeling supportive behavior and valuing high standards.

Strengths-based leadership is knowing each team member and coaching to improve the strengths either measured or displayed during their performance. Careful observation generally entails more active listening than "telling" to identify team strengths. Initiating the conversation, utilizing free or inexpensive assessment tools, can open the door to self-reflection by the team and growth as each person becomes more self-aware. Being more self-aware leads to an increased awareness of "other" when dealing with the stresses of the complex human side of healthcare. Identifying personal strengths and coaching team strengths leads to optimal care delivery and successful advancement in the organization.

# POSITIVE LEADERSHIP

Positive leadership is an emerging leadership practice, evolving with the field of positive psychology. It refers to the performance in which leaders facilitate optimistic transformations, cultivate favorable organizational cultures, and bring out the best of human conditions (Cameron, 2012). Positive leadership focuses on building human relationships and well-being and creating *abundance gaps*, the difference between ordinary and extraordinary performance (Cameron, 2010). Positive leadership strategies and practices have the potential to foster positivity and meaningful work and inspire followers to perform and accomplish best outcomes (Cameron, 2010, 2014). The following discussion will provide some positive leadership strategies and practices that can support exceptional leadership performance.

# LEADING WITH A CLEAR VISION

Leaders are like bus drivers, determining the directions buses go. In addition to having the right people on the "bus," an organization needs to have the right leader in driving the "bus." The right leaders know where to take their teams. Positive leaders act as translators and unifiers for their teams. They translate organizations' visions for their team members and align organizational goals and visions with the team and individual goals, facilitating the achievement of the organizational vision (Ashkenas & Manville, 2019; Wei, Corbett et al., 2020). Practices for leading with a clear vision include inspiring teams with organizations' missions, visions, and goals; fostering a higher sense of ownership and purpose; and creating channels for two-way communication, top-down and bottom-up, such as shared governance.

# CULTIVATING CARING RELATIONSHIPS

Leadership is a relationship, setting the tone of a team (Anderson, 2012). There is a saying that people will leave their jobs because of poor managers. Research shows that leaders have the power to make or break a team (Wei, Sewell et al., 2018). Leaders need to practice caring and accountability with their teams at the same time. Focusing more on responsibility and accountability and less on caring may lead to a less humanistic environment and decreased motivation. Yet, if leaders only focus on caring and not on accountability, productivity may suffer. It is essential to find a balance between the two (Wei & Watson, 2019). Practices of cultivating caring relationships include building a caring culture to promote nurse-patient, nurse-nurse, and nurse-healthcare professional relationships and foster nurses' sense of ownership and belonging.

## INSPIRING AND EMPOWERING FOLLOWERS

Positive leaders are inspiring and empowering. They are like a fuel station, supplying energy to followers by treating them with positive regard. Positive leaders understand the power of appreciation and recognition has on their teams (Clifton & Harter, 2019; Wei, King et al., 2020). Great leaders should be brave on approval and generous on praise, inspiring and empowering (Salas-Vallina et al., 2020; Wei et al., 2019). Leaders' using effective recognition, such as praise, can be an energy source or a refresher for followers struggling with a task. It is a skill set that leader can learn and practice. Practices include identifying what's right, finding opportunities to praise, empowering followers to take on new adventures, turning complaints into opportunities, promoting personal and professional development, and ensuring authenticity in recognition.

## REFOCUSING ON MEANING AND PURPOSE

Purpose guides leaders' vision and action. There is a common saying that you find purpose and meaning (which is sometimes hard to find) during difficult and hazy times. Thus, the purpose and meaning of work may need to be created instead of found, serving as a compass and an energy source for actions and performance (Wei, Kifner et al., 2020; Wei & Wei, 2020). Positive leaders need to frequently evaluate their own purpose and meaning of work and help team members create or refocus on their purpose and meaning of work. Positive leadership suggests that people get burnout from what they do, not why they do (Gordon, 2017). The purpose and meaning of work can shine a light on our actions. Practices include encouraging team members to reflect on why they initially chose the work they're doing, formulate meaning from what they do, listening to them, understanding them, and guiding them to refocus on purpose and meaning.

# LEADERSHIP'S ROLE IN DEALING WITH WORKPLACE POLITICS

*Politics*, often thought of in a negative context, is defined by Merriam-Webster (n.d.) as "the art or science of guiding or influencing government." In the context of healthcare, politics is vital in guiding and influencing policy and practice. The study of politics is divided into two levels; structures that support policy changes on the state and national level, the big "P"; and organizational politics, the little "p" (Patton et al., 2015). Involvement in big "P" politics includes participation with coalitions, lobbyists, and politicians who influence policy at the formal legislative level. Staying abreast of current state or national policy issues is a professional responsibility.

## BIG "P" POLITICS

Involvement in one's state or national professional organization provides an opportunity to be aware of policy issues affecting one's practice. Volunteering to be on the legislative committee and interacting with legislators provides a more direct level of involvement. Professional organizations offer education regarding lobbying and ways to contact influential legislators. Nursing leaders are encouraged to volunteer to reach and educate legislators on healthcare issues important to nursing or healthcare in general. Professional organizations usually provide a day to meet legislators at the state level and support internships at the national level to educate nurses on becoming more politically astute.

Involvement with political campaigns provides the opportunity to meet and influence political candidates or their staff. Building such relationships provides an avenue to supply insight from a nursing perspective and help provide the clinical evidence needed to support policy issues under consideration. Taking time to email or write letters to legislators and their staff on important issues can significantly influence legislators' votes.

The National Academy of Medicine's *Future of Nursing* report (Institute of Medicine, 2011) identified the need to increase the voice of nurses in healthcare by increasing nursing's presence on governing boards and executive-level decision-making teams. To support this recommendation, the Nursing on Boards Coalition was formed and exceeded the goal to have 10,000 nurses sit on boards by 2020, demonstrating how professional involvement can achieve a significant professional milestone (Nurses on Boards Coalition, n.d.). As Disch (2020) indicates, nurses bring a unique perspective from working within all levels of healthcare, making decisions from the bedside to the boardroom in policy development, dealing with regulatory agencies, and creating coalitions to implement change. Nurses bring a pragmatic view and expert knowledge of care delivery to identify and mitigate unintended consequences of well-intended policy decisions.

## LITTLE "P" POLITICS

In organizational leadership, politics receives little attention in nursing education programs but is a fact of life in all healthcare organizations. Understanding organizational politics and how to negotiate within the political structure can help career advancement. Attaining a senior leadership position allows one to influence change and develop a harmonious culture with one's vision for healthcare delivery. Intelligence and hard work are not enough to advance a career, whether in business or healthcare organizations.

Being heard by the right people at the right table and building support encompasses a political process. While those who choose nursing as a career do so for more altruistic reasons than to become a manager or chief nursing officer, preparation to negotiate for resources or changes to processes important for high-quality care delivery systems will require one to master the skill of politics. When interviewed regarding the role of power and politics play in work settings, an executive coach stated that women, as a rule, do not push for higher positions in the workplace, as power is not what they seek in their professional careers. In an example provided from her coaching of a female leader in healthcare, the executive coach identified a reluctance to climb the career ladder due to organizational politics. The executive coach helped this leader understand that changing the culture and reaching a more senior-level position involved understanding and using organizational politics to support a more positive culture. Pfeffer (2010) noted in a study of 509 leaders from education and finance managers that political skill was associated with higher performance evaluations and higher ratings on effectiveness.

Understanding the politics of an organization entails being observant of colleagues and paying attention to the actions of other leaders who are successful in eliciting support for resources or process changes. New leaders should be encouraged to ask successful leaders what contributed to their ability to secure initiatives they were proposing. Leaders usually feel honored to be asked and are willing to mentor new leaders, helping others gain insights on navigating the political environment. Such advice often includes being observant when entering a new organization, noticing who has the ear of senior leadership, and presenting their proposals. In addition, seeking advice from someone successful is crucial to identify the formal and informal (shadow) systems used to accomplish change, contributing to success. Shadow systems exist in organizations and comprise those staff who support the formal leaders, such as clinical staff who are respected and regarded as leaders because of their tenure or expertise within the organization and knowledge of how to "get things done." An excellent example of a shadow system is the administrative assistants who support senior leaders. This group often has a long tenure in their organizations and knows the processes and procedures to accomplish tasks. Identifying and using the shadow system can be crucial in successfully implementing change and navigating the political environment.

Frame your proposals while considering the organization's strategic priorities and prepare with data and evidence supporting the identified needs. It is essential to know how senior leaders measure success within the organization to frame persuasive and successful strategies. For example, if a strategic goal is to increase satisfaction with patient experience, identify how a proposal may improve patients' experience. An additional strategic plan of healthcare organizations is financial solvency. Thus, determining how a proposal improves the bottom line via cost avoidance can contribute to success. Proposal success may be dependent upon setting the stage with a decision-making body before a formal request. Establish a time to talk with colleagues whose support may be essential or other stakeholders whom the proposal will impact. Always prepare and elicit support from one's direct supervisor to avoid surprises and ensure support in decision-making groups.

## HUMAN CAPITAL

Building human capital contributes to organizational success. There are several types of human capital: intellectual capital, social capital, and political capital. *Intellectual capital* is knowledge acquired by an individual or group through experience or evidence. When a long-term employee leaves, the intellectual capital they take with them may disrupt operations or quality measures in the short term, because it is challenging to capture everything that needs to be handed over to replacements. In some instances, the person leaving the organization may be reluctant to share their acquired knowledge.

*Social capital* is developed through relationships and can be built by volunteering to work on a task force or project with other leaders or disciplines. Assisting with an operational issue in another department can build social capital with the leadership in that department or division. Social capital is built on honesty and trust in dealing with both senior leaders and the team that reports to you. Building a social network by being friendly and listening to others supports your team and other leaders.

*Political capital* comes from advocacy and the development of coalitions to support an objective. It may entail informal meetings before the significant decision is made and may include negotiation with affected stakeholders before the final decision to ensure their support. Political acumen can make a difference in your success and is vital in developing a power base to move things forward in your area of responsibility. Dealing with people in the political structure of organizations requires a skill set that takes time and experience to develop. Personalities can sometimes be challenging to navigate. Kathleen Reardon's book, *It's All Politics* (2005), provides an in-depth approach and strategies to deal with organizational politics and complex people situations.

# POWER

Kanter's (1993) early work on power structures in organizations has been the impetus for continued research on how power is used, acquired, and lost within organizations. In her early work, Kanter defined *power* as the ability to mobilize resources and get things done using whatever was needed to reach a goal. She was one of the first who identified the lack of women in senior positions and how power played a role in the social structure of organizations. Later work by researchers (Pfeffer, 2010, 2015; Reardon, 2005) provided additional insight into power sources and strategies for developing power. Understanding how to acquire and use power is essential for leaders in the complex health organizations of today and into the future. Sherman (2018) noted that nurses should seek power and influence because both are important to the success of their work. Power combined with politics provides the ability to influence decisions.

Sources of power vary from individual attributes as well as association with others who hold power. Disch (2020, p. 5) listed the various types of power encountered in organizations:

1. *Coercive power*—a perceived or actual fear of one person by another

2. *Reward power*—the belief that someone may bestow a reward or favor

3. *Legitimate (or positional) power*—power associated with an organizational position

4. *Expert power*—the power derived from an individual's expertise or unique talents

5. *Referent power*—the power generated from association with another

6. *Information power*—the belief that one has power based on particular information the person has

7. *Connection power*—the power derived from being connected with an individual or organization

8. *Empowerment*—a source of power when one in power shares authority and/or influence

Understanding how power is used facilitates the acquisition and use of power to influence decisions, an important role for leaders.

# BUILDING A POWER BASE

Positional power, while important, is not always effective in solidifying a power base. Pfeffer (2010) suggests that most power bases start small, such as assisting others as needed and taking advantage of reward power. Sharing your expertise increases your expert power by becoming the go-to person in the area (Pfeffer, 2010). Referent power is developed by associating with leaders in higher positions or those known to have expert power. Volunteering on a task force with persons viewed as having power can improve perceived power due to the social capital gained by the association with those perceived as powerful. Do not hesitate to volunteer to participate in projects or develop new services and programs as such work interactions may contribute to building a power base. As a person has more responsibility, their information power and connection power will increase. Empowering others contributes to one's overall power base, reflecting on the leader's ability. Ideally, as Porter O'Grady and Malloch (2018) noted, power is no longer concentrated at the top level of healthcare organizations, as today's successful leaders support the empowerment of team members to initiate change and improve care at all levels.

Understanding the role of power and politics is an essential element of leadership. As we move forward in nursing, embracing the concepts and developing the skills needed to influence change should be incorporated into leadership training. The goal of developing power is to be heard and influence decision-making. Thoughtful leadership actions facilitate achieving a power base and influencing decisions.

# EFFECTIVE COMMUNICATION

Today's healthcare environment is considerably complex and encompasses a culturally diverse workforce. Additionally, healthcare services have become decentralized to locations across regions and time zones. Healthcare environments often incorporate various forms of technology for patient care and data management and operate within complex organizational structures, with patient care services modeled on multiple layers/systems and work processes. Nursing leaders are under pressure to secure high-quality patient care outcomes while keeping their organizations fiscally solvent. During their daily work, nursing leaders interact with those around them through some form of communication. Communication is one of the most fundamental aspects of human relationships. Northouse (2022) defines leadership as "a process whereby an individual influences a group of individuals to achieve a common goal" (p. 6), and communication is the main tool leaders utilize to be influential in their roles. Ruben and Gigliotti (2016) state that *communication* is "a mechanism or strategic tool through which planned and intentional leadership outcomes occur" (p. 467). To effectively lead teams, a leader must understand the importance of communication and be an effective communicator.

Communication has been cited as an essential skill for nursing leaders. The American Organization for Nursing Leadership (AONL) designated it as the first competency in the Nurse Executive Competency tool (AONL, 2015). Failure to master the skill of communication can lead to loss as a leader. Effective communication requires knowledge of the communication process and its components. Secondly, mastering communication skills requires understanding and practicing techniques of effective communication. Everyone has their own style of communication that has been learned from social interactions and past experiences. The classical Linear Model of communication describes it as a process in which a message is sent from a sender to a receiver, interpreting and acting upon it (Ruben & Gigliotti, 2016). The Interactional Model of communication states that other variables come into play during the sending/receiving message process. This model says that nonverbal and verbal cues are involved, and the receiver provides communication back to the sender during the same process (Ruben & Gigliotti, 2016).

A third model, the Systems Model, views communication as "the way people create, convey, select, and interpret the messages that inform and shape their lives" (Ruben & Gigliotti, 2016, p. 471). Essentially, this model factors in life experiences such as culture, values, aspirations, and education, which can influence communication between two individuals. The model explains that the sender and receiver carry those factors with them during communication, and they must make a "match" during the messaging. The more significant the difference between the messenger and receiver, the greater the chances of a mismatch between the messenger and receiver, leading to a failed communication outcome (Ruben & Gigliotti, 2016). Leaders can greatly influence followers by understanding and adapting the communication models and their components while mastering techniques for effective communication.

## COMMUNICATION TIPS

Business communications have developed over the last century. Earlier forms of business communications involved direct face-to-face interaction, evolving to include the memo or other written forms of communication and audio use via the telephone. Today, digital communication has exponentially grown to include internal/external emails and audio/video and social media platforms. Leaders would be wise to understand the impact and role various forms of communication have on their followers to choose the correct communication method for their message. For example, the millennial generation grew up with technology in their daily lives. Thus, they are most comfortable using and prefer instant messaging and social media platforms as a means of communication (Waltz et al., 2020). Sherman (2021) provides five key areas leaders should consider before sending messages:

1. The target audience

2. The message

3. Time and frequencies to send the message

4. Potential impacts on the target audience

5. The best communication method

The importance of efficient and effective communication is an essential skill for nursing leadership, and it is one of the top competencies cited by AONL (2015). Through communication, nurse leaders can influence the care environment to provide the highest quality of patient care, help followers navigate complex healthcare systems, prepare for and negotiate change, and retain an experienced workforce. Nursing leaders need to understand the components of communication and develop strategies to become effective communicators.

# CONFLICT MANAGEMENT

In today's healthcare environment, teams must function in a complex system with multiple layers of leadership, services, and a diverse workforce. As with any other team, healthcare teams are vulnerable to conflict stemming from the complexity of their environments and the high demands placed upon them. Conflict is a basic human trait that exists, at some point, in all relationships. In healthcare teams, conflicts are sometimes labeled as "horizontal violence" or "incivility" (Reinhardt et al., 2020). Conflicts can evolve from differences between team members based on gender, culture, ethnicity, race, income, education, personal beliefs, or ethics and can be influenced by team members' mental health, intelligence, and emotional maturity (Porter-O'Grady & Malloch, 2011). Healthcare environments that contain such conflict have been linked to staff nurses' intent to leave their positions, resulting in costly turnovers and impacting patient care quality (Reinhardt et al., 2020; Wei, Sewell et al., 2018). In response to this concern, the American Association of Critical-Care Nurses (AACN) promoted a Healthy Work Environment (HWE) framework in 2001. In February 2019, the AACN released a report from a survey of nurses demonstrating that focus on an HWE has had an impressive impact: 66% of nurses reported a higher quality of care; 24% reported a decrease in moral distress; and 61% reported an intention to remain in their positions (Implementing Healthy Work Environment Standards Makes a Difference, 2020). Thus, managing team conflict is a significant component of establishing an HWE and should be a priority of nursing leaders.

Conflict does not have to be "unhealthy" for a team. When managed appropriately, conflict can enhance a team's cohesion as team members work through their differences. Furthermore, conflicts can help drive a team's innovation and critical thinking for problem-solving (McKibben, 2017). Teams that manage their differences gain trust among their membership and learn to work cohesively on problems and issues, leading to recognition as a high-performing team (Pipas, 2020). Lencioni (2002) noted that high-performing teams have five key behaviors: trust, conflict, commitment, accountability, and results. A team must utilize trust to manage differences to achieve commitment, accountability, and results. Nurse leaders must help manage team dynamics by guiding the team to establish trust and manage their conflict. Using an approach to managing conflict is important. Prause and Majtaba (2015) proposed five modes for conflict management:

- **Competing:** placing one's concerns ahead of others'
- **Accommodating:** placing others' concerns over your own
- **Avoiding:** not dealing with the conflict
- **Collaborating:** working together to come to a resolution
- **Compromising:** solving the conflict through partial fulfillment of one another's needs

Conflict is a basic human condition that is common among all teams. However, if pervasive, conflict can impact a team's ability to trust, debilitating quality of care. Low-performing teams are at risk for losing team members through attrition, resulting in further stress on the patient care team. Nursing leaders must understand conflict and how to mitigate it. Utilizing a model for conflict resolution is a crucial tool for nurse leaders as they work with their teams to establish cohesion and harmony to evolve into a high-performing team.

# TEAM-BUILDING

The human dynamics that occur with individuals working in groups have been recognized going back to the earliest history of humanity. Whether working as a "team" for hunting game for food, building the pyramids of Egypt, or working to win the Super Bowl in football, teams have demonstrated their power for accomplishment. Healthcare environments comprise various types of teams, including those working on short-term projects or teams that regularly meet to review and act on quality metrics. Today's nursing leaders need to lead, mentor, and support teams to meet organizational goals, including high-quality patient care. With the growth in technology, teamwork has moved from face-to-face encounters to virtual ones, challenging nursing leaders to apply their leadership skills to the virtual realm.

The cohesion of the group is essential for team members to work together to reach a common goal. A *team* refers to "a group composed of a small number of people, with complementary skills who are committed to a common purpose, set of performance goals and approach for which they hold themselves mutually accountable" (Hakanen et al., 2015, p. 44). An essential aspect of cohesion is trust (Hakanen et al., 2015). To build trust, leaders must support team members to gain familiarity with one another, foster healthy communication, resolve conflict, and encourage openness, honesty, and mutual respect (Hakanen et al., 2015).

Sherman (2021) identified that "the best teams do the following:

- Have a common purpose that they work to achieve.

- Communicate openly and clearly.

- Have trust among team members.

- Respect the role and contributions of every team member.

- Provide team back up to one another when needed.

- Make it safe to ask questions and make mistakes.

- Appreciate the value of diversity and successfully navigate conflict.

- See their work as having an impact.

- Recognize that different team members have different work styles on teams, and each is important." (Sherman, 2021, p. 124)

# VIRTUAL TEAMS

The use of virtual technology has been increasing for the last several decades and offers new and exciting platforms for teams to do their work. With the advent of the COVID-19 pandemic of 2020, most work teams moved from in-person interactions to working strictly from a virtual platform; and the popular thought is that virtual teams are here to stay (Prashara & Das-Monfrais, 2021). Nursing leaders must recognize the difference the virtual world encompasses from the in-person one and utilize their leadership skills in this new setting. Nursing leaders should cultivate trust within virtual teams as they foster it with in-person teams— by maintaining contact with each team member. Additionally, nursing leaders can cultivate trust by several key tactics: helping to establish the vision and goals of the group; practicing consistency and reliability with timely responses to inquiries from members of the team; maintaining informational transparency with the group; resolving conflict; celebrating successes; and establishing frequent "check-ins" with the team and each team member (Ford et al., 2017). When communicating with virtual teams, the nursing leader should maintain the professional milieu and be cautious of using virtual communication methods in a "personal" style. Instead, keep communication professional by spellchecking all messages before sending and using emojis sparingly and decisively. Furthermore, messages should be to the point, business-oriented, and not take on a personal style by avoidance of encoding emotions and use of sound effects (Darics, 2020).

Nursing leaders should support the infrastructure of the virtual teams, which includes the equipment (hardware and software) and any organizational policies that would affect the team. The importance of reliable, modern hardware and software to support the team's work is essential for performance. Collaboration between nursing leaders and Information Technology departments is critical. The partnership can advocate for reliable, easy-to-use equipment that offers features conducive to various team needs (i.e., whiteboard use during brainstorming, task management platforms to keep team members on track, etc.).

While established procedures provide step-by-step instruction on how to complete a task, policies offer philosophical guidance to solve issues confronting team members. Both are essential to maintain structure in organizations. Many policies and procedures were written to accommodate in-person situations. With the change to virtual work, nursing leaders will need to review applicable organizational policies and procedures to ensure they encompass virtual work and advocate for changes to such policies and procedures if they are not supportive (Ford et al., 2017). Teamwork is essential to healthcare organizations for meeting patient care and operational targets. Nursing leaders must support and guide teams to cultivate a high-performing working unit to accomplish identified goals. Understanding the dynamics of teamwork and understanding what comprises high-performing teams is essential for nursing leaders.

# TIPS TO IMPROVE LEADERSHIP INFLUENCE

Today's nurse leader is responsible for supporting the goals of the organization in which they practice; one of the most critical goals includes the outcome of high-quality patient care. Nurse leaders need to use all the leadership tools available to achieve success with this high-stakes responsibility. One crucial tool the nurse leader has is *influence,* which has been defined as "the ability to persuade others based on authority, communication traits, knowledge-based competencies, status and timing" (Johnson & Costa, 2019, p. 108). Recognizing the importance of influence on the healthcare environment, the AONL included it as a sub-competency in the Nurse Executive Competencies (AONL, 2015). Understanding strategies to enhance performance through influence is essential for nurse leaders in today's complex healthcare environment.

# LEADERSHIP STYLE

Cultivating influence is an essential step to enhancing leadership and its impact on organizational outcomes. Ruben and Gigliotti (2017) state that "leaders are presumed to be responsible for initiating the workplace and stakeholder relationship, creating communication linkages, and carrying the burden for providing the direction necessary to maintain these relationships" (p. 17). Leadership style has been determined to enhance influence within a nursing team (Wei, King et al., 2020). A transformational leadership style has been determined to be the relationship-based leadership style that most significantly influences teams (Cummings et al., 2018; Majeed & Jamshed, 2021; Waltz et al., 2020; Wang et al., 2017). Transformational Leadership is a process in which leaders focus on team emotions, values, and ethics to help reach long-term goals. This leader is attentive to the needs of followers and cultivates their well-being and professional goals through encouraging creativity, building trust, setting a vision, and recognizing achievements (Northouse, 2022).

# EMOTIONAL INTELLIGENCE AND AUTHENTICITY

The ability to influence others is dependent on the relationship between the leader and the follower; to cultivate that relationship, leaders must understand themselves from both an emotional intelligence perspective and the perception of authenticity they demonstrate. One of the most consistent traits found among successful leaders was emotional intelligence. *Emotional intelligence* is "the ability to understand and manage your own emotions, as well as recognize and influence the emotions of those around you" (Landry, 2019, para. 3). There are four components of emotional intelligence: self-awareness, self-management, social awareness, and relationship management. Successful leaders must learn to develop their approaches based on these domains as applied to interactions with followers and constituents. Internet-based, free tools exist, which leaders can use to assess each domain and build skills to enhance their interactions (Johnson & Costa, 2019).

An essential aspect of this relationship is the perception of the "authenticity" of the leader by the followers. The state of *authenticity* involves "three aspects: a match between conscious awareness and experience, being true to oneself in most situations, and living by one's values and beliefs" (Zheng et al., 2020). Zheng et al. studied authenticity and its relationship to followers through influence. They discovered that for leaders to have influence, they must be authentic in what they say and do and help their followers develop a sense of "belongingness" in the leader-follower relationship.

# LEADERSHIP MODEL TO GUIDE PRACTICE

The complexity of today's healthcare systems demands a leadership approach that is not reliant on a hierarchical model, but rather one that allows followers to interact with and be influenced by their leaders to cultivate a healthy work environment and accomplish the organization's goals. To meet this need, nurse leaders must have a relationship-based leadership style (such as Transformational Leadership) to interact, support, mentor, and be vulnerable with their staff. The demands from nursing staff, patient care, and the internal and external industry requirements can challenge even the most experienced nurse leader. Using a leadership model would be a helpful tool for nurse leaders facing such complex, high stakes demands. The Human-Centered Leadership Model "seeks to address complexity through upholding, awakening, and connecting the people who care for the people with an ultimate goal of nurturing cultures of care, excellence, and trust" (Kennedy et al., 2020). The model focuses on the relationship the leader has with followers by cultivating a "fair and just" culture, a learning environment for staff, supporting innovation from those who are doing the work, and helping to enhance the care experience for both the staff and patients (Kennedy et al., 2020; Leclerc et al., 2020).

Nursing leaders must cultivate the influence they exhibit in the healthcare environment. Understanding one's emotional intelligence and perceived authenticity can lay the foundation of influence. Additionally, adapting one's leadership style to a more relationship-based approach, such as Transformational Leadership, can further add to a nurse leader's impact. The use of leadership models, such as the Human-Centered Leadership Model, can guide nurse leaders while using these approaches and tools to help navigate the complexity of the many needs of today's healthcare systems.

# IMPLICATIONS FOR PRACTICE

Leadership requires an understanding of key components regarding organizations. Identification and focus on personal strengths support effective coaching of the interprofessional team needed to deliver the quality care that has become an expectation. Understanding, developing, and using power and political structures is necessary to advance to positions of influence within organizations, thus ensuring that voices from a nursing perspective can be heard at the highest decision-making levels. Rather than harboring reluctance to get involved with organizational politics, one should embrace, learn, and practice what is needed to be successful. Building a professional and social network is an important aspect of the leadership role. Relationships are often crucial to success in moving toward the empowered workforce important to a successful organization. Complexity in healthcare and the pace of change are unavoidable, underscoring the need for ongoing self-development to support the best outcomes.

One of the most important tools used by leaders is the ability to communicate. Through communication, leaders impart their vision, provide direction, and give feedback that molds and strengthens their teams. Leaders must familiarize themselves with the different communication modalities today, including the written word, audio (i.e., telephone), and visual (internet-based), including social media. Learning to use each modality to its full potential would give leaders a powerful tool to build and lead teams. Teams come in many forms (e.g., in-person and virtual) and in many settings in which leaders must adapt their leadership approach for success. Conflict within teams is common and can provide opportunities to solve problems and strengthen innovation and trust within the team. Leaders must learn to recognize and solve conflict when it arises. The transformational, strengths-based, and positive leadership styles are paramount to the effectiveness of leaders with their teams. Leadership plays a significant role in teams' success.

# SUMMARY

This chapter goes beyond the age-old question about whether leaders are made or born, providing strategies to improve leadership skills and capacities. However, leadership is not just the information in the book but requires leaders' motivations and actions. Learning to lead takes a willing heart and serving motivations. Understanding strategies to enhance performance is essential in today's complex healthcare environment.

# REFLECTIVE QUESTIONS

1.  What are factors critical to the development of strengths-based leadership for nurse leaders?

2.  Please describe the sources of power in organizations.

3.  What are the key components of effective communication for leaders?

4.  Please describe the five modes to solve conflicts.

5.  What is positive leadership?

---

## NARRATIVE

One Monday morning, when Megan, the nurse manager of a surgical unit, stepped into the unit, she saw that everyone was busy. She noticed that the unit code cart was parked outside Room 1, and the code team was in the room. She was informed that a new nurse administered the wrong dose of medicine to the patient in Room 1. The patient was transferred to the ICU after the code. Once things had calmed down, Megan called the nurse to her office and asked, "What happened?" The nurse said, "I was very busy with my patients and heard other nurses talking about me. I kept thinking about what they had said about me. I was upset. I was distracted and pulled the wrong dose of medicine." Megan could tell the nurse felt terrible, and then she mumbled, "I want them to like me. I should not be distracted by them." Megan did not understand what the nurse meant and questioned the nurse, "What are you talking about?"

In the following few days, the nurse called out sick. A few weeks later, the nurse submitted her resignation letter to Megan and left the unit. A few other nurses also left the unit consecutively. Megan started to realize the necessity to evaluate the unit's work environment. She recognizes a need for a change in culture in her unit.

# AUTHOR BIOGRAPHIES

**Nancy M. Ballard, PhD, RN, NEA-BC,** is an Assistant Professor at Kennesaw State University in Kennesaw, Georgia, and a Nurse Researcher and Coordinator of the MSN in the Leadership in Nursing-Nursing Administration Track. Prior to her current position, after starting in critical care, she held hospital and system leadership roles as Cardiac Rehabilitation Coordinator, Nurse Manager, Clinical Nurse Specialist, Cardiac Outcomes Coordinator, and Director of the Center for Nursing Excellence for WellStar Health System. Serving as an appraiser and team leader for the ANCC Magnet Designation program for more than a decade has provided insight into excellence in nursing leadership and practice in both national and international settings. Research interest in the practice environment and shared governance has led to presentations of her research at national and international conferences with publications in the *American Journal of Critical Care*, *Journal of Nursing Administration*, *Journal of Emergency Nursing*, and *Western Journal of Nursing Research*.

**Todd E. Tussing, DNP, RN, CENP, NEA-BC,** is Assistant Professor of Clinical Nursing for the College of Nursing at The Ohio State University. He has over 34 years of nursing experience, of which 30+ years have been in some type of leadership role. Tussing began his nursing career as a staff nurse in various intensive care units with experience in caring for critically ill medical and surgical patients. Tussing began his leadership career as charge nurse progressing to nursing supervisor, nurse manager, director of nursing and administrative director of nursing. Additionally, he has been actively involved in educating nurses. He has taught in pre-licensure programs, RN to BSN completion programs, masters, and doctoral programs. A diploma in nursing graduate, he furthered his education by completing his BSN, Master of Science, and Doctor of Nursing Practice degrees. He is currently dual certified as a nurse executive.

**Holly Wei, PhD, RN, NEA-BC, FAAN,** is a Professor and Assistant Dean for the PhD program at the University of Louisville School of Nursing. Her overarching research focuses on healthcare organizational culture, leadership development, clinician well-being, stress genomic biomarkers, and patient care quality. She is known nationally and internationally for her nursing practice models and a Convergent Care Theory. Multiple healthcare systems have used Wei's nursing models to guide practice and promote organizational culture and patient care with significant improvements in nursing practice and patient care quality.

# REFERENCES

American Organization for Nursing Leadership. (2015). *Nurse executive competencies*. https://www.aonl.org/system/files/media/file/2019/06/nec.pdf

Anderson, D. (2012). Is building relationships the key to leadership? Performance improvement, *International Society for Performance Improvement, 51*(2), 15–21. https://doi.org/10.1002/pfi.21245

Ashkenas, R., & Manville, B. (2019, April 4). You don't have to be CEO to be a visionary leader. *Harvard Business Review*. https://hbr.org/2019/04/you-dont-have-to-be-ceo-to-be-a-visionary-leader

Cameron, K. (2010). Five keys to flourishing in trying times. *Leader to Leader, 2010*(55), 45–51. doi:10.1002/ltl.401

Cameron, K. (2012). *Positive leadership: Strategies for extraordinary performance.* Berrett-Koehler.

Cameron, K. (2014). Activate virtuousness. In J. E. Dutton & G. M. Spreitzer (Eds.), *How to be a positive leader: Small actions, big impact* (pp. 79–89). Berrett-Koehler.

Clifton, J., & Harter, J. (2019). *It's the manager: Moving from boss to coach.* Gallup Press.

Cummings, G. G., Tate, K., Lee, S., Wong, C. A., Paananen, T., Micaroni, S. P. M., & Chatterjee, G. E. (2018). Leadership style and outcome patterns for the nursing workforce and work environment: A systematic review. *International Journal of Nursing Studies, 85,* 19–60.

Darics, E. (2020). E-leadership or "How to be boss in instant messaging?" The role of nonverbal communication. *International Journal of Business Communications, 57*(1), 3–29.

Ding, H. & Yu, E. (2020). Follower strengths-based leadership and follower innovative behavior: The roles of core self-evaluations and psychological well-being. *Journal of Work and Organizational Psychology, 36*(2), 103–110. https://doi.org/10.5093/jwop2020a8

Disch, J. (2020). Nursing leadership in policy formation. *Nursing Forum, 55,* 4–10. doi: 10.1111/nuf.12375

Ford, R. C., Piccolo, R. F., & Ford, L. R. (2017). Strategies for building effective virtual teams: Trust is the key. *Business Horizons, 60,* 25–34.

Gordon, J. (2017). *The power of positive leadership: How and why positive leaders transform teams and organizations and change the world* (1st ed.). John Wiley & Sons, Inc.

Gottlieb, L. N., Gottlieb, B., & Shamian, J. (2012). Principles of strengths-based nursing leadership for strengths-based nursing care: A new paradigm for nursing and healthcare for the 21st century. *Nursing Leadership, 25*(2), 38–50. doi: 10.12927/cjnl.2012.22960

Hakanen, M., Hakkinen, M., & Soudunsaari, A. (2015). Trust in building high-performing teams – conceptual approach. *Electronic Journal of Business Ethics and Organizational Studies, 20*(2), 43–53. http://ejbo.jyu.fi/pdf/ejbo_vol20_no2_pages_43-53.pfd

Implementing healthy work environment standards makes a difference. (2020). *AACN Bold Voices, 12*(1), 18–19.

Institute of Medicine (US) Committee on the Robert Wood Johnson Foundation Initiative on the Future of Nursing, at the Institute of Medicine. (2011). *The future of nursing: Leading change, advancing health.* National Academies Press. PMID: 24983041.

Johnson, J. E., & Costa, L. L. (2019). *The DNP nurse in executive leadership roles.* DEStech Publications.

Kanter, R. M. (1993). *Men and women of the corporation.* Basic Books.

Kennedy, K., Campis, S., & Leclerc, L. (2020). Human-centered leadership: Creating change from the inside out. *Nurse Leader, 18*(3), 227–231.

Landry, L. (2019, April 3). *Why emotional intelligence is important in leadership.* Harvard Business School Online. https://online.hbs.edu/blog/post/emotional-intelligence-in-leadership

Leclerc, L., Kennedy, K., & Campis, S. (2020). Human-centered leadership in health care. *Nursing Administration Quarterly, 44*(2), 117–126.

Lencioni, P. (2002). *The five dysfunctions of a team.* Jossey-Bass.

Linley, A., Willars, J., & Biswas-Diener, R. (2010). *The strengths book: Be confident, be successful, and enjoy better relationships by realising the best of you.* CAPP Press.

Majeed, N., & Jamshed, S. (2021). Nursing turnover intentions: The role of leader emotional intelligence and team culture. *Journal of Nursing Management, 29,* 229–239.

McKibben, L. (2017). Conflict management: Importance and implications. *British Journal of Nursing, 26*(2), 100–103.

Merriam-Webster. (n.d.). *Politics*. In Merriam-Webster.com dictionary. https://www.merriam-webster.com/dictionary/politics

Northouse, P. G. (2022). *Leadership theory & practice* (9th ed.). Sage Publishing.

Nurses on Boards Coalition. (n.d.). *Our story*. Retrieved from https://www.nursesonboardscoalition.org/about/

Patton, R., Zalon, M., & Ludwick, R. (2015). *Nurses making policy*. American Nurses Association & Springer Publishing.

Peterson, G., & Seligman, M. E. P. (2004). *Character strengths and virtues: A handbook and classification*. Oxford University Press.

Pfeffer, J. (2010). *Power: Why some people have it and others don't*. HarperCollins Publishers, Inc.

Pfeffer, J. (2015). *Leadership B.S.* HarperCollins Publishers, Inc.

Pipas, C. F. (2020). Two habits of a health team: Managing conflict and practicing gratitude. *Family Practice Management, 27*(4), 11–16.

Porter-O'Grady, T. & Malloch, K. (2011). *Quantum leadership advancing innovation, transforming health care* (3rd ed.). Jones & Bartlett Learning.

Porter-O'Grady, T., & Malloch, K. (2018). *Quantum leadership: Creating sustainable value in health care* (5th ed.). Jones & Bartlett Learning.

Prashara, S., & Das-Monfrais, C. (2021). The new leadership dynamics. *PM Network, 35*(2), 18–46.

Prause, D., & Majtaba, B. G. (2015). Conflict management practices for diverse workplaces. *Journal of Business Studies Quarterly, 6*(3), 13–22.

Reardon, K. K. (2005). *It's all politics*. DoubleDay.

Reinhardt, A. C., Leon, T. G., & Amatya, A. (2020). Why nurses stay: Analysis of the registered nurse workforce and the relationship to work environments. *Applied Nursing Research, 55*. https://doi.org/10.1016/j.apnr.2020.151316

Roberts, L. M., Dutton, J. E., Spreitzer, G. M., Heaphy, E. D., & Quinn, R. E. (2005). Composing the reflected best-self-portrait: Building pathways for becoming extraordinary in work organizations. *The Academy of Management Review, 30*, 712–736. doi: 10.5465/AMR.2005.18378874

Ruben, B. D., & Gigliotti, R. A. (2016). Leadership as social influence: An expanded view of leadership communication theory and practice. *Journal of Leadership & Organizational Studies, 23*(4), 467–479.

Ruben, B. D., & Gigliotti, R. A. (2017). Communication: Sine qua non of organizational leadership theory and practice. *International Journal of Business Communication, 54*(1), 12–30. https://doi.org/10.1177/2329488416675447

Salas-Vallina, A., Simone, C., & Fernández-Guerrero, R. (2020). The human side of leadership: Inspirational leadership effects on follower characteristics and happiness at work (HAW). *Journal of Business Research, 107*, 162–171. https://doi.org/10.1016/j.jbusres.2018.10.044

Sherman, R. (2018). Leadership influence and power. *Nurse Leader, 16*(1), 6–7.

Sherman, R. O. (2021). *The nuts and bolts of nursing leadership. Your toolkit for success*. Rose O. Sherman Publisher.

Waltz, L. A., Munoz, L., Johnson, H. W., & Rodriguez, T. (2020). Exploring job satisfaction and workplace engagement in millennial nurses. *Journal of Nursing Management, 28*, 673–681.

Wang, L., Tao, H. T., Bowers, B. J., Brown, R., & Zhang, Y. (2017). When nurse emotional intelligence matters: How transformational leadership influences intent to stay. *Journal of Nursing Management, 26*, 358–365.

Warren, R. (2017). Strengths-based leadership assessments miss the target – and the species. *Development and Learning in Organizations, 31*(6), 1–3. doi:10.1108/DLO-06-2017-0060

Wei, H., Corbett, R. W., Ray, J., & Wei, T. L. (2020). A culture of caring: The essence of healthcare interprofessional collaboration. *Journal of Interprofessional Care, 34*(3), 321–334. https://doi.org/10.10 80/13561820.2019.1641476

Wei, H., Kifner, H., Dawes, M. E., Wei, T. L., & Boyd, J. M. (2020). Self-care strategies to combat burnout among pediatric critical care nurses and physicians. *Critical Care Nurse, 40*(2), 1–11. https://doi. org/10.4037/ccn2020621

Wei, H., King, A., Jiang., Y., & Lake, D. (2020). The impact of nurse leadership styles on nurse burnout: A systematic literature review. *Nurse Leader, 18*(5), 439–450. https://doi.org/10.1016/j.mnl.2020.04.002

Wei, H., Roberts, P., Stricker, J., & Corbett, R. (2019). Nurse leaders' strategies to foster nurse resilience. *Journal of Nursing Management, 27*(4), 681–687. doi:10.1111/jonm.12736

Wei, H., Sewell, K. A., Woody, G., & Rose, M. A. (2018). The state of the science of nurse work environments in the United States: A systematic review. *International Journal of Nursing Sciences, 5*(3), 287–300. https://doi.org/10.1016/j.ijnss.2018.04.010

Wei, H., & Watson, J. (2019). Healthcare interprofessional team members' perspectives on human caring: A directed content analysis study. *International Journal of Nursing Sciences, 6*(1), 17–23. https://doi. org/10.1016/j.ijnss.2018.12.001

Wei, H., & Wei, T. L. (2020). The power of self-care: An ENERGY Model to combat clinician burnout. *American Nurse, 15*(10), 28–31." *15*(10), 28–31. https://www.myamericannurse.com/wp-content/ uploads/2020/09/an10-Energy-916.pdf

Welch, D., Grossaint, K., Reid, K., & Walker, C. (2014). Strengths-based leadership development: Insights from expert coaches. *Consulting Psychology Journal: Practice and Research, 66*(1), 20–37. doi: 10.1037/ cpb0000002

Zheng, M. X., Yuan, Y., van Dijke, M., De Cremer, D., & Van Hiel, A. (2020). The interactive effect of a leader's sense of uniqueness and sense of belongingness on followers' perceptions of leader authenticity. *Journal of Business Ethics, 164*, 515–533.

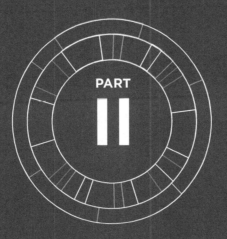

# FOSTERING HEALTHY WORK ENVIRONMENTS

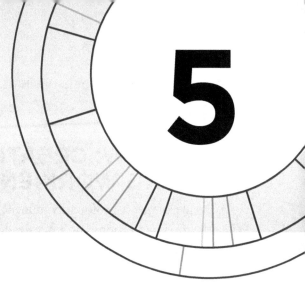

# 5

# NURTURING HEALTHY AND HEALING WORK ENVIRONMENTS

Wanda J. Borges, PhD, RN, ANP-BC
Gisela H. van Rensburg, DLitt et Phil
Chelsie Monroe, MSN, APRN, PMHNP-BC
Sara Horton-Deutsch, PhD, RN, PMHCNS, FAAN, ANEF

## LEARNING OBJECTIVES

After completing this chapter, the learner will be able to:

- Identify characteristics of both healthy and healing work environments

- Describe intentional and iterative leadership practices that lead to authentic care of self, others, and the environment

- Apply theoretical, philosophical, and research knowledge that guides nursing leaders in developing intentional and iterative practices to transform healthcare environments

- Develop strategies for application in practice

# OVERVIEW: CREATING HEALTHY AND HEALING WORK ENVIRONMENTS

Work environments profoundly influence how nurses feel about their jobs. Thus, healthcare organizations and nurse leaders must do their part to create safe spaces where everyone is valued, included, and held accountable for creating a healthy and healing work environment. Healthy environments improve job satisfaction, support retention, influence patient and student experiences, enhance teamwork, and improve patient outcomes (Wei et al., 2018). On the contrary, when nurses suffer, patients, families, and organizations suffer as well. This chapter will explore what a healthy and healing environment is; explain theoretical, philosophical, and research knowledge that guides nurse leaders to develop one; and describe intentional practices to build and enhance healthy, healing environments for leaders and others. Finally, we will prioritize nurse leader actions for regenerating them through actions intended to renew and restore.

# BACKGROUND

The Occupational Health and Safety Act was passed in the United States in 1970. The Occupational Safety and Health Administration, established in 1971, developed the first standards for the health of workers (US Department of Labor, n.d.). Johnson & Johnson developed a worksite wellness program, Live for Life, in 1979, and subsequent studies demonstrated a positive impact on employee health with a decrease in healthcare expenditures and employee absenteeism (Isaac, 2001). The Live for Life program was spread throughout the company, and other organizations used the model to implement worksite wellness programs in the 1980s. In 1990, Occupational Safety and Health was included in the Healthy People 2000 priority areas, with health promotion services offered to 75% of employers with 50 or more workers (Centers for Disease Control [CDC], 1999). One of the Healthy People 2010 and 2020 objectives for Occupational Safety and Health was that 50% of employers with 50 or more workers would have a worksite stress reduction program (CDC, n.d.). Of note is that in 2010 the number of worksite wellness programs decreased.

Studies in the 1970s of job satisfaction in nursing demonstrated that organizational variables affected satisfaction and turnover (Alspach, 2009). Identifying the factors associated with work environments that attract and retain nursing staff, the study that described the "Forces of Magnetism" that started the American Nurses Credentialing Center (ANCC) Magnet Recognition program was completed in 1983 (ANCC, n.d.). In 2008, the Commission on Magnet developed a conceptual model with five key components:

1.  Transformational Leadership

2.  Structural Empowerment

3.  Exemplary Professional Practice

4.  New Knowledge, Innovations & Improvements

5.  Empirical Outcomes

Within the key components, the original 14 organizational attributes remained the same. Kramer et al. (2010) conducted meta-analyses of two sets of publications that included publications from professional organizations and regulatory bodies that advocated for healthy work environments and publications from the Essentials of Magnetism studies. They identified the nine most influential structures for a quality work environment, which are listed below (Kramer et al., 2010, p. 10):

- Quality leadership at all levels of the organization

- Availability of and support for education, career, performance, and competence development

- Administrative sanction for autonomous and collaborative practice

- Evidence-based practice education and operational supports

- Culture, practice, and opportunity to learn interdisciplinary collaboration

- Empowered, shared decision-making structures for control of the context of nursing practice

- Generation and nurturance of a patient-centered culture

- Staffing structures that take into account RN competence, patient acuity, and teamwork

- Development and support of intradisciplinary teamwork

Other professional nursing organizations also developed models and advocate for healthy work environments (Association of Critical-Care Nurses [AACN, 2016; ANCC, 2018; American Organization for Nursing Leadership, 2019). The factors associated with healthy work environments have many similarities and are multidimensional and interrelated (Alspach, 2009). While most factors influencing healthy work environments are organizational, affecting nurses throughout the organization, they are often operationalized at a unit level. Those elements that operate at the individual nurse level are not included. The American Nurses Association (ANA) Code of Ethics (2015) was revised and serves as a framework to create optimal professional practice, a guide for peer review, quality assurance, a method to educate nursing students in professional conduct, and further professional goals. The revised Code of Ethics also includes elements that define nurses' duties for self-care and workplace ethics and responsibilities for research and scholarly inquiry. It is paramount to understand that the nurse owes the same duties to self as to others, including the responsibility to promote health and safety, preserve wholeness of character and integrity, maintain competence, and continue personal and professional growth. Self-care becomes paramount to ethical practice as a nurse.

While the models for creating healthy work environments to improve patient safety and quality have been described in the literature for decades, medical errors remain high in the US (Makary & Daniel, 2016). In addition, burnout rates in the healthcare professions remain high: 51% of physicians (Shanafelt et al., 2012) and 54% of nurses, with 28% reporting experiencing high levels of burnout (Kelly et al., 2020). Wei et al. (2018) noted that most studies reviewed were descriptive in their systematic review of the literature. Further research is needed to design and test interventions to create healthy work environments.

There is a difference between healing and health. "While health is an outcome, healing is a choice" (Georgiou in McMorrow, 2017, para. 11). Healing involves a process that can be physical but also spiritual, emotional, and psychological. Healing involves action to engage in behaviors that will lead to health. A healing environment has a nurturing and therapeutic effect that promotes a sense of well-being (Montefiore Medical Center, 2021). The Institute for Healthcare Improvement advocates for the Quadruple Aim after adding joy to the Triple Aim in 2017. Joy is not just about reducing burnout. "Joy in work is an essential resource for the enterprise of healing" (Perlo et al., 2017, p. 4). Ultimately, attending to the healing process is what will result in a healthy and healing work environment. This change in focus requires examining the elements of healing spaces, emphasizing creating healing environments, leading to healthy work environments. By expanding on our understanding that a healthy environment must be healing, healing requires a commitment to self-care as a foundation for healing others.

# THEORETICAL, PHILOSOPHICAL, AND RESEARCH KNOWLEDGE NEEDED FOR NURSING

At the core of the landscape of nursing is a healthy workforce and a healthy and healing work environment. An organizational culture that empowers and supports skilled communication, collaboration, and respect are characteristics of a healthy and healing work environment. As a result, employees feel emotionally and physically safe (Kupperschmidt et al., 2010). Safety is a crucial component to developing a therapeutic and healing environment. If the nurse is safe, only then can they step up and support and care for those in need. Safety involves understanding the culture within the environment, including a culture of respect, caring for self and others, and reporting. Within an environment that fosters caring relationships lies an underlying belief that the patient always deserves the best. A nurse who feels safe develops a deepened understanding, empathy, and compassion for others, supporting the development of a healthy workplace where conflict is viewed as transformative, and open communication and civility flourish (Griffin et al., 2021). The personal responsibility to take care of our health and healing is influenced by professional knowledge based on theoretical, philosophical, and research knowledge.

We are currently in an era of theory utilization in that nurses use philosophies, theories, and models for nursing practice (Alligood, 2018). Research conducted by Bond et al. (2011) indicated that theories are essential for our progress as a profession and applying theory to practice. Philosophies, theories, and models of nursing guide logical reasoning, thoughtful action, and efficient information processing. The question that then arises is: "What is the nature of the theoretical, philosophical, and research knowledge needed for the practice of nursing?" Such questions have driven professional nursing. The ability to resolve struggles between what nursing is and what nurses do orders the profession's existence (Smith et al., 2013). More so, the quality of care is directly influenced by the absence of structure provided by knowledge. Therefore, theory utilization is directly aligned with goals for quality healthcare. Nevertheless, so are all role players/individuals rendering the care.

Ensuring a healthy workforce requires a healing environment that fosters reflective practices, intentional practices to enhance self-care, mindfulness, and well-being in general. Often, proposed solutions to health workforce problems compromise a deeper, philosophical, values-based profession where self-care is essential. The hallmark of a philosophy that underpins and understands the wholeness of a person's needs and situations is based on trust, knowledge, skills, and the ability to manage all these elements simultaneously, with both a theoretical and a practical side (Austgard, 2008). According to social exchange theories (Worchel et al., 1991), when individuals (nurses) interact with others (patients), there is a *cost* involved. At the same time, there are *rewards* involved. To make the interaction worthwhile and considering one's responsibility towards personal health and healing, careful consideration for one's well-being is essential. Interaction requires purposeful and intentional communication.

The Theory of Human Becoming by Parse (1992) describes nurses as being on a pathway to becoming skilled communicators. Nurses interact with the environment and with people in the environment to co-create meaning between and among them. In doing so, nurses are responsible for the significances of relationships and how they evolve and relate to each other. Parse highlights the importance of being present when interacting with others to enhance the quality of work and life both for themselves and for others. Furthermore, good communication skills that enhance respectful interaction are an ethical mandate necessary to reach and maintain healthy work environments.

Parse's theory provides a transformative approach to all levels of nursing. Therefore, the focus is not on solving problems but rather on providing perspectives that acknowledge different viewpoints of different role players (e.g., nurses and patients). Such perspectives allow for presence and opportunities to co-create goals. The focus is on the art of human becoming present with the unfolding of meaning, harmonizing rhythms, and wholeness. The theory provides research methodologies and a framework to guide inquiry. For research, it includes the *simultaneity paradigm*, which states that man is a unitary being in continuous, mutual interaction with the environment.

The Caring Science philosophy by Watson (2008) posits that an environment promotes healing if it includes the physical and psychological safety of both patient and nurse or care provider. Nurse leaders who practice within the Watson Caring Science framework promote an environment where caring and healing are intentional. This framework teaches nurses how to use heart-centered practices and caring-healing modalities to create compassionate healing environments for themselves and others (Norman et al., 2016; Watson, 2008). In such an environment, mindfulness not only of one's own emotions and feelings but also of those of the patients is evident by how you present yourself authentically. Authentic presence in a healthy and healing environment recognizes the uniqueness of every moment one encounters in the workplace.

To create and regenerate healthy and healing environments, theory-based skills, self-regulatory skills, and tools are important. Skills in offering compassion with a balanced approach, both for oneself and others, require relational-based care. Relational-based care involves new ways of understanding the deeper meaning of the pressure experienced in the workplace by putting yourself in the other person's position. Learning how to be more humane towards oneself and others within complex situations also helps one learn how to deal with impasses. Finding solutions through knowledge creation, translation, and uptake draw on Watson's embodiments of heart-centered practices, which increase access to higher consciousness, engaged communication, care, compassion, intellect, and practices that enhance authentic presence. To decrease stress in the workplace, nurses must collaborate with the patient and family, meeting their basic needs and increase the likelihood of co-creating safe and healing environments.

Within the context of knowledge development, the dynamic processes of a quest for feasible truths about reality begin with creative approaches from multiple perspectives to knowledge and knowing. The potential effects of self-care techniques on increasing nurses' effectiveness and influencing positive patient care outcomes have often been underestimated (Crane & Ward, 2016). With the current increased stress because of a global pandemic, longer working hours, and changes in patient composition, disease patterns, and illness severity, the need has increased to educate nurses on self-care and creating safe spaces for self-care to flourish. Studies show that knowledge of individual response patterns in the work environment is vital to learning more effective coping mechanisms. Self-care is a deeply rooted process that requires presence, authenticity, and intentionality that nurses use to provide the highest form of care for themselves and others.

Watson's Theory of Caring Science (2008) guides nurses to enhance mindfulness and expand their caring literacy by embracing connections with self and others and building resiliency, which contributes to creating a healthy and healing work environment. It provides a framework for how nurses can reflect, listen, and connect with self and others more deeply. Self-care is essential to effective coping mechanisms related to body, mind, emotions, and spirit. Such a holistic approach asks for experimenting with creative techniques and not relying on superficial and external actions.

Self-care is a way of being. Research and knowledge about self-care techniques and practical self-care exercises need to be explored, implemented, and reinforced. The development of such a knowledge base is an iterative and ongoing process requiring intermittent analysis and synthesis of the relevant body of knowledge.

Acquiring theoretical knowledge is based on sound scientific research. Although throughout the years, nurses have often relied on traditions, trial and error, authoritative experience, borrowing, intuition, and logical reasoning, the scientific method of acquiring knowledge ensures the generation of evidence around relevant issues to the nursing profession. We use this inquisitive, scientific method in our process towards self-care until it becomes a way of being.

Nurses are increasingly expected to understand and conduct a high standard of research to base their practice on sound research evidence. Scientific knowledge provides a particularly solid basis for evidence-based practice. Not only is research an integral part of self-development (including self-care practices), nursing leadership, nursing practice, education, and management, it includes the pursuit for "research-mindedness" that nurse leaders should foster to create awareness for evidence-based practice and evidence-informed decision-making (Brink et al., 2018). Research should not merely refer to information-gathering, excavating, or conversing of facts from one source to another but must ensure an exploration, discovery, and careful study of unexplained phenomena (Bowling & Ebrahim, 2005).

A healthy and healing work environment requires a knowledgeable and critically conscious workforce. Nurses are educated to be problem-solvers. One might argue that the similarities between problem-solving and research would prepare nurses well for research. However, the differences between them are quite significant. When referring to problem-solving, the focus is on looking for a solution to a direct problem that exists at that time and for a person or persons in a certain setting. The purpose of scientific research is wider, with its broad aim towards solutions and obtained knowledge that can be generalized.

For example, research fatigue has become a reality in the academic and clinical environment. Often individuals experience an attitude of indifference or apathy brought on by overexposure to a repeated series of similar events or requests to participate in research. Individuals feel exhausted by engaging in research resulting in resistance to and avoidance of participation in any further research (Clark, 2008).

A practical way to engage in more research on the health and healing of nurses could be autoethnography, which is often used to investigate the healing capacity of clinical environments. It allows one to critically reflect on the multiple roles as a compassionate care provider, service-user, and health professional (Liggins et al., 2013). The ability to "speak" personal and professional experiences and theory become mutually intertwined concerns potentially stretching the healing landscape concept.

A landscape that fosters healthy and healing working environments provides beneficial practice innovations where nurses are likely to engage in research activities along a continuum of participation. At one end are consumers of research who utilize research findings by reading reports and executive summaries of completed studies to stay abreast of the latest developments in terms of best evidence. At the other end of the continuum are the producers of research findings, the nurse researchers. Between the two opposite points of the research continuum, a variety of research activities are undertaken. These activities may range from contributions to research topics or ideas by identifying gaps in the knowledge base, field workers who are engaged in data collection or advocacy for their patients/study participants, assisting in literature searches, clinical roles in research that is conducted in the clinical field, and by participating in journal clubs or capacity development sessions. While the focus is often on the research topic and research process, the well-being of the persons involved is neglected. Little is said about how it impacts the well-being of participants, researchers, field workers, and nurses in general. Given this, it is not surprising that much of the resiliency work in healthcare is aimed at quantitative surface-level interventions rather than an iterative process that involves an authentic connection to self and others.

As nurses, we have come to accept that we need a working environment that accepts the desirability of incorporating research and research evidence in nursing practice. Changes to nursing practice and the nursing profession now occur frequently because of evolving theoretical knowledge and best evidence because of research. However, do we spend as much time on evolving self-care techniques? The integration of self-care practices is becoming more essential and requires an environment that fosters healing and well-being.

## INTENTIONAL AND ITERATIVE PRACTICES TO CREATE HEALTHY AND HEALING WORK ENVIRONMENTS

There is value in generating intentional self-care practices to build resilience in the workplace. Self-work is not limited to our lives' personal or professional side but is integrated into our whole being. Theoretical perspectives function as a guide for nurses to reach beyond nursing tasks and establish a way of *being* within the profession. With higher acuities and advancement in the medical field than ever before, the focus within nursing is easily consumed with didactic scientific knowledge and skill. However, the demands and stress of the current healthcare workforce increase the need to translate and implement these theories into practice. This transition from practice to praxis has been described throughout the literature in various interventions including mindfulness, gratitude, connection with others, equanimity, values work, and self-awareness (Horton-Deutsch et al., 2020). With society becoming more and more consumed with expediency, technology, and achievement, there is a growing movement within positive psychology to slow down and develop intrinsic abilities to cope with these ongoing pressures. This expansion of knowing is not new rhetoric but a calling to return to an inner state of knowing and spiritual connection.

The topic of self-care is often presented in the literature and mainstream media as interventions that require additional time, effort, and doing more to be "enough." The next best method to feel "good enough" and less stressed relies on external resources that never fill the cup of personal wholeness. Instead, self-care is not about going about what we are already doing but is about being present and spiritually connected. Achieving personal healing, contentment, and the ability to withstand life's stressors comes from a knowing deep within. This knowing is a personal connection to presence, authenticity, and just *being* without the need for judgment and evaluation. Instead of focusing on the outside noise of doing, one feels a state of personal integration and healing through the constant iterative practices that connect mind, body, and spirit to self and others. Self-care is challenging, requires ongoing effort to develop and refine, and is an iterative process. It may feel uncomfortable and out of the ordinary. However, it begins with a surrender of perfection and expectations and accepting possibilities and vulnerability within oneself while being steadfast to personal authenticity. Just being and caring for oneself is not a forced intervention. It is a voluntary, daily choice to live in the real from a heart-centered space and expands out to others and the organization when done with intention and reverence. Embracing self-development and engaging in intentional practices with others and throughout the organization are key to creating healthy and healing work environments.

# DEVELOPING THE SELF

Developing the spiritual self is manifested through intentional self-care practices that connect mind, body, and spirit. Mindfulness is one of the most widely researched tools for generating this experience. *Mindfulness*, a "moment to moment awareness and presence of one's own experience without judgment" (Davis & Hayes, 2011, p. 198), is utilized to address both internal capabilities and affect work environments by facilitating adaptive appraisal of stressful events in the workplace. This becomes a cumulative effect and can change cultures, thus leading to healthier work environments and increased nurse engagement (Horton-Deutsch et al., 2020). Mindfulness does not require a specific set of interventions to reach this state. It's pure awareness without future forecasting or past rumination. Mindfulness in the healthcare environment impacts the well-being of staff, reduction in errors and poor outcomes, and increased patient satisfaction scores (Monroe et al., 2021). Learning to be mindful takes practice without expectations or judgment. Many mindfulness-based interventions have been studied throughout the literature to reduce burnout in nurses. Well-studied programs such as Mindfulness-Based Stress Reduction are encouraged for healthcare workers to implement in their lives and weave throughout everyday practice (Kabat-Zinn, 2004). A qualitative study on a mindfulness practice within a nursing unit notes that participants found themselves feeling enriched at work, experiencing authentic presence with their patients, and being a part of something bigger, which created a ripple effect on the unit and resulted in a healthier work environment. This intervention was further reinforced by improved job satisfaction in the quantitative study that followed (Horton-Deutsch et al., 2020; Monroe et al., 2021).

Fostering self-awareness is another tool for integrating our state of being. Becoming aware of the environment, one's roles and reactions within that environment, and seeing concepts from a broader perspective are necessary to widen the lens of self-awareness. This skill develops with thoughtful reflective practice in both personal and professional environments. Reflective practice is the art of tapping into things deeply human, our knowledge, experience, and understanding of others. It begins with listening, observing, and noticing what is happening within ourselves and others (Horton-Deutsch & Sherwood, 2017). Through engaging in this practice, we more readily see where there is a need. When a need is recognized, appreciating and integrating all ways of knowing (personal, empirical, aesthetic, ethical) into our response provides the most accurate, desirable, and compassionate care. Reflective practice can be done individually as a personal inventory, or including others in professional supervision and group settings. Reflective practice helps create personal meaning out of work and realigns our values with the present, everyday experiences.

Building one's knowledge base and understanding of oneself allows one to become more aware of possible self-deception. As nurse leaders, managing one's emotions and effectively managing interpersonal relationships are major aspects of the leader's effectiveness. Research on leadership illustrates how self-deception could be regarded as one reason contributing to organizational disruption (Pienaar, 2016). A leader can only raise the level of consciousness of others to that which they possess. Therefore, self-awareness becomes the key to combating self-deception. Pienaar (2016) further argues that there should be a stronger focus on developing processes to help individuals in general and nurse leaders in particular to understand the underlying motivation for their behaviors to become more self-aware. Self-care develops from self-awareness that drives an understanding of one's values, goals, and dreams.

Intentional self-care practices that bring presence to our lives are not limited. Any practice that connects one's body, mind, and spirit shifts us into a state of being that creates a healing environment. The responsibility of creating healing spaces lies with all nurses working within the environment. Watson (2008) emphasizes the need for authenticity and intentionality in nursing practice. Nurses may cause harm unintentionally if they are not authentic and intentional in their practice. Watson (2008) developed touchstones to guide nurses to set intentions for caring and healing throughout the day.

Parker Palmer (2004) describes living an undivided life—living our ethics and values in our work environment and not compromising. While not everything can be reconciled, healing environments provide safe spaces for us to ask questions and encourage discourse about complex issues. They teach us to listen with compassion, treat each other with kindness and respect, honor each person's experience, and trust we evolve the discourse through these practices and create new possibilities.

A connection to self is imperative to foster self-reflection and maintain an ongoing healthy connection with others. This connection begins with self-compassion and staying true to authenticity without internal division (Neff, 2011). Connection with self is a spiritual, heart-centered process that can be self-directed or include a spiritual connection with something outside of oneself. When nurses cannot provide care and compassion to themselves as a result of internal depletion, the capacity to give to others is diminished. Therefore, the nurse-patient relationship or nurse-team relationship is affected. However, we know the reciprocal is true; the more direct self-healing and presence can occur from within healthcare providers, the greater the impact on the team, work environments, engagement, and interactions with patients (Horton-Deutsch et al., 2020).

# INTENTIONALITY WITH OTHERS

If all nurses took personal responsibility to develop a connection with self and manifest personal healing, a ripple effect might occur in the environment. By taking our inner work into the outer worlds, the environment develops a shift in its consciousness. Attending personal work is one way to show up in the community. Circle work and sharing stories are other approaches to further develop a connection with self and others. Healing circles assert that we heal best in a community and deepen the capacity to heal through accessing one's inner guidance in witness with others (Healing Circles Global, 2021). Working within circles allows communities to experience wholeness together and can regenerate internal healing practices and awareness (Baldwin & Linnea, 2010; Palmer 2004).

Gratitude is another intentional practice that supports well-being and can be used individually or with others. *Gratitude* is defined in the literature as "a generalized tendency to recognize and respond with grateful emotion to the roles of other people's benevolence in the positive experiences and outcomes that one obtains" (McCullough et al., 2002, p. 112). This is a common strategy within the positive psychology movement that is relatively easy to understand and complete. Gratitude can be applied to the actions of others, as well as impersonal and nonhuman subjects such as God or mother nature. Interventions of gratitude in research have shown an increase in positive emotions and smiling while reducing anger and other negative emotions, facial tension, and heart rate variability (Emmons & McCullough, 2003). Gratitude enhances coping with stress through positive thinking; increases accessibility to positive memories, which is linked to alleviating depression; improves relationships with others; and enhances spiritual well-being (Cheng et al., 2015).

Giving energy to and caring for others is a spiritual process and energy exchange within the profession of nursing. Jean Watson asserts that one must show up authentically and develop boundaries with the self and others in order to give fully without resentments or expectations. Boundaries are not always clearly understood nor taught. Boundaries within the healthcare environment can be challenging to practice given the demands faced every day. However, boundaries help us and others grow through the delicate balance of self and others. The nurse is not required to choose caring for self vs. others, but to provide care in a balanced way, honoring self and others, being mindful not to prohibit others' self-efficacy and growth by over-caring. A reciprocal exchange of energy creates an environment of respect and collaboration within groups and teams.

# ORGANIZATIONAL PRACTICES

The above skills and intentional self-care practices are versions of mind, body, and spirit connections. Each individual nurse is responsible for creating their internal environment, which then affects the team and greater community or organization. However, organizations themselves have responsibilities to maintain these standards at a community level and create and hold spaces for their members to foster these skills. A systematic review of an organization or whole system interventions demonstrated positive effects on the health and well-being of healthcare staff and improvement of health behaviors (Brand et al., 2017). However, only 11 studies met the criteria, and the level of quality of the studies were low to medium, indicating a need for further research with validated outcome measures. Targeting the organization itself is impossible without self-motivation at the individual level to carry out this magnitude of change. At the same time, a self-motivated individual needs an organization to create a supportive and caring environment.

Several organizational interventions have been studied and implemented throughout healthcare organizations. Hinsley et al. (2016) worked as an interprofessional team and used the American Association of Critical-Care Nurses (AACN) Healthy Work Environment standards to develop a tool to learn how staff viewed the work environment. Staff was asked to anonymously complete the REAL Indicator Survey (Relative Environment Assessment Lens) monthly, with results shared at monthly meetings. While initially piloted on one unit, the REAL Indicator Survey has been spread to other hospital areas, with quality issues identified and resolved based on the survey results.

One mindfulness project that captures many of the individual and group practices mentioned above and demonstrates practice to praxis in an organization is Project7 Mindfulness Pledge. The program was rooted in a caring/healing philosophy (Polkinghorne, 2004; Watson, 2008) and scholarly works in mindfulness (Kabat-Zinn, 2004; Thich Nhat Hanh, 2012). The voluntary mindfulness project developed by a unit charge nurse combines practice with self-compassion, gratitude, and reflective practice to sustain resilience in the workforce. The pledge (see Table 5.1) serves as a reminder to connect with self and others using an iterative process (Varney, 2012). Each month an agreement is selected and becomes the lens to foster self-awareness and appreciation. Inspirational quotes related to the pledge, a sign-in sheet, and a visual board to celebrate accomplishments and express gratitude encourage participation and foster self-awareness in the unit. The structure of the pledges and visuals on the unit serve as reminders to integrate mindfulness and self-awareness. No formal training is required, and the pledges are recirculated throughout the year in an ongoing manner to regenerate mindfulness and resilience within the team (Horton Deutsch et al., 2020; Monroe et al., 2021).

## TABLE 5.1   Project7 Mindfulness Pledge

### 1. I pledge to be here

I recognize it can be difficult to separate work and home life. I've agreed to work here and to perform to the best of my ability. I will focus on being present in body, mind, and heart. Work isn't just a warm body taking up physical space in a room. It's me fully present and engaged in the unfolding challenges right here, right now, at this moment.

### 2. I pledge to be prepared

I strive to be successful. It's easier to be successful when I'm prepared. A good sleep, right attitude, nourishment, knowledge, and professional growth are examples of my responsibility toward preparedness here at work. I will aim to be prepared for my success at work.

### 3. I pledge to be humble

I don't know everything. I will ask for help when I face something unknown to me. I will actively listen and obtain feedback from coworkers who express concerns about safety. I will be open to coworkers who come to me for my own expertise and welcome constructive feedback. I recognize that all levels of experience add to our team as well as the patient and family experience.

### 4. I pledge to look at what I have

I recognize there is an infinite number of problems in the world, and work is part of the world. I will spend more time being optimistic about what I have to work with and less time seeking out what is missing. I will be a proactive team member and offer solutions. I'm more likely to find solutions at the moment if I focus on the good that surrounds me right here, right now. I pledge to look at what I have.

### 5. I pledge to look at how I can help

I recognize I have an internal dialog with myself all the time. With pledge 4 in mind, I will start asking myself these two questions: How can I help? Is there something I can do to make this better? I'm bound to find solutions if I look for ways to help.

**6. I pledge to aim for excellence**

I recognize excellence when I see it. It's my priority to be empowered to achieve professional excellence. When I aim for excellence, I'm bound to surpass the average and reach excellence. I will aim for excellence and trust. I aim to be supportive of my coworkers' goals to reach excellence in their work as well.

**7. I pledge to have strength and courage**

I recognize it's my responsibility to find enjoyment and fulfillment in my work. When I feel unchallenged, I pledge to have courage and push myself towards personal and professional growth. I will remain positive and seek out opportunities to be an active member of our team. I will grow and remain fulfilled in my work here.

---

*Varney, 2012*

The iterative process of practice to praxis allows individuals, teams, and organizations to heal and shift into healthy work environments. The next section describes the standards and attributes of nursing leaders who create and regenerate healthy and healing work environments.

# NURSING LEADERSHIP AS THE FOUNDATION OF HEALTHY AND HEALING WORKPLACES

At the heart of every healthy and healing workplace is a leader who creates an environment where others want to belong. As an art and a science, leadership requires a leader to engage others in envisioning and enabling the creation of a preferred way of being. In support of this, the AACN (2016) landmark document identified six standards for creating and sustaining healthy work environments for nurses and a quality and safe environment for patients: authentic leadership, skilled communication, meaningful recognition, true collaboration, effective decision-making, and appropriate staffing.

Authentic leadership requires knowing oneself, managing personal emotions, aligning values to work, and harnessing personal strengths. Emotional reactivity can impact resilience and influence how others perceive a nurse leader. Leaders need to know themselves, be aware of what triggers an emotional overreaction, and notice and respond to triggers earlier to remain calm and effective at work.

Values represent what a leader believes is important in life and work, and misalignment can influence resilience. If leaders cannot live their values, it often negatively impacts their work and relationships with others. On the contrary, leaders who live their values at work are often more resourced, and in turn, able to support others. Barrett's Values Assessment (https://www.valuescentre.com/tools-assessments/pva) is one tool that can facilitate learning and articulating values. When leaders can gain clarity on values, notice what they have reacted to at work that demonstrates an important value, maintain values when compromised or under pressure, and consistently live values at work, they are more effective at leading themselves and others, and representing the organization.

One aspect of resourcefulness, knowing and harnessing personal strengths, is engaging and satisfying for the leader and those who follow. Considering how to craft a position to maximize each person's strengths goes a long way toward creating a healthy and healing environment. Leaders who align inherent strengths with different aspects of their role and do the same for followers maximize each member's contributions and build relational capacity. Strengths-Based Leadership (Rath, 2008) is a valuable tool to discover one's professional strengths.

Skilled communication is key to effective leadership and a healthy workplace. As a skilled communicator, a leader works with others to creatively seek solutions and achieve desired outcomes, advance collaboration, seek and listen to all perspectives, build consensus and a common understanding, model congruence between words and actions, and request input from others and remain open to the need for continuous improvement. Beyond holding this as a personal attribute, effective nurse leaders ensure those that follow receive the coaching and education needed to develop critical communication skills. Some of the essential communication skills include self-awareness, listening, dialogue, negotiation, conflict management, and advocacy.

In healthcare, working effectively together in teams is essential for providing quality and safe care. Nurse leaders and their interprofessional partners modeling and fostering true collaboration and holding others accountable create safe and supportive work environments. When a culture of collaboration is absent, visionary leaders seek investment in education to improve communication, build processes, and evaluate operational structures. Building and sustaining a collaborative culture is often an iterative, relentless, and fulfilling pursuit for nurse leaders.

As the messenger between an organization and individual members, nurse leaders model effective decision-making by building an accountable leadership team with the necessary skills, including accurately assessing situations, sharing factual information, communicating clearly, and actively inquiring for a deeper understanding. These skills are vital to creating environments that empower nurses. Fortified with these skills, nurse leaders and their members are prepared to make policy, direct and evaluate patient care, and lead organizational functions.

A healthy work environment recognizes members for the value they bring to the organization through meaningful recognition. Often defined as the acknowledgment of a nurse's contribution to the organizational outcomes, meaningful recognition is most readily identified as the existence of organizational programs and awards. Since these awards typically only acknowledge a few nurses, knowing what nurses find meaningful is vital to avoid burnout and remain engaged. Studies have found reflective practice an effective way to recognize and appreciate oneself for work well done (Cherian, 2016, 2017). Nurse leaders who model and encourage reflective practices co-create work cultures that embrace the outcomes of their work together. Recognition is most meaningful when it is relevant to the nurse's values and goals, and reflective practices create environments where these critical foundations are explored (Sherwood et al., 2018).

Finally, ensuring members have the resources, including adequate staffing, to ensure patient needs are met is essential to creating a healthy and healing work environment. This has been especially difficult in recent years and potentially into the future with more nurses retiring and leaving the profession. Influential nurse leaders advocate for their members to be involved in the staffing process to ensure patient needs match nursing skills.

The one study that moves beyond the focus of health to healing is Hernandez's dissertation (2020) which explored how nurse leaders create caring, healing environments. She discovered that nurse leaders who create caring, healing environments for others embody a caring-loving consciousness and engage in informed, moral actions through practice. They do this by attending to physical and psychological safety and aesthetic surroundings for staff. In addition, they repattern the environment through theory-guided practice, openness, and accessibility. Notably, nurse leaders who create caring, healing environments remain intentional, purposeful, and responsible for their leadership practices through ongoing personal and professional development.

# IMPLICATIONS FOR PRACTICE: INSPIRING ACTION

The Press Ganey White Paper on Nursing Manager Impact (2017) identified frontline leaders as the key to nurse retention. Importantly, these leaders embrace the essential elements of healthy and healing work environments through courageous actions that model compassionate care and support for nurses. More specifically, nurse leaders who provide safe spaces for nurses to share their individual and collective stories intentionally create space for new stories of healing. Deepening and softening our ways of being with one another creates the critical consciousness needed to align our behaviors and structures. Leaders who embrace critical, deep, and authentic connections weave a thread that can be pulled to support resilience and evolution (Brown, 2017).

However, it is essential to note that formal leaders are not the only people in an organization who create healing spaces that lead to a healthy work environment. It takes individuals to mobilize the organization and take accountability for their healing journey starting with self-care and developing mind, body, and spirit connections with others. Creating healthy work environments must involve the engagement of individuals, groups/teams, and the organization creating intentional healing environments for everyone in the organization.

# SUMMARY

Creating healing spaces and engaging in healing practices are fundamental and essential to creating healthy work environments. Leaders and organizations can no longer expect the individual nurse to carry this burden alone. Collectively, individuals, leaders, teams, and organizations must work together to integrate healing at all levels. All healthcare professionals need safe spaces where they can express their deepest truths, be honored, heard, and included in co-creating solutions that lead to healthy and healing work environments.

# REFLECTIVE QUESTIONS

1. Reflect on theoretical nursing knowledge and your values and strengths as a nurse. How are they visible and invisible in your role as a nurse leader?

2. What intentional healing practices do you use that demonstrate care for yourself? For others?

3. How do you currently use reflective practice in your personal and professional life? What more can you do? Why does it matter?

4. Describe the landscape of your current healthcare environment. What is the most important step you can take, as a leader, to integrate healing practices into the environment?

5. How does your well-being influence you and your role as a nurse leader who develops and applies nursing knowledge?

# NARRATIVE

You are a nurse manager on an inpatient medical-surgical unit and have been in your position for two years. While the clinical environment is beginning to settle into a new normal after COVID-19, you have lost a number of staff and experience changes at the bedside at a more rapid pace than before. At the same time, the organization is requesting you start a number of new quality and safety initiatives, and you are faced with competing priorities. In addition to a stressful environment, you have very little time to yourself or to check in with staff due to being in meetings all day long. You get home to receive a call that the unit is short-staffed with three nurses for 24 patients. You have a six-month-old baby at home and want to spend time with your family but feel guilty leaving your nurses short-staffed. These types of situations are occurring more and more frequently at work. What intentional practices will help you to navigate care for yourself and others, and influence the organization to create a more healing environment?

# AUTHOR BIOGRAPHIES

**Wanda J. Borges, PhD, RN, ANP-BC,** is a Professor and Associate Director of Graduate Programs in the School of Nursing at New Mexico State University. In her current role she oversees a Nursing Leadership and Administration MSN program, a Population Health Leadership DNP program, and an FNP and PMHNP program. She has worked as a nurse for more than 20 years in a wide variety of settings including director and management positions. She continues her work to establish intentional Academic Practice Partnerships with healthcare agencies that have a shared mission and values with NMSU and provide students the opportunity to learn to solve real world problems. Partnering with community-based health centers to improve healthcare outcomes, she has provided external evaluation and continues her work in evaluation of healthcare interventions

**Gisela H. van Rensburg,** Professor, University of South Africa, is actively involved in teaching, supervision, and research in the field of reflective practices in Caring Science, creating a healthy and healing teaching and learning environment using creative student support activities and supervision practices, currently focusing on the disruptive space as a result of the global COVID-19 pandemic. van Rensburg is engaged in a variety of projects on research capacity development and teaching of research methodology. Her educational interests lie in health sciences education, individual differences in the learning process, and student support. Her clinical interests are in orthopedic nursing and ensuring a conducive practice environment where quality care is rendered through sound teaching and learning practices. She has been involved in several national and international research projects in these fields and has published on them widely. These projects included research on innovative student support strategies, child-headed households, and children's rights within the context of a pandemic.

**Chelsie Monroe, MSN, APRN, PMHNP-BC,** is a board-certified Psychiatric Mental Health Nurse Practitioner and founder of Balanced Mental Wellness in Englewood, Colorado. She has been in various healthcare and academic institutions for the last 11 years. She is an integrative psychiatry specialist and incorporates the mind, body, and spirit in her work. Monroe uses approaches from Internal Family Systems, Emotions Focused, and psychodynamic therapies to treat complex trauma and PTSD. She is also the co-founder of Better Together Healing LLC, a holistic practice partnership that specializes in an integrative approach to heal the self, build collaborations, and create healthy and bounded healthcare communities.

**Sara Horton-Deutsch, PhD, RN, PMHCNS, FAAN, ANEF,** is a Caritas Coach and a Professor and the Director of the Kaiser Permanente/USF Partnership at the University of San Francisco, where she mentors the next generation of nursing leaders through the lens of Caring Science and values-based leadership. She also serves as a Faculty Associate with the Watson Caring Science Institute. In 2021, she co-created and initiated the Caritas Leadership Program, a uniquely customized six-month program guiding participants through executive Caring Science leader dialogues, interactive circles, and participant transformation projects. She is also a founding partner of Better Together Healing, LLC, a holistic practice partnership specializing in an integrative approach to heal the self, build collaborations, and create healthy and bounded communities. As a therapeutic practitioner and Caritas leadership coach, she collaborates with healthcare professionals and organizations seeking balance and growth who are open to engaging in innovative approaches to healing. Her comprehensive approach includes certifications in professional coaching and training through the Leadership Circle and Working with Resilience, providing comprehensive profiles and assessments to raise the conscious practice of leadership and build regenerative success at work.

# REFERENCES

Alligood, M. R. (2018). *Nursing theorists and their work* (9th ed.). Elsevier.

Alspach, G. (2009). Craft your own healthy work environment. *Critical Care Nurse, 20*(2), 12–21.

American Association of Critical-Care Nurses. (2016). *AACN standards for establishing and sustaining healthy work environments: A journey to excellence* (2nd ed.). https://www.aacn.org/~/media/aacn-website/nursing-excellence/healthy-work-environment/execsum.pdf?la=en

American Nurses Association. (2015). *Guide to the code of ethics for nursing* (2nd ed.). Author.

American Nurses Credentialing Center. (n.d.). *About Magnet.* https://www.nursingworld.org/organizational-programs/magnet/about-magnet/

American Nurses Credentialing Center. (2018). *American Nurses Credentialing Center (ANCC) program verification & evaluation.* http://www.cgfns.org/services/credentials-evaluation/ancc/

American Organization for Nursing Leadership. (2019). *Elements of a healthy practice environment.* https://www.aonl.org/system/files/media/file/2020/02/elements-healthy-practice-environment_1.pdf

Austgard, K. I. (2008). What characterizes nursing care? A hermeneutical philosophical inquiry. *Scandinavian Journal of Caring Science, 22,* 314–319.

Baldwin, C., & Linnea, A. (2010). *The circle way: A leader in every chair.* Berrett-Koehler.

Bond, A. E., Eshah, N. F., Bani-Khaled, M., Hamad, A. O., Habashneh, S., Kataua, H., al-Jarrah, I., Kamal, A. A., Hamdah, F. R., & Maabreh, R. (2011). Who uses nursing theory? A univariate descriptive analysis of five years' research articles. *Scandinavian Journal of Caring Science, 25,* 404–409. doi: 10.1111/j.1471-6712.2010.00835.x

Bowling, A., & Ebrahim, S. (2005). *Handbook of health research methods.* McGraw Hill Education.

Brand, S., Thompson, C., Fleming, L. E., Carroll, L., Bethel, A., & Wyatt, K. (2017). Whole system approaches to improving the health and well-being of healthcare workers: A systemic review. *PLoS One, 12*(12), E0188418. doi: 10.1371/journal.pone.0188418

Brink, H., van der Walt, C., & van Rensburg, G. (2018). *Fundamentals of research methodology for healthcare professionals* (4th ed.). Juta.

Brown, A. M. (2017). *Emergent strategy. Shaping change, changing worlds.* A. K. Press.

Centers for Disease Control and Prevention, National Center for Health Statistics. (n.d.). *Occupational safety and health.* https://www.cdc.gov/nchs/data/hpdata2010/hp2010_final_review_focus_area_20.pdf

Centers for Disease Control and Prevention, National Center for Health Statistics. (1999, November 19). *Occupational safety and health objective status.* https://www.cdc.gov/nchs/data/hp2000/safety/sumtable.pdf

Cheng, S., Tsui, P., & Lam, J. (2015). Improving mental health care in practitioners: A randomized controlled trial of a gratitude intervention. *Journal of Consulting and Clinical Psychology, 83*(1), 177–186.

Cherian, U. (2016). *Impact of meaningful recognition on nurses' work environment in ICU: A comparative exploration of nurse leaders' and staff nurses' perception* [Unpublished DNP scholarly project]. University of North Carolina at Chapel Hill School of Nursing.

Cherian, U. (2017). *Describing the impact of meaningful recognition on nurses' work environment: Comparing nurse leaders' and staff nurses' perceptions* [Oral presentation]. Creating Healthy Work Environments Conference, Sigma Theta Tau International, Indianapolis, IN.

Clark, T. (2008). We're over-researched here!: Exploring accounts of research fatigue within qualitative research engagements. *Sociology, 42*(5), 953–970. doi: 10.1177/0038038508094573

Crane, P. J., & Ward, S. F. (2016). Self-healing and self-care for nurses. *AORN Journal, 104*(5), 386–400.

Davis, D. M., & Hayes, J. A. (2011). What are the benefits of mindfulness? A practice review of psychotherapy-related research. *Psychotherapy, 48*(2), 198.

Davis, D. E., Choe, E., Meyers, J., Wade, N., Varjas, K., Gifford, A., Quinn, A., Hook, J. N., Van Tongeren, D. R., Griffin, B. J., & Worthington, E. L. (2016). Thankful for the little things: A meta-analysis of gratitude interventions. *Journal of Counseling Psychology, 63*(1), 20–31.

Emmons, R. A., & McCullough, M. E. (2003). Counting blessings versus burdens: An experimental investigation of gratitude and subjective well-being in daily life. *Journal of Personality and Social Psychology, 84*(2), 377–389.

Griffin, C., Nowacki, K., & Woodroof, A. (2021). Creating safe and healing environments: Innovative curriculum to support team members during patient and family escalations in a quaternary care pediatric hospital. *Archives of Psychiatric Nursing, 35*(2), 200–205.

Healing Circles Global. (2021, July 9). *Healing circles.* https://healingcirclesglobal.org/

Hernandez, G. (2020). *The lived experience of nurse leaders practicing within Watson Caring Science framework creating a caring, healing environment for staff* [Unpublished dissertation]. University of Colorado Anschutz Medical Campus. https://hdl.handle.net/10968/6024

Hinsley, K. E., Marshall, A. C., Hurtig, M. H., Thornton, J. M., O'Connell, C. A., Porter, C. L., Connor, J. A., & Hickey, P. A. (2016). Monitoring the health of the work environment with a daily assessment tool: The REAL-Relative Environment Assessment Lens-Indicator. *Cardiology in the Young, 26*, 1082–1089. doi: 10.1017/S1047951115001808

Horton-Deutsch, S., Monroe, C., Varney, R., Loresto, F., Eron, K., & Kleiner, C. (2020). Moving from practice to praxis: A qualitative descriptive study revealing the value of Project7 Mindfulness Pledge. *Journal of Nursing Management, 28*(3), 728–734.

Horton-Deutsch, S., & Sherwood, G. (2017). *Reflective practice: Transforming education and improving outcomes* (2nd ed.). Sigma Theta Tau International.

Isaac, F. (2001). Leaders of a new frontier. *American Journal of Health Promotion, 15*, 365–367.

Kabat-Zinn, J. (2004). Mindfulness-based interventions in context: Past, present and future. *Clinical Psychology: Science and Practice, 10*(2), 144–156. https://doi.org/10.1093/clipsy/bpg016

Kelly, L., Gee, P., & Butler, R. (2020). Impact of nurse burnout on organizational and position turnover. *Nursing Outlook, 69*(1), 96–102. doi: 10.1016/j.outlook.2020.06.008

Kramer, M., Schmalenberg, C., & Maguire, P. (2010). Nine structures and best leadership practices essential for a magnetic (healthy) work environment. *Nursing Administration Quarterly, 33*(4), 4–17.

Kupperschmidt, B., Kientz, E., Ward, J., & Reinholz, B. (2010). A healthy work environment: It begins with you. *The Online Journal of Issues in Nursing, 15*(1). doi: 10.3912/OJIN.Vol15No01Man3

Liggins, J., Kearns, R. A., & Adams, P. J. (2013). Using autoethnography to reclaim the 'place of healing' in mental health care. *Social Science and Medicine, 91*, 105–109.

Makary, M. A., & Daniel, M. (2016). Medical error – the third leading cause of death in the U.S. *British Medical Journal, 353*. https://doi.org/10.1136/bmj.i2139

McCullough, M. E., Emmons, R. A., & Tsang, J. A. (2002). The grateful disposition: A conceptual and empirical topography. *Journal of Personality and Social Psychology, 82*, 112–127.

McMorrow, P. (2017, Sept. 20). *The difference between health vs. healing.* https://www.caringbridge.org/resources/health-vs-healing/

Monroe, C., Loresto, F., Horton-Deutsch, S., Kleiner, C., Eron, K., Varney, R., & Grimm, S. (2021). The value of intentional self-care practices: The effects of mindfulness on improving job satisfaction, teamwork and workplace environments. *Archives of Psychiatric Nursing, 35*(2), 189–194.

Montefiore Medical Center. (2021). *Creating a healing hospital environment.* https://www.montefiore.org/healingarts-healing-environment

Neff, K. (2011). *Self-compassion: The proven power of being kind to yourself.* HarperCollins.

Norman, V., Rossillo, K., & Skelton, K. (2016). Creating healing environments through the theory of caring. *AORN Journal, 104*(5), 401–409.

Palmer, P. (2004). *A hidden wholeness: The journey toward an undivided life.* Jossey-Bass.

Parse, R. R. (1992). Human becoming: Parse's theory of nursing. *Nursing Science Quarterly, 5*(1), 5–42.

Perlo, J., Balik, B., Swensen, S., Kabcenell, A., Landsman, J., & Feeley, D. (2017). *IHI framework for improving joy in work* [White paper]. Cambridge, Massachusetts: Institute for Healthcare Improvement.

Pienaar, C. (2016). The role of self-deception in leadership ineffectiveness: A theoretical overview. *South African Journal of Psychology, 39*(1), 133–141. doi: 10.1.1.879.7070

Polkinghorne, D. (2004). *Practice and the human sciences. The case for a judgment-based practice of care.* SUNY Press.

Press Ganey. (2017). *2017 nursing special report—the influence of nurse manager leadership on patient and nurse outcomes and the mediating effects of the nurse work environment.* https://healthcare.pressganey.com/2017-Nursing-Special-Report?s=White_Paper-Web

Rath, T. (2008). *Strengths based leadership*. Gallup Press.

Shanafelt, T. D., Boone, S., Tan, L., Dyrbye, L. N., Sotile, W., Satele, D., West, C. P., Sloan, J., & Oreskovich, M. R. (2012). Burnout and satisfaction with work-life balance among US physicians relative to the general US population. *Archives of Internal Medicine, 172*(18), 1377–1385. doi: 10.1001/archinternmed.2012.3199

Sherwood, G., Cherian, U., & Horton-Deutsch, S. (2018). Reflective practices: Meaningful recognition for healthy work environments. *Nursing Management, 24*(10), 30–34. doi: 10.7748/nm.2018.e1684

Smith, M. C., Turkel, M., & Wolf, Z. R. (2013). *Caring in nursing classics: An essential resource*. Springer Publishing Company and Watson Caring Science Institute.

Thich Nhat Hanh. (2012). *Peace is every breath: A practice for busy lives*. Harper One.

US Department of Labor. (n.d.). *About OSHA*. https://www.osha.gov/aboutosha

Varney, R. (2012). *Project7 Mindfulness Pledge*. [Mindfulness Pledge]. https://project7pledge.com/blog/p7p

Watson, J. (2008). *The philosophy and science of caring* [Revised edition]. University Press of Colorado.

Wei, H., Sewel, K., Wood, G., & Rose, M. (2018). The state of the science of nurse work environments in the United States: A systematic review. *International Journal of Nursing Sciences, 5*, 287–300.

Worchel, S., Cooper, J., & Goethals, G. R. (1991). *Understanding social psychology*. Thrift Books.

Zeller, J. M., & Levin, P. F. (2013). Mindfulness interventions to reduce stress among nursing personnel: An occupational health perspective. *Workplace Health & Safety, 61*, 85–89. doi:10.3928/21650799-20130116-67

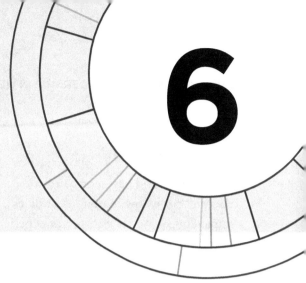

# 6

# LEADERSHIP ROLES IN PROMOTING A RESILIENT WORKFORCE

Christine Griffin, PhD, RN, NPD-BC, CPN
Katherine Reed, LPC
Jennifer Reese, MD

## LEARNING OBJECTIVES

After completing this chapter, you should be able to:

- Review the concept of compassion fatigue, its prevalence, and the impact it has on healthcare

- Describe what is needed to build a resilient organizational culture at the leadership level

- Review evidence-based programs for building resiliency for health-care providers

- Share the implications of a resilient workforce in healthcare

# OVERVIEW

As witnesses and healers, healthcare professionals step into their patients' lives in the midst of intense emotions of illness, pain, suffering, trauma, and sometimes impending death. These are not experienced in the abstract but in each tangible moment of care and compassion. Those at the bedside become the constant and stalwart companions of their patients and loved ones through some of the most difficult moments of life. The reality is these professionals, who are called to care for others, quite often experience intense pain and suffering as they cope with the complexities of caring for others. In current hospital settings, there is a continual demand for healthcare professionals to stay compassionate and maintain the humanity of the care offered to patients. What is missing is the understanding that those providing the care are also human. What they give to the patients will eventually run out if there is not a meaningful practice of recovery and replenishment. The absence of such practice comes at a cost not just for the patient and care provider but also for the organization. Stressed employees are inherently less empathetic, more likely to make a mistake, and very likely to leave the organization. All of these have a cost. Poor patient satisfaction, patient harm, and turnover are huge expenses for healthcare organizations (Branch & Klinkenberg, 2015; Drury et al., 2013; Meadors & Lamson, 2008; Moss et al., 2016). Conversely, prioritizing programs that help the healthcare professional manage stress, stay connected to their mission as a healthcare professional, and know their purpose in helping patients will improve the quality of care and keep the staff thriving in their roles.

Recent efforts to promote resilience in the healthcare environment have focused on moving beyond alleviating burnout and instead promoting flourishing and thriving. Just as we provide healthcare to our patients, our focus is beyond eliminating illness and disease; we aim to see our patients experience wellness. Eckleberry-Hunt et al. highlight the importance of this topic, stating that "it is time to move beyond burnout into positive psychology that focuses on strength, resilience, growth, and happiness rather than the absence of burnout" (2018, p. 369). We need to ask ourselves if the end goal is to reduce burnout or to promote wellness.

The study of positive psychology aims to understand what factors contribute to an individual thriving and promote a sense of well-being. These factors are valuable for all individuals working in the stressful healthcare environment and should be considered to address the system drivers of burnout and distress. By understanding the causes of burnout (and what is causing a negative impact) is important, we might be able to provide opportunities to promote flourishing even amid those environments and circumstances.

This chapter will review the costs professional caregivers are faced with and offer strategies for organizations and their leaders as they seek to support their staff to ensure they can care for each of their patients and flourish within their chosen profession.

# THE CONCEPTS OF ORGANIZATIONAL RESILIENCE

There is not a shortage of terms used to describe the emotional costs of caring for others. Compassion fatigue, secondary traumatic stress, burnout, vicarious trauma, emotional labor, caregiver stress, and post-traumatic stress disorder have all been attributed to the effects of working with patients (Adriaenssens et al. 2014; Beck, 2011; Berger et al., 2015; Branch & Klinkenberg, 2015; Cricco-Lizza, 2014; Czaja et al., 2012; Joinson, 1992; Mealer, 2014). Along with the continuous exposure to suffering, care providers are faced with organizational stressors like increasing workload, insufficient rewards, and lack of control (Moss et al., 2016). In turn, they report poor job satisfaction, have high absenteeism, and increasingly poor retention rates (Brunero et al., 2008).

*Compassion fatigue*, defined as the inability to form nurturing relationships with the patient and the resulting distress caregivers experience, is well documented in healthcare (Johnson, 2013; Mealer et al., 2012; Zerach & Shalev, 2015). The psychological symptoms associated with compassion fatigue have long-term effects, including post-traumatic stress disorder, anxiety, hopelessness, and depression

(Beck, 2011; Berger et al., 2015; Johnson, 2013; Moss et al., 2016). Compassion fatigue also diminishes the altruistic satisfaction care providers desire, highlighted in current healthcare shortages and poor retention rates (Flarity et al., 2013; Johnson, 2013; Quinn et al., 2003; Sinclair et al., 2017).

The opposite experience to compassion fatigue is known as *compassion satisfaction* This is the gratification caregivers feel when caring for others stays in balance, allowing them to embody the positive aspects of altruism (Berger et al., 2015). *Altruism*, acting on behalf of others instead of for personal reasons, is a core characteristic of competent healthcare professionals (McGaghie et al., 2002). Compassion and empathy are the driving force behind compassion satisfaction when the professional is moved to alleviate suffering and feels good about making a difference in another person's life. This increases optimism and hope and gives the impetus to continue in the caregiver role (Sacco & Copel, 2017). Compassion satisfaction is linked to the ability of the professional to be caring and has a positive correlation between increased work meaningfulness and improved patient satisfaction (Burston & Stichler, 2010).

*Burnout*, often associated with inefficient or imbalanced organizational practices, is the syndrome of emotional exhaustion, depersonalization, and reduced personal accomplishment (Beck, 2011; Gentry, 2002; Mealer, 2014). Committed professionals begin their careers with energy, dedication, and efficacy, but poor organizational environments cause them to become cynical, ineffective, and less caring (Bush, 2009). *Secondary trauma* is attributed to feeling overwhelmed due to the constant exposure to extreme events or suffering experienced by another (Beck, 2011; Gentry, 2002).

*Emotional labor* is a new concept that depicts the unique demand on healthcare providers as they manage the intricacies of caring for others in the complexities of a hospital setting. Importantly, emotional labor considers the quantity of emotional demand on healthcare professionals and the quality of the experience and environments where the care occurs (Brotheridge, 2002). It considers the nature of compassion, the experience of suffering, and the effects of moral distress often reported by healthcare professionals. Suffering is unavoidable in healthcare; as Figley (2002) explains, "In our effort to view the world from the perspective of the suffering we suffer" (p. 1434). Moments of authentic compassion demand presence, vulnerability, and empathy. The very nature of this compassion puts the professional at risk as they foster care for another within the openness that it demands. Lewin (1996) illustrated the complexities of a caregiver's compassion as being able to stay in personal balance while holding a patient's despair in one hand and hope in the other. When these are not held in balance, either due to individual incapacity or practicing in an unsupportive environment, the same level of compassion will indubitably lead to fatigue (Figley, 2002; Lewin, 1996).

*Moral distress* is described as the suffering experienced when a healthcare provider knows the right thing to do but cannot carry it out because of institutional constraints (Leggett et al., 2013). The threat to a professional's physical and psychological safety combined with an unethical climate contribute to the degree of moral distress (Leggett et al., 2013). Psychological safety is affected when constraints are found in policies or cultures that create a disequilibrium between the care provider's core values and ethical obligations. Unsafe physical environments directly contribute to moral distress because a healthcare provider understands the organization lacks respect and care for their employees yet demands they provide safe environments for the patients (Meadors & Lamson, 2008).

# BUILDING RESILIENT ORGANIZATIONAL CULTURES AT THE LEADERSHIP LEVEL

With the increase in compassion fatigue and burnout in healthcare, it is important for organizations to focus on their staff. While there will always be a degree of inherent stress in these roles, organizations can create built-in support that honors the emotional labor endured by their employees and work to support resiliency and recovery as part of the job. Just as the risks are widespread and complex, the programs to combat it must be extensive and layered. Resilient organizations recognize the nature of caring, manage the suffering experienced by those at the bedside, and create morally conscious environments. It begins with a collective recognition and normalization of the stress within healthcare. Recognizing emotional labor as a normal component of the job sets the stage to prioritize and focus on managing the resources needed. Programs that focus on recovery, integrating work and life, and building communities to discuss the job pressures will all aid in this normalization.

As with any problem we face in addressing resilience in healthcare, it is essential to measure the impact of challenges and interventions and track these data over time. One approach is to create a "resilience index," a measure of resilience among healthcare providers (Reese & Ziniel, 2018). This can be done by using standardized instruments (e.g., Maslach Burnout Inventory, Mind Garden assessments, Mayo Physician Well-Being Index), which often require payment for the use of their surveys. Another approach is to use existing data and validated analysis tracked over time within the organization's regularly occurring staff or faculty satisfaction or engagement surveys. Creating and measuring a resilience index allows evaluation within certain roles, departments, and disciplines. This can lead to specific interventions in areas that may be struggling and the study of best practices in consistently thriving areas. Specific interventions that can be employed based on these data will be discussed later in this chapter.

Organizational resiliency also relies on the individual healthcare provider's willingness to address their capabilities and expand their practices to ensure they have the personal skills and knowledge to sustain their capacity to care. As mentioned, resilient organizations see this as part of the work and not outside work. In the next section, we focus on how an organization builds resiliency through leadership, paying attention to work environments, and prioritizing individual growth and recovery.

# RESILIENT LEADERSHIP

Leadership matters. In a meta-synthesis of compassion fatigue research, it is evident that the medical environments and cultures directly contribute to the experience of stress and burnout among healthcare professionals. The prevalent oppressive nature of current medical and business models does not leave much room to focus on the healthcare providers' perspectives and values. Healthcare professionals define healthy work environments by leadership recognition of emotional labor, allowing time to connect meaningfully with patients, structures for peer support, ethical environments, and prioritizing self-care and recovery (Cricco-Lizza, 2014; Drury et al., 2013; Maytum et al., 2004; Morrison & Morris, 2017; Shimoinaba et al., 2015). There is also a call to incorporate meaning in work, autonomy, work-life integration, and resources needed to meet the demands of the job (Shanafelt et al., 2012).

Dyrbye et al. (2020) and Shanafelt and Noseworthy (2017) have published findings on leadership behaviors, qualities, and tactics related to burnout and satisfaction. Behaviors that are associated with burnout/satisfaction include holding career development conversations, empowerment to do the job, encouraging suggestions for improvement, treating employees with respect and dignity, providing helpful feedback and coaching on performance, recognition for a job well done, keeping people informed about changes taking place, encouragement to develop talents and skills, and leaders who inspire others to do their best and are interested in others' opinions.

Leaders seeking to promote resilience in healthcare should understand and employ known strategies to enhance individual, organizational, and team well-being and satisfaction. To describe how important leadership is to build organizational resiliency, it may be easiest to describe what happens when positive leadership is missing. Poor or lacking leadership creates and contributes to environments filled with toxicity, stress, insecurity, and even sometimes violence (Byrne, 2015; Ganster & Rosen, 2013). Research reveals distress when workers are motivated by fear rather than intrinsic motivators like making a difference or for the simple love of doing the job (Byrne, 2015). On the job, these environments do not motivate workers to go above and beyond. Instead, they set them up to function in survival mode (Byrne, 2015). Stress from the job can then spill over into home life, decreasing the professional's ability to recover and return with enough energy to do the work (Barber & Santuzzi, 2015). Often the leader is unaware of how they contribute to these situations. Take incivility, for example. A leader who does not create or enforce policies on psychological safety can create a workplace where subtle violence like gossiping, rankism, or bullying prevails. The research has shown that these environments will suffer from poor job satisfaction and high turnover rates (Byrne, 2015).

On the other side is a leader who creates environments that focus on resiliency and consider not just traditional occupational health concerns but include wellness and well-being of the employees. Employees look for leaders who do not just care about their effectiveness on the job but are concerned about them as individuals. Employees are less at risk of burnout when they can build a strong relationship with their leaders, one that allows them to feel connected and inspired by whom they work for (Byrne, 2015). There are numerous approaches to leadership practices that can impact healthcare providers' well-being. According to Ryan and Deci (2000), factors that contribute to individual well-being are three innate psychological needs: competence, autonomy, and relatedness. When these needs are satisfied, self-motivation and mental health are enhanced. When leaders discuss their employees' satisfaction, they should address topics such as opportunities for professional development and personal growth, meaningful work, autonomy, and personal culture and values (Hartzband & Groopman, 2020).

When considering organizational strategies to promote well-being, leaders need to address factors such as logistical support to work well, organizational learning (how does the team as a group get better and better over time), close connection to mission and purpose, and how people cooperate in developing and applying new ideas (Shanafelt et al., 2000).

# LEADERSHIP STYLE

Leadership style is a crucial component of creating positive environments that help staff thrive and know their organization is focused on what matters to them. A leader's ability to build relationships and foster trust is directly related to the level of burnout among healthcare teams (Shanafelt et al., 2012). Creating safety, building relationships, and giving permission for innovation and growth set the stage for engaging and happy professionals. Leaders must also pay attention to both extrinsic and intrinsic motivators. Simply giving more money or reward for the job doesn't increase healthcare employee engagement (Byrne, 2015). This means that leaders must work harder to discover what motivates each individual. It is also crucial for leaders to understand what the professional needs to recover and rejuvenate throughout their career. This requires the leader to spend time and understand the employee individually. This relational leadership style is described in most emerging leadership styles, including transformational, servant leadership, and authentic leadership. These leaders inspire their teams by modeling resiliency practices; focus on the wellness and flourishing of their teams; and invest time in getting to know the unique skills, needs, and motivations of each employee (Byrne, 2015). Inherent in these leadership styles is the willingness of the leader to share their own strengths and weaknesses. This transparency and perceived vulnerability creates an environment of trust, fairness, and equity and inspires employees to follow suit. The study of positivity (Fredrickson, 2009) has also revealed practices that lead to success in leadership. The negative screams at you, but the positive whispers—a call to mind that we are hardwired to scan our environment for the negative. Leaders who attempt to offer five positives for every one negative comment or action are more successful (Losada & Heaphy, 2004).

The hallmark of resilient leadership lies within the relationships leaders form with their teams. Healthcare organizations fall short of this when focusing more on technology, research, and profit and overlooking how to support employees to stay connected to helping people heal. The science of medicine requires expertise and knowledge of pathophysiology, pharmacology, innovation, and technology, but none of that happens without a relationship between a patient and the health-care provider. While other organizations sell commodities and products, health-care is selling relationships, and it is only within a caring relationship that another person can receive what they need to heal. On one side of the relationship is the person in need; many times, their very lives are at stake. On the other side is a person who has to navigate all the empirical knowledge and care enough to be safe, competent, and compassionate. The challenge in healthcare is not just hiring staff who are competent and in it for the right reasons, but then knowing how to support them so they have the capacity to provide all the aspects of care. In health-care, this requires leaders who understand that caring people need to be cared for. Those who listen as part of their job also need to be heard. True listening honors the professional's unique gifts and the strength they bring to their role and does not shy away from asking what they need to recover and thrive in their profession. Scholars have shown that the relationship with the leader is a key component to help each individual know why they do what they do, see their unique contribution to the organization, and thrive in their roles (Anger et al., 2015; Byrne, 2015; Sauter & Hurrell, 2017). When their leaders take the time to know them, it helps the professionals remember who they are and what they do matters. This contributes to their drive and passion for helping others and helps decrease the risk of compassion fatigue and burnout.

# ENVIRONMENTS OF CARE

Leaders need to develop a new style of leading for healthcare, but they also need to pay close attention to the environments where care is happening. The ideal leader is concerned with the organization's culture and climate in which the employees are spending their time. If we cannot recover from the high-stress environments and the demands placed on us, then we run the risk of lowering our capacity to be kind, attentive, and civil. Of utmost importance is the feeling of safety (Byrne, 2015). Humans need to feel physical and psychological safety, or we will revert to survival mode. In this state, it is near impossible to be caring, innovative, or even efficient because stress blocks the use of higher cognitive functioning.

This cortical inhibition decreases the caregiver's access to emotional regulation, planning, reasoning, and engaged communication. In this state, it is impossible to function at a high capacity because of the drain on the body, both physically and emotionally. Environments of care need attention to both types of safety and need to consider the patient/care provider relationship and experiences among peers.

We know that workplace violence in healthcare settings is at a crisis point in the United States. Reports show that healthcare organizations have almost as many serious injuries from violence as all other industries combined (OSHA, 2013; Phillips, 2016). Even worse, due to cultural issues and lack of institutional support, many of the assaults and threats go unreported, especially incidents of incivility among colleagues. The costs of workplace violence have reached a crescendo, provoking a response from several leading healthcare organizations, including the Center for Disease Control, Occupational Safety and Health Administration (OSHA), American Organization of Nursing Leadership, American Nurse Association (ANA), and the Joint Commission. They have all prioritized workplace violence initiatives.

Team climate and culture are also essential drivers of resilient organizations. It is important to address and promote collegiality. Safety is increased when collectively the team believes "my teammates have my back," and "we are all in it together." Teams have psychological safety by knowing "mistakes have led to positive changes here" and "we cooperate in developing new ideas at work," and that staff will be recognized for accomplishments. In a resilient hospital culture, all professionals must believe that they matter. Regardless of role or placement in the hierarchy, each team member is equally important. To measure an individual's experience of safety, consider asking them to answer what we call the steering wheel test. When sitting in their car just before they get out to start their shift, ask what their experience is. Do they get out with confidence that regardless of what they are about to face, they know that they will be okay? This equates to an understanding that the shift may be hard but that they will have the resources they need to provide the type of care they want to; regardless of the outcome, they will feel supported and know they will be okay. It speaks to their personal reserve and capacity, the culture and climate in which they are working. If, on the other hand, they sit a little while longer because they are unsure of what they will face and whether they will have the resources to do their job, then their well-being may be at risk. Again, this includes their personal reserves to care for their patients but mostly speaks to the climates they are working in, which does not allow them what they need physically, emotionally, or psychologically. To get a quick gauge of what is happening, a leader can use the steering wheel test as a litmus test to see how the unit is functioning.

# RECOVERY

To understand how healthcare professionals recover, first, let's understand what occupational stress looks like. Work-related stress, while not a new concept, is gaining more attention today. In a general sense, *stress* is a perceived experience of not having what you need in a given moment to get your job done, leading to the feeling of being overwhelmed. It could be having too many tasks and not enough time or not enough experience or knowledge to complete a task. Maybe you have the resources and knowledge but don't feel safe, so psychologically, you are stressed and unable to perform. Byrne (2015) defines *occupational stress* as job-related triggers that "force employees to deviate from their normal feelings or behaviors" (p. 171). Studies highlight that physical stressors like workload, shift work, high expectations combined with psychological stress associated with conflicts, ambiguity, or job insecurity increase stress on the employee (Byrne, 2015; Ganster & Rosen, 2013). We have already highlighted how the complexities of healthcare contribute even more to these job stressors. It is also important to consider the individual factors that each person brings to work, paying attention to the whole person with all their characteristics and needs (Anger et al., 2015; Ganster & Rosen, 2013). If an employee is dealing with a situation at home or has a mental health issue, stress can be compounded.

Recovery from stress needs to be a layered approach, recognizing that the amount of recovery needed is directly related to the stress experienced. In healthcare, stress is a daily occurrence, so employers have to pay attention to both accumulative stress and shifts that include an unusually intense amount of stress. We know that any amount of stress, no matter how small, will eventually exceed the employee's capacity if not interrupted by recovery (Ganster & Rosen, 2013). Leaders need to pay close attention to their employees' level of stress as it may be subtle at first. This again requires building a relationship with each employee to know their own personal signs and symptoms of overload. One employee may get frustrated and lash out as a sign, while another employee may become introverted and quietly shut down. The leader also needs to empower each employee to build in recovery while at work to manage their stress—for instance, using micro-practices throughout the shift to build in recovery within the job. Anger et al. (2015) cited several studies finding that integrating stress management, coping techniques, meditation, and exercise within work hours increased overall worker health. This approach reframes the concepts of work-life balance to focus more on work-life integration, bringing small amounts of recovery from stress throughout the day so that employees are not surviving work and hoping to have enough recovery at home. Designated time to recover and have joy, or incorporating moments of play during a shift increase energy and help workers thrive even while at work (Anger et al., 2015). One way is to create a community at work that helps employees recover during work hours by feeling connected and supported amid the daily doses of stress. Maslow's hierarchy recognizes belonging to a group as a prerequisite to self-esteem. Most of the new leadership theories include attention to relationships and building community at work (Byrne, 2015). If the leader understands the type of stress that affects their staff and works to create an environment that addresses these stresses as they happen, then both leader and healthcare professional win.

Along with integrating these programs within the workday, organizations must also pay close attention to how employees recover after work hours. Do employees often answer emails on vacation or during off-hours? Are they always on call regardless of the time of day? Do they report (or are leaders asking about) sleep patterns? These are important questions that can get to the root of increases in stress and highlight the individual's antecedents to compassion fatigue and burnout (Barber & Santuzzi, 2015; Ganster & Rosen. 2013). Policies that honor time away from work as sacred recovery time can be essential. Disconnecting with work and reconnecting with family and activities or hobbies that help a worker recover from stress is crucial. There is some tension with these suggestions, as they sometimes go against where healthcare organizations have historically focused. Organizations often reward and recognize employees who go above and beyond to get the work done. Unfortunately, the individual and organizational costs related to burnout have risen to the level that we have to reprioritize recovery and low stress as the new attributes to recognize. Suppose the paradigm is *not* shifted to focus on flourishing and thriving metrics. In that case, organizations will continue to contribute to compassion fatigue and burnout and must deal with the mounting repercussions as discussed.

# BUILDING RESILIENT ORGANIZATIONAL CULTURE BY SUPPORTING THE INDIVIDUAL

So far, we have focused on the responsibilities of healthcare organizations to build a resilient culture through leadership and support for healthcare professionals. It is crucial that programs are available and seen as part of the job, requiring dedication from the healthcare professionals themselves. Resiliency will only be realized if the individual professional is committed to their own growth and recovery. This cannot be a prescriptive process. Each professional has unique needs, skills, motivators, and practices that will help them stay connected to their purpose as a care provider. This means there need to be various offerings and tools so each professional can build their own personal growth recovery package. Organizations must offer a wide variety of opportunities and support both during and after work hours and create a culture that prioritizes recovery by using incentives for wellness. Below, we have included a wide variety of resources using evidence-based practices to help the healers heal and continue to have the capacity to do the work they yearn to do.

# POSITIVE PSYCHOLOGY PRACTICES

As previously mentioned, the study of positive psychology can offer insight into promoting flourishing and thriving among those working in the healthcare environment. As Sin and Lyubomirsky (2009) report, psychological well-being is the absence of mental disorders and the presence of positive psychological resources such as positive affect, life satisfaction, and happiness. Positive psychology interventions are treatment methods or intentional activities that aim to cultivate positive feelings, behaviors, or thoughts. Numerous studies of the impact of these positive psychology interventions are shown to increase happiness and decrease depression and anxiety, with sustained benefits over time, long after the intervention has ceased. Positive psychology interventions include regular gratitude practices, the Three Good Things exercise (see sidebar below; Seligman et al., 2005), socializing, and random acts of kindness. Seligman and colleagues (2005) have found that being kind is the most reliable immediate boost in well-being leading to a positive change in mood. Resilient organizations do their part by recognizing and promoting activities of this nature on a regular basis.

---

## THREE GOOD THINGS

This only takes about 10 minutes a day and the research has shown a sustained increase in happiness and significant decrease in depressive symptoms.

| Part 1 | Part 2 |
|---|---|
| Every day for one week | |
| Write down three good things that happened that day. These don't have to be grand events—small experiences also count. | Next to each good thing write: |
| | 1. Why did this good thing happen? |
| Give the event a title "I received a compliment on a project I am working on." | 2. What did this mean to you? |
| | 3. How did it make you feel when it happened and as you are remembering it? |
| Write exactly what happened including as many details as you can recall. | 4. How can you have more of this good thing in the future? |
| (Seligman et al., 2005) | |

# THE ARTS IN HEALING

One primary resource in hospitals that varies depending on staffing and programmatic structure is using the expertise of art therapists to help care providers heal. A vital creative arts therapy program, including music, art, dance/movement, and drama therapies, can provide essential clinical services to patients, from children to adults to seniors. Since 1960, when art therapy was initially integrated into the medical field as a viable treatment modality for diagnostic symptomology (including depression, anxiety, suicidal ideation, dysthymia, cognitive distortions, rehab complications, etc.), creative clinical approaches have become more and more common. Creative arts therapists can do more than improve patient outcomes, but their expertise is significantly underutilized in most healthcare settings. Clinical creative arts therapists can play a major role in building internal resilience structures designed to support a healthcare organization's emotional, psychological, and social vitality. Arts-based encounters have been shown to reduce stress and burnout in healthcare workers, specifically increasing participants' self-esteem, stimulating personal growth, reducing work-related fatigue, improving communication and relationships, and promoting a sense of community at work (Huss & Sarid, 2014; Karpaviciute & Macijauskiene, 2016; Repar & Reid, 2014).

So how can engagement in the arts create these positive effects? This question has been studied for centuries among different populations and after global traumas. When language fails us to represent or process acts so horrific or unspeakable, we often turn to the arts for many reasons. Primarily, the arts can reflect emotion to match its intensity, whether through color, rhythm, tone, or movement, that surpasses the ability of language. As an example, the catalysts for the Civil Rights Movement in the United States in the 1960s were often images, poetry, and song, which seemed to capture and galvanize groups of citizens in ways that newspaper articles or even television could not.

Similarly, the level of trauma experienced by healthcare professionals is often deeper than words convey, especially because there is so little time to emotionally process events that move through a typical day in a working hospital. So as the nurse holds the hand of a dying COVID-19 patient because no family is allowed on the unit, the next patient waits in the next room, and the next, and the next. After a shift in this unprecedented pandemic era, this nurse goes home to a family that cannot comprehend the level of loss they have witnessed. Where do we put that pain? Who holds the hand of these sacred witnesses as they shed so many unshed tears? Who cares for the caregivers of our massive healthcare establishments?

The arts can hold this pain. They can illuminate the sadness, capture the shock, sing back to the worry until it abates. Dance can help the trauma move through the body until it is reprocessed, digested, transformed, and released. Within communities of healthcare professionals and under the direction of creative arts therapists, narratives can be expressed in metaphor that allows the pain of the experiences to be transmuted through a story, through song, image, or movement. New meaning can be woven from individual and collective traumas, especially if it is shared in communities of people who learn to trust their vulnerabilities and allow authentic expressions to emerge. This concept can in itself be revolutionary in typical Western medical environments.

Beyond processing trauma, the arts can also help to create a sense of community. Though medical teams work together day after day, oftentimes, there is no inherent opportunity to know each other. The sense of isolation can be emphasized by the lack of authentic emotional expression in fast-paced medical units. Symptoms of stress and burnout can be exacerbated if not allowed to be expressed or communicated within a medical community. The arts can provide a doorway into that expression. In one children's hospital, a large exhibition was planned to feature murals made by different teams across the hospital. These murals were created with the caps to medicine vials, which come in many colors. Working for a full year, the

21 teams that participated experienced increased feelings of belonging, a renewed sense of purpose, and enjoyment in the process of working on a shared creative goal. When the exhibition was installed, each team included an "artist statement" to summarize both the process and the design. One group of medical interpreters chose to create a scene of butterflies out of their medicine caps. They wrote:

> We originally chose the monarch butterflies as the theme for our department because they are representative of migrants and their incredible journey. Our Medical Interpreters Department is made up of team members from Latin America, Spain, United Kingdom, and the USA. Each one of us has a unique story of what brought us here. As interpreters, we work in all areas of patient care in the hospital, where we have met many providers, each with their own journeys around the country and the world while pursuing their careers or providing healthcare. Through our language services, we serve a very rich and diverse community of families who have migrated from every corner of the world. When a new diagnosis or a tragic accident brings them here, this is where we all meet. Every day within the walls of this hospital, we bear witness to their stories of adversity and resiliency, each one of them a survivor. These butterflies represent the survivors that exist in all of us. It is within our nature to fight against the odds and retain our inner beauty through life's challenges, beating our wings and looking for warmer climates to replenish our souls.

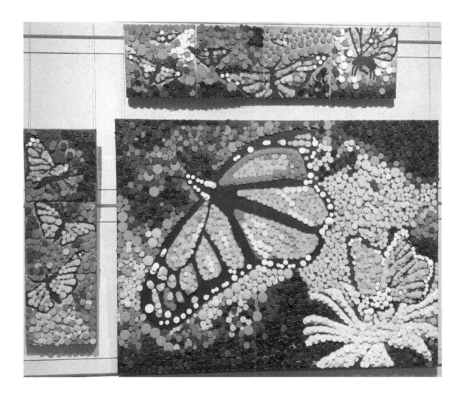

# A TEAM-BASED APPROACH TO RESILIENCY

A team-based approach to improving team function and resilience can also be employed. Pierce and colleagues (2019) published their findings, and this approach has been used in numerous settings to address dissatisfaction and burnout among teams. The approach is to identify a team, using organizational resilience index data, that is languishing or struggling with engagement and satisfaction. Then a stepwise approach is taken to prepare for and conduct a team retreat. The preparation typically includes a deeper dive into the team's drivers of dissatisfaction using surveys, focus groups, and leadership input. A retreat (typically half-day to full-day) is conducted with the entire team, including leadership members.

After identifying goals, objectives, and ground rules and reviewing the data that is known, the team is taken through a series of actions to:

1.  Identify core values using a "peak experiences exercise"

2.  Prioritize values among the entire team (identify four to six values that the team agrees on to promote their best work)

3.  Create a list of action items that are necessary to do work more aligned with each value

4.  Create a road map for action to achieve the most important/top priority action items that the team agrees to enact

This approach gives teams the time to build connection and camaraderie, align around shared and prioritized values, and agree upon a road map for action with measurable change to attain their goals.

## COMPASSIONATE COMMUNITIES

The need for recovery for our team members has never been more important. Using the framework of compassion circles, a series of small group gatherings have brought a unique process that infuses support for each other with compassion and healing. Based on the work of Bradley and Scott (2021), the intention is to create a safe space where healthcare providers are invited to recover, be heard, be held up, and seek healing. Each compassion circle follows the same structure and flow, including checking in, first thought, thinking rounds, partner connection, commitment rounds, and appreciation rounds. This format has been adjusted to support healthcare providers in different settings and experience levels. It can be used for small group mentoring sessions or for a drop-in session for healthcare professionals as needed. It is also used in the new graduate nurse residency program as part of the curriculum throughout the year in regular intervals. For new nurses, a trained facilitator guides the small groups through the same practices each session, creating space to discuss topics ranging from the transition from school to bedside, creating a safe community for support, self-compassion, and the realities of being a nurse.

# THEORY-GUIDED PRACTICES/CARING SCIENCE

Offering classes that focus on theory-guided practices promoting self-care and re-covery is another doorway into helping healthcare professionals flourish. To offer a deeper dive into theory, specifically Jean Watson's Caring Science, we created a program called Caritas Circles. This six-month curriculum allows care providers to pause and reconnect to why they chose the profession of caring. These sessions used both self-reflection practices and time to connect with other professionals to create a theoretical foundation that they can stand on as they work through the complexities of their roles. The reflections and exercises experienced in the Caritas Circle offer skills and practices to help healthcare professionals pause, be present, and find peace within their day-to-day experiences. Caring Science does not have all the answers to magically fix the complexities of working in healthcare. It cannot change the acuities of patients or take away the inadequacies of medicine as an imperfect science. It does not attempt to minimize the pain and suffering of the experiences to create a false sense of "just do this, and it will be easy." Caring Science begins by honoring all these intricacies and giving voice to the deep connection the professionals have to be the best caregiver possible. It unabashed-ly reminds medical models that caregivers at the bedside offer expertise that no other part of healthcare understands or attempts to provide. Watson herself draws on concepts like consciousness, oneness, vulnerability, the dignity that at times seem intangible to modern medicine but are a perfect description of what these professionals offer their patients. The results of the Caritas Circles classes show a significant increase in these professionals' ability to treat themselves with lov-ing-kindness, to practice self-care as a means to meet their own basic needs, and to be able to pause in a moment so they can re-center and bring their best self to the encounter with the patient (Griffin et al., 2021).

# PEER-TO-PEER SUPPORT

Peer support is essential to respond to adverse events that happen in healthcare. Virtually every healthcare provider has experienced an event at work that leaves them feeling adversely impacted. The response to the events can lead to adverse emotional, physical, cognitive, and behavioral outcomes (Scott et al., 2009; Seys et al., 2013). Shapiro & Galowitz (2016) found that "creating a peer support program is one way forward, away from a culture of invulnerability, isolation, and shame and toward a culture that truly values a sense of shared organizational responsibility for clinician wellbeing and patient safety" (p. 1204).

The most desired form of support among healthcare professionals after an adverse clinical event is a "trusted peer" to talk to. (Burlison et al., 2018). Every organization should develop a peer support program (Sexton et al., 2021). Peer supporters should be identified by their leaders and peers as someone colleagues are comfortable talking to and receiving support from. Peer supporters should be trained using a consistent approach to teaching basic skills of active and reflective listening, emotional support, and availability. Peer supporters should be trained to recognize concerning behaviors in colleagues that require further referral for support and should be trusted to maintain utmost confidentiality. Peer support is essential to supporting colleagues' recovery from inevitable adverse events and contributes to a sense of team culture, safety, and organizational well-being.

Each of these evidence-based recovery practices meets the needs of healthcare professionals in unique ways. Resilient organizations understand the need to offer a variety of programs, during and after work, so that each individual staff member has the opportunity to flourish even when the demands of the job are difficult.

# IMPLICATIONS FOR PRACTICE

The implications of building a resilient workforce in healthcare are vast. The most important population it serves is the patients seeking care. When compassion fatigue and burnout are prevalent, it is almost impossible for patients to get the care they need. The literature shares the risks of this type of healthcare, conveying the dehumanization of patients or the regression of a healing environment to a toxic environment void of healing potential (Halldorsdottir, 2008; Swanson, 1993). However, imagine if all caregivers are flourishing in their role, how different the experiences of the patient will be.

Promoting a resilient workforce can also transform the care provider. Remember, compassion fatigue is not only about the inability to form caring relationships but also the resulting distress this causes the care provider. Being able to care for a patient is why individuals get into this profession. When their capacity is low, the suffering is not just felt by the patient. Working in an organization that recognizes this type of suffering and promotes cultures and training that offer support is the key to thriving in these environments. It helps ensure each nurse, doctor, respiratory therapist, social worker, clinical assistant, etc. has the capacity to live out their caring values. More importantly, it honors that care providers deserve to be whole themselves. All healthcare organizations must agree that no one should suffer because they choose to care as a profession. Also, we must agree that no one should feel dehumanized because they find themselves unable to care anymore. Instead, using the principles and practices outlined in this chapter, organizations and individuals can create a road map to ensure that flourishing and thriving as a healthcare professional is prioritized.

# SUMMARY

Working in healthcare is complex, and so the interventions to sustain care providers must meet many demands. In this chapter, we have illustrated the vital role leadership plays in promoting and supporting a resilient workforce. It begins with recognizing the emotional labor that healthcare providers deal with on a day-to-day basis. Until the stress is recognized as a normal and often profound side effect of working in healthcare, the professional's need for support is minimized. This chapter also highlighted the need for resiliency to be managed at an organizational level and recognized as part of the job, not side work. This includes having resiliency-focused leaders who pay attention to the environments where the care is provided and are committed to supporting each individual. As these leaders honor each individual's recovery process and needs, they can ensure the professional can live out their life's purpose while still flourishing as a human. Finally, we outline some evidence-based interventions that offer a wide variety of support to help healthcare professionals walk toward their personal wholeness as they continue to help their patients heal. The benefits of having a flourishing healthcare team affect the organization, the care providers, and each patient in their care. Choosing to be a healthcare provider necessitates a unique commitment to serving others. To share in another person's suffering and see this as a privilege and not a burden. To step into the stress of illness and want to make a difference. To continually offer dignity and respect to another while often putting aside personal needs. It is time to honor these professions by supporting their resiliency practice so they can continue to care for others without paying too high of a cost for themselves

# REFLECTIVE QUESTIONS

1. Describe the effects that compassion fatigue can have on caregivers, patients, and organizations.

2. Discuss why leadership is important to resiliency when self-care is a personal practice/decision.

3. List three attributes of a leader who is focused on care provider resiliency.

4. Describe the difference in healthcare providers' experience when working on a unit that prioritizes support, resiliency, and recovery vs. a unit that does not.

5. What are some offerings that an organization can prioritize to help build a resiliency culture in healthcare?

## NARRATIVE

Behavioral Health Specialists are responsible for direct patient care and safety, including supervision and management of children and adolescents who may be experiencing a psychiatric crisis. Behavioral Health Specialists work in diverse environments, including inpatient psychiatric units, partial hospitalization or day treatment programs, and medical floors. One Behavioral Health Specialist named Neena, working in the psychiatric department of a large children's hospital, participated in a 12-week workshop designed to create community and develop resilience using artmaking. This workshop was facilitated by an art therapist, using a sequential curriculum within a peer-reviewed research protocol. Each week, Neena attended the group, looking forward to the chance to focus on herself, her creativity, and new relationships with other providers with similar self-care goals. Neena practiced different therapeutic skills and art-making techniques, building her confidence as well as her ability to be vulnerable. On the seventh week, she was asked to visually represent an especially challenging day at work, one that she may not be able to forget. Neena created an image of the day she was physically assaulted by a patient in distress. The image included red prison bars, representing her feeling of being trapped in the situation, and a red pool of blood at the bottom, which was her own. The image itself brought Neena to tears as she shared it with the group, recounting the story that she had not shared with anyone since it happened 12 weeks prior.

The group witnessed her courage and vulnerability in this process, offering her words of support and understanding. Neena left that day exhausted but relieved to have let this trauma pour out of her onto paper. She came back the following week feeling refreshed and rejuvenated, with new purpose and perspective on her professional worth.

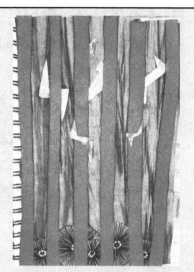

In the last few weeks of the group, participants were asked to share artwork and writing for a collaborative book, with the goal of sharing their voices beyond the intimate setting of the group. Neena wrote the following to accompany another artwork she had created, depicting another intense day:

Behind the mask, tears are streaming down my face and my adrenaline is pumping harder than it has in my entire life. I can hear my own heartbeat, and the pounding in my ears is terrifying. One of my coworkers starts counting down from 3, and I know that once we get to 1, we're releasing our grip on the door handle and entering our patient's room to put them into a supine hold. This step, while traumatic for both the patient and for staff, is necessary at this moment to maintain the safety of our patient and everyone else on our unit. Knowing that doesn't make it any easier. Once we get to 1, I have to face the reality that I may witness one or more of my coworkers getting hurt. I have to accept that I may no longer have control and could get hurt myself. I have to be the most aware and present I have ever been to ensure our patient remains safe. 3, 2, 1. I take a deep breath, and I step forward.

Behind the mask, I am a Behavioral Health Specialist working on a psychiatric unit during a global pandemic. Sometimes my job is rewarding beyond what I could ever imagine. Feeling the impact we have on our patients and witnessing the changes they can make is amazing. At the same time, I have left work countless times crying, dehydrated, bruised, bleeding, or covered in bodily fluids. I've continually surprised myself with my ability to step up to the plate but being the holder of someone's else's pain and trauma is never easy and always weighs on you. Something I've taken away from our art group is that this is a shared sentiment among healthcare workers, yet we never back down. We continue to show up, day in and day out, for our patients and for our coworkers. We find ways to build resilience and we lean on each other. We step up to the plate in hard or scary situations, and that makes us brave. Throughout this group experience and my reflections on the past year of working in healthcare during a pandemic, I've been reminded that despite everything, hope and courage still persist.

After reading through the experience of the healthcare provider in the narrative, what can you appreciate about a resiliency approach that includes different creative modalities to help staff process their trauma and reconnect to their individual purpose?

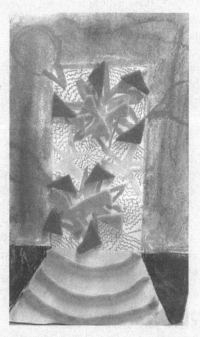

# AUTHOR BIOGRAPHIES

**Christine Griffin, PhD, RN, NPD-BC, CPN,** Caritas Coach, is a board-certified nurse in professional development at Children's Hospital Colorado, matching expertise in adult learning with a passion to heal the healers in healthcare. For the past 10 years Griffin has developed resiliency curriculum, presented at national and international conferences, and offered workshops with healthcare organizations around the country. In her PhD program, Griffin studied how the essential truths of Caring Science can inform interventions to understand compassion fatigue, decrease burnout, mediate secondary trauma, and increase compassion satisfaction for healthcare providers. As a Caritas Coach, CCEP Faculty Member, and HeartMath Trainer, she hopes to bring theory-guided practices to those working in healthcare so they can experience Compassion without Fatigue.

**Katherine Reed, LPC,** has been Program Manager for the Ponzio Creative Arts Therapy Program since its inception in 2005 and has dedicated her team's expertise to the resilience efforts at Children's Hospital Colorado through workshops, conferences, art exhibitions, and system-wide integration of the arts into the daily experience of healthcare providers. Reed is the co-PI, along with Marc Moss, MD, on the Colorado Resilience in the Arts Lab (CORAL) research team, funded by the National Endowment of the Arts. Reed authored "Creative Arts Therapy as a Potential Intervention to Prevent Burnout and Build Resilience in Health Care Professionals," published in the *AACN Advanced Critical Care Journal* in 2020, as a preliminary study to the clinical trials created and facilitated by CORAL therapists and writers. The trials involve 12 weeks of sequential workshops in art, music, dance, and writing for healthcare professionals to develop communities of expression and support.

**Jennifer Reese, MD,** is an Associate Professor of Clinical Pediatrics at the University of Colorado School of Medicine. She is the Section Head of the Pediatric Hospital, Medicine. She also serves as the leader for provider well-being at Children's Hospital Colorado and the Department of Pediatrics, University of Colorado School of Medicine. Her clinical time is spent as a pediatric hospitalist, and her administrative duties include quality and process improvement and clinical leadership, as well as developing and promoting programs that support wellness and resilience for healthcare providers. Her undergraduate and medical school were completed at University of Washington, in Seattle, Washington, and her pediatric internship and residency were completed at the University of Colorado School of Medicine and Children's Hospital Colorado. Since finishing residency, she has worked at Children's Hospital Colorado.

# REFERENCES

Adriaenssens, J., DeGicht, V., & Maes, S. (2014). Determinants and prevalence of burnout in emergency nurses: A systemic review of 25 years of research. *International Journal of Nursing Studies, 52*, 649–661.

Anger, W. K., Elliot, D. L., Bodner, T., Olson, R., Rohlman, D. S., Truxillo, D., Kuehl, K., Hammer, L. B., & Montgomery, D. (2015). Effectiveness of total worker health interventions. *Journal of Occupational Health Psychology, 20*(2), 226–247.

Barber, L. K., & Santuzzi, A. M. (2015). Please respond ASAP: Workplace telepressure and employee recovery. *Journal of Occupational Health Psychology, 20*(2), 172–189.

Beck, C.T. (2011). Secondary traumatic stress in nurses: A systematic review. *Archives of Psychiatric Nursing, 25*(1), 1–10.

Berger, J., Polivka, B., Smoot, E. A., & Owens, H. (2015). Compassion fatigue in pediatric nurses. *Journal of Pediatric Nursing, 30*, 11–17.

Bradley, A., & Scott, A. (2021). Compassion practices: Enabling us to be kinder. *Coaching Perspectives.*

Branch, C., & Klinkenberg, D. (2015). Compassion fatigue among pediatric healthcare providers. *MCN Healthcare, 40*(3), 160–166.

Brotheridge, C. M. (2002). Emotional labor and burnout: Comparing two perspectives of "people work." *Journal of Vocational Behavior, 60*, 17–39.

Brunero, S., Cowan, D., & Fairbrother, G. (2008). Reducing emotional distress in nurses using cognitive behavioral therapy: A preliminary program evaluation. *Japan Journal of Nursing Science, 5*, 109–115.

Burlison, J. D., Scott, S. D, Browne, E. K., Thompson, S. G., & Hoffman, J. M. (2018). The second victim experience and support tool (SVEST): Validation of an organizational resource for assessing second victim effects and the quality of support resources. *Journal of Patient Safety, 13*(2), 93–102.

Burston, P. L., & Stichler, J. F. (2010). Nursing Work environment and nurse care: relationship among motivational factors. *Journal of Advanced Nursing, 66*(8), 1819–1831.

Bush, N. J. (2009). Compassion fatigue: Are you at risk? *Oncology Nursing Forum, 36*(1), 24–28.

Byrne, A. (2015). *Organizational psychology & behavior: An integrated approach to understanding the workplace.* Kendall Hunt Publishing Company.

Cricco-Lizza, R. (2014). The need to nurse the nurse: Emotional labor in neonatal intensive care. *Qualitative Health Research, 24*(5), 615–628.

Czaja, A. S., Moss, M., & Mealer, M. (2012). Symptoms of post-traumatic stress disorder among pediatric acute care nurses. *Journal of Pediatric Nursing, 27*(4), 357–365.

Drury, V., Craugue, M., Francis, K., Aoun, S., & Hegney, D. G. (2013) Compassion satisfaction, compassion fatigue, anxiety, depression, and stress in registered nurses in Australia: Phase 2 results. *Journal of Nursing Management,* 1–13.

Dyrbye, L. N., Major-Elechi, B., Hays, J. T., Fraser, C. H., Buskirk, S. J., & West, C. P.(2020). Relationship between organizational leadership and health care employee burnout and satisfaction. *Mayo Clinic Proceedings, 95*(4), 698–708.

Eckleberry-Hunt, J., Kirkpatrick, H., & Barbera, T. (2018). The problems with burnout research. *Journal of the Association of American Medical Colleges, 93*(3), 367–370.

Figley, C. (2002). Compassion fatigue: Psychotherapists' chronic lack of self-care. *Psychotherapy in Practice, 58*(11). 1433–1441.

Flarity, K., Gentry, J. E., & Mesnikiff, N. (2013). The effectiveness of an educational program on preventing and treating compassion fatigue in emergency nurses. *Advanced Emergency Nursing Journal, 35*(3), 247–258.

Frederickson, B. (2009). *Positivity: Top-notch research reveals the 3-to-1 ratio that will change your life.* Harmony.

Ganster, D. C., & Rosen, C. C. (2013) Work stress and employee health: A multidisciplinary review. *Journal of Management, 39*(5), 1085–1122.

Gentry, E. (2002). Compassion fatigue: A crucible of transformation. *The Hawthorne Press, 1*(3/4), 37–61.

Griffin, C., Oman, K. S., Ziniel, S. I., Kight, S., Jacobs-Lowry, S., & Givens, P. (2021). Increasing the capacity to provide compassionate care by expanding knowledge of Caring Science practices at a pediatric hospital. *Archives of Psychiatric Nursing, 35,* 34–41.

Halldorsdottir, S. (2008). The dynamics of the nurse-patient relationship. Introducing a synthesized theory from the patient's perspective. *Scandinavian Journal of Caring Science, 22,* 643–652.

Hartzband, P., & Groopman, J. (2020). Physician burnout, interrupted. *The New England Journal of Medicine.* https://www.nejm.org/

Huss, E., & Sarid, O. (2014). Visually transforming artwork and guided imagery as a way to reduce work related stress: A quantitative pilot study. *Arts Psychotherapy, 41,* 409–412.

Joinson, C. (1992). Coping with compassion fatigue. *Nursing,* 116–121.

Johnson, K. M. (2013). *Prevalence of compassion fatigue among pediatric nurses.* [Unpublished doctoral dissertation]. University of Colorado, Denver, Colorado.

Karpaviciute, S, & Macijauskiene, J. (2016). The impact of arts activity on nursing staff wellbeing: An intervention in the workplace. *International Journal of Environmental Res. Pub Health. 13,* 435. doi:10.3390/ijerph13040435.

Leggett, J. M., Wasson, K., Sinacore, J. M., & Gamelli, R. L. (2013). A pilot study examining moral distress in nurses working in one United States burn unit. *Journal of Burn Care & Research, 34*(5), 521–528.

Lewin, R. A. (1996). *Compassion: The core value that animate psychotherapy.* Jason Aronson.

Losada, M., & Heaphy, E. (2004). The Role of positivity and connectivity in the performance of business teams. *American Behavioral Scientist, 47*(6), 740–765. doi:10.1177/0002764203260208

Maytum, J., Heiman, M. B., & Garwick, A. W. (2004). Compassion fatigue and burnout in nurses who work with children with chronic conditions and their families. *Journal of Pediatric Health Care, 18,* 171–179.

McGaghie, W. C., Mytko, J. J., Brown, N., & Cameron, J. R. (2002). Altruism and compassion in health professions: a search for clarity and precision. *Medical Teacher, 24*(4), 374–378.

Meadors, P., & Lamson, A. (2008). Compassion fatigue and secondary traumatization: Provider self-care on intensive care units for children. *Journal of Pediatric Health Care.* 22(1), 24–34.

Mealer, M. (2014). *Individual and group factors that affect resilience and mediate the relationship between resilience and the development of post-traumatic stress disorder in ICU nurses.* [Unpublished doctoral dissertation]. University of Colorado, Denver, Colorado.

Mealer, M., Jones, J., Newman, J., McFann, K., Rothbaum, B., & Moss, M. (2012). The presence of resilience is associated with a healthier psychological profile in ICU nurses: Results of a national survey. *International Journal of Nursing Studies, 49*(3), 292–299.

Morrison, C. F., & Morris, E. J. (2017). The practices and meaning of care for nurses working on a pediatric bone marrow transplant unit. *Journal of Pediatric Oncology Nursing,* 1–8.

Moss, M., Good, V. S., Gozal, D., Kleinpell, R., & Sessler, C. N. (2016). A critical care societies collaborative statement: Burnout syndrome in critical care healthcare professionals. *American Journal of Respiratory and Critical Care Medicine, 194*(1), 106–113.

Occupational Safety and Health Administration. (2013). *Caring for our care givers.* https://www.osha.gov/dsg/hospitals/documents/1.2_Factbook_508.pdf

Phillips, J. P. (2016). Workplace violence against healthcare workers in the United States. *The New England Journal of Medicine, 374*(17) 1661–1669.

Pierce, R. G., Diaz, M., & Kneeland, P. (2019). Optimizing well-being, practice culture, and professional thriving in an era of turbulence. *Journal of Hospital Medicine, 14*(2), 126–128.

Quinn, J. F., Smith, M., Ritenbaugh, C., Swanson, K., & Watson, J. (2003). Research guidelines for assessing the impact of healing relationships in clinical nursing. *Alternative Therapies, 9*(3), 65–79.

Repar, P. A., & Reid, S. (2014) Creatively caring: Effects of arts-based encounters on hospice caregivers in South Africa. *Journal of Pain Symptom Management, 47,* 946–954.

Reese, J., & Ziniel, S. (2018). Diving into the data: Using a metrics to evaluate ca comprehensive program as a larger academic pediatric medical center. *Inaugural National Summit on Promoting Well-being and Resilience in Healthcare Providers.* Oral presentation, Columbus, Ohio.

Ryan, R. M., & Deci, E. L. (2000). Self-determination theory and the facilitation of intrinsic motivation, social development and wellbeing. *American Psychologist.* https://doii.org/10.1037//0003-066x.55.1.68

Sacco, T. L., & Carman-Copel, L. (2017). Compassion satisfaction: A concept analysis in nursing. *Nursing Forum.* 1–8.

Sauter, S. L., & Hurrell, J. J. (2017) Occupational health contributions to the development and promise of occupational health psychology. *Journal of Occupational Health Psychology, 22*(3), 251–258.

Scott, S. D, Hirschinger, L. E, Cox, K. R, McCoig, M, Brandt, J., & Hall, L. W. (2009). The natural history of recovery for the healthcare provider "second victim" after adverse patient events. *Quality & Safety in Health Care, 18*(5), 325–330.

Seligman, M. E., Steen, T. A., Park, N., & Peterson, C. (2005). Positive psychology progress: Empirical validation of interventions. *American Psychologist, 42,* 874–884.

Sexton, J. B., Adair, K. C., Profit, J., Milne, J., McCulloh, M., Scott, S., & Frankel, A. (2021). Perceptions of institutional support for "second victims" are associated with safety culture and workforce well-being. *The Joint Commission Journal on Quality and Patient Safety, 000,* 1–7.

Seys, D., Wu, A., W., Van Gerven, E., Vleugels, A., Euwema, M., Panella, M., Scott, S. D., Conway, J., Sermeus, W., & Vanhaecht, K. (2013). Health care professionals as second victims after adverse events: A systematic review. *Evaluation and the Health Professions, 35*(2), 135–162.

Shanafelt, T. D., Boone, S. B., Tan, L. T., Dyrbye, L. N., Sotile, W., Satele, D., Wets, C. P., Sloan, J., Oreskovich, M. R. (2012). Burnout and satisfaction with work-life balance among US physicians relative to the general US population. *Achieves Internal Medicine, 172*(18), 1377–1385.

Shanafelt, T. D., Gorringe, G., Menaker, R., Stora, K.A ., Reeves, D., Buskirk, S. J., Sloan, J. A., Swensen, S. J. (2000). Impact of organizational leadership on physician burnout and satisfaction. *Mayo Clinic Proceedings, 95*(4), 698–708.

Shanafelt T. D., & Noseworthy, J. H. (2017). Executive leadership and physician well-being: Nine organizational strategies to promote engagement and reduce burnout. *Mayo Clinic Proceedings, 92*(1) 129–146.

Shapiro, J., & Galowitz, O. (2016). Peer support for clinicians: A programmatic approach. *Academic Medicine, 91*(9).

Shimoinaba, K., O'Connor, M., Lee, S., Kissane, D. (2015). Nurses' resilience and nurturance of the self. *International Journal of Palliative Nursing, 21*(10), 504–510.

Sin, N. L., & Lyubomirsky, S. (2009) Enhancing wellbeing and alleviating depressive symptoms with positive psychology interventions: A practice-friendly meta-analysis. *Journal of Clinical Psychology, 65*(5), 467–487.

Sinclair, S., Raffin-Bouchal, S., Venturato, L., Mijovic-Kondejewski, J., & Smith-MacDonald, L. (2017). Compassion fatigue: A meta-narrative review of the healthcare literature. *International Journal of Nursing Studies, 69,* 9–24.

Swanson, K. (1993). Nursing as informed caring for the wellbeing of others. *Journal of Nursing Scholarship, 25*(4). 352–357.

Zerach, G., & Shalev, T. B. (2015). The relations between violence exposure, post-traumatic stress symptoms, secondary traumatization, vicarious post traumatic growth and illness among psychiatric nurses. *Archives of Psychiatric Nursing, 29*(1), 135–142.

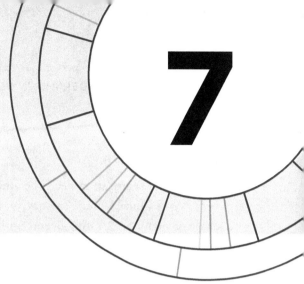

# 7

# LEADERSHIP ROLES IN MITIGATING ORGANIZATIONAL TRAUMA

Sonya R. Hardin, PhD, CCRN, NP-C, FAAN
Karen J. Foli, PhD, RN, FAAN

---

## LEARNING OBJECTIVES

After completing this chapter, the learner will be able to:

- Describe how organizational trauma occurs from devastating events

- Discuss the cumulative impacts of organizational trauma on leadership and organizational culture and behaviors

- Relate destructive organizational despair and rapid turnover of personnel, large miscalculations resulting in financial loss, budget cuts, and layoffs

- Critique supervisor/middle manager's interactions with nurses who experience secondary traumatic stress

- Convey ways of using caring consciousness and actions to promote organizational caring-healing system environments

- Examine the goals of a trauma-informed and healing organization

- Defend the Sanctuary Model as a viable approach to trauma-informed institutional change and problem-solving

- Analyze ways to enhance organizational post-traumatic growth

- Select implications for nursing leaders within a trauma-informed context

---

# OVERVIEW

What kind of organization needs healing? Typically, an organization that has experienced trauma will die or survive. Organizational trauma may result from a single or many devastating events and from a pattern of events that results in a culmination of persistent unhealthy organizational dynamics. Organizational trauma may occur through four different avenues:

1.   Sudden event that destabilizes an organization such as a natural disaster, embezzlement, death of an employee

2.   Cumulative effects of oppression, authoritative leadership, hostile relationships, individuals constantly feeling under attack emotionally

3.   Nature of the work, which can be overwhelming due to the type of work, amount of work, or team members displaying toxic hostility

4.   Level of empathetic work required in the organization, such as caring for others through emotional or physical labor that creates an intensity

High-intensity work can impact communication on teams (Vivian & Hormann, 2013) and lead to moral injury or burnout. *Moral injury* can occur when you fail to intervene or prevent harm, or experience transgressions against deeply held beliefs. Individuals who constantly experience moral injury may find themselves in a state of burnout. *Burnout* has physical, emotional, and behavioral symptoms. When many individuals are in this state, an organization needs healing as a whole.

# PATTERNS OF TRAUMA IN ORGANIZATIONS

Organizational trauma is emotionally overwhelming for individuals impacted day after day. The cumulative impact can result in various symptoms: collusion, groupthink, scapegoating, closed boundaries, stress and anxiety contagion, organizational amnesia, unrecognized wounding, unproductive relationships, narrowing worldview, and depression. Within the discipline of nursing, an example of each may help shed light on how an organization becomes unhealthy.

*Closed boundaries* occur when there is an "us vs. them" mentality. An example is when critical care nurses do not answer the phone when they hear it ringing as the caller ID on the phone is the emergency department. A conversation will go like this: "Surely they cannot be calling to give reports on another patient. We haven't got this one admitted." Or, "They always wait until 6pm and try to transfer all the patients out of the emergency department before the next shift comes in. They let the patients sit for hours in the ED, but as soon as 6pm is on the clock, they jump into action." Feelings of being overwhelmed and overworked facilitate closed boundaries.

*Stress and anxiety* become a contagion infecting every individual in a unit. Destructive forms of communication erupt when stress, anxiety, and fear occur day after day. Without constructive approaches for communication, a cascade of toxicity can erupt: blaming, backstabbing, undeserved credit, name bashing, workplace violence, and complaining without identifying solutions or addressing the issue. A contagion can infect every cell of an organization through gossiping and spreading rumors (Bragg, 2001). Sources of stress can be the intensity of the patient cases, time constraints, lack of control, and conflict with leadership or coworkers. Workplace violence can appear as rudeness, incivility, interpersonal conflict, bullying, relational aggression, or being set up, undermined, sabotaged, ignored, marginalized, or degraded (Berquist et al., 2017), and emotional abuse. These behaviors are often discussed in terms of "joy stealing" or "mean girl games." Stress and anxiety can lead to burnout, which can be seen in employees arriving late for work, calling out of work, or a lack of vigilance in delivering care or thoroughness in the documentation.

*Organizational amnesia* is when we do not talk about or process an event. Yet, the impact of the event continues to influence the organization. For example, many years ago, a nurse who was well respected made a medication error that resulted in the death of a patient. The organization fired the nurse. The medication error by a well-respected nurse and the organizational response of firing the nurse sent waves of fear and doubt through the other employees. Employees were told not to discuss the incident. Each week that went by, the more anxious nurses became. Eventually, half the nurses resigned or transferred from the unit over six months. The organization provided no interventions, and the nurses did not seek trauma-informed care.

*Unrecognized wounding* occurs when employees do not believe that their organization has been impacted. For example, when the trauma is caused by racism or oppression (Griffith et al., 2007), individuals may want to deny that the organization is harmed. An example is when a person from an underrepresented minority group is more qualified than the other candidates for a position and does not get the job. This type of decision sends a message through the organization that results in traumatization.

*Unproductive relationships* between an organization and an entity outside the organization can result in trauma. For example, a local hospital had an antagonistic relationship with the local newspaper. The owner of the newspaper sits on the board of the competitor's hospital. The employees of the hospital felt that the newspaper always reported favorable information about the hospital in the back pages while the competitor had news on the front page. Years of this form of behavior by the local newspaper impacted the way employees saw themselves. They could often be heard making comments that insinuated that they were the underdogs in the community.

A *narrowing worldview* occurs when beliefs invade the minds of employees. For example, if a home health agency has several poor outcomes, nurses will be hesitant to recommend the agency or respond to patients about the agency. This narrowing of a worldview of an organization has resulted in some organizations changing their name to improve the community's attitude toward the services they offer.

*Depression* or despair of an organization can emerge due to rapid turnover of personnel; large miscalculations resulting in financial loss, budget cuts, layoffs; or when employees have one merger after another. For example, despair happens when a unit has a new manager every year for the last five years. There is a sense of impermanence about the organization. Such an environment sets up a lack of trust, inconsistent expectations, and feelings of helplessness. Depression can result in less energy to be innovative and on the cutting edge. These organizations often lack best practices and are struggling to maintain services. Many studies find that rapid and frequent change in an organization result in employees experiencing acute emotions such as anger, anxiety, disorientation, and depression (Marquitz et al., 2016; Smollan, 2014; Zell, 2003).

The characteristics discussed are often seen in combination within traumatized organizations. These organizations will have deeply rooted patterns of dysfunction with an inability to fulfill their mission and have poor quality outcomes. There is groupthink and reactivity due to stress and anxiety. Emotion guides individuals instead of logic and rational thought processes. Organizations with persistent traumatization have individuals who cannot change their behavior, resulting in any new change causing high drama regardless of how minor the change. Employees are extra sensitive to each other's moods, and a leader can expect outbursts and those who feel paralyzed and cannot speak for fear of retribution. Employees may find it easier not to talk rather than assume trustworthiness and take risks speaking. Ultimately a leader will see a lack of engagement and time lost from work. Individuals report feeling physically ill reporting to the workplace. A past reality of unresolved pain can quickly emerge if triggered.

Tafoya (2018) indicated that there are three elements to keep in mind when preparing interventions in a traumatized organization: 1) understand how the disruption creates confusion, 2) understand employees' responses, and 3) investigate how the adverse impact has affected services, productivity, quality, and cost.

A new leader in a traumatized organization runs the risk of being swept up into the system's internal dynamics and losing perspective (Norman et al., 2016). This risk increases as exposure lengthens and the work deepens. When a new leader comes into a traumatized organization, the day-to-day operations can be overwhelming as the organization will be in chaos. Be careful not to take sides on issues, as entering into an organization requires listening and not blaming prior leaders.

# THE ROLE OF THE SUPERVISOR/MIDDLE MANAGER

Let's take a more micro view of trauma within an organization. Supervisors need to support the overall aims of *trauma-informed organizations*, defined as organizations that "infuse and sustain trauma awareness, knowledge, and skills into their organizational cultures, practices, and policies" (National Child Traumatic Stress Network [NCTSN], 2020, para. 1). There is a saying in the workplace: "People don't quit their jobs. They quit their supervisors." In organizations in which individuals (such as nurses) are continually exposed to the trauma of those they serve, a trauma-informed, competent supervisor can make a significant impact.

One type of trauma is especially relevant because of its influence on nurses: *secondary traumatic stress* (STS), which is the emotional toll and distress resulting from co-experiencing the firsthand trauma expressed by another. Post-traumatic stress disorder (PTSD)-like symptoms were found to be defining attributes of STS and included avoidance, intrusion, and arousal (Arnold, 2020). Trauma-informed supervisors may be able to mitigate such symptoms when knowledgeable support is offered to the bedside nurse experiencing STS.

By the nature of what it means to be a nurse and render compassionate care to others, nurses in organizations are at risk for STS. The good news is that supervisors have the tools necessary to mitigate the impact of STS on their nursing staff.

The STS core competencies for trauma-informed supervision (NCTSN, 2018) provide a framework for a knowledgeable approach (see sidebar below).

> Let's take the case of Kristen, a five-year veteran of a community hospital medical-surgical unit. She is newly married and has weathered the COVID-19 pandemic, contracting the virus herself, and is now fully recovered. Kristen works the night shift, 1800 to 0600, and has a history of outstanding performance. However, Kristen's supervisor, Jenna, has recently noticed Kristen displays a flat affect and calls off work more frequently. So, Jenna seeks Kristen out to explore and verify her observations.

---

### SAMPLE SECONDARY TRAUMA STRESS (STS) CORE COMPETENCIES

- Knowledge of signs, symptoms, and risk factors
- Capacity to self-assess and monitor personal STS
- Skills to assist employees in emotional re-regulation
- Knowledge of Psychological First Aid (PFA)
- Ability to model and coach employees
- Ability to structure resilience-building

*Reference: National Child Traumatic Stress Network [NCTSN], 2020.*

---

The first core competency of trauma-informed supervision recognizes the signs and symptoms of STS and its impact on nursing staff. Embedded in this competency is also the knowledge of referral resources when the team is assessed to need more than what the nurse supervisor can offer (NCTSN, 2018).

> During their conversation, Kristen mentions that she's "okay, but struggling a bit." Jenna gently presses further and learns that Kristen reports

feeling a lack of empathy toward the patients at times, which scares her, and intrusive thoughts of patients who passed alone during the COVID-19 pandemic. Kristen says she is feeling tired a lot but recently had a check-up with her nurse practitioner, and she's okay physically. Kristen adds how much the psychological experiences of the pandemic has lingered.

The second core competency is the ability of the nurse supervisor to recognize their own STS and how it may affect behaviors (NCTSN, 2018). Part of being trauma-informed is being able to process emotions and behaviors born from traumatic events, which may result in misinterpretation of behaviors without this lens. For example, avoidance, exaggerated anger, and apathy are examples of trauma-induced behaviors commonly misread by others.

Jenna offers support to Kristen and shares that she may be experiencing STS effects, observing that her symptoms are congruent with STS. Jenna shares that she was also a bedside nurse during the pandemic, had a history of STS, and questioned her spirituality at times. They continue to talk about shared experiences and emotions.

An individual's ability to feel psychological safety is at the heart of trauma-informed care. Aligning with this, the supervisor's ability to listen and encourage nursing staff members to share the emotional labor of caring for patients is the third competency. Examples of supervisor skills include a strengths-based approach, educating about common emotional responses in experiencing others' trauma, and operationalizing therapeutic communication to provide a sense of safety (NCTSN, 2018).

Jenna uses body language and other nonverbal cues to convey psychological safety. She listens nonjudgmentally as Kristen begins to tell her stories of when she cared for patients early in the pandemic, the shortage of personal protective equipment, and her anger at the organization for putting her life at risk. She also conveys how empathizing with patients has been exhausting. She is scared that this ability is being "shut down" inside her.

The supervisor's skills and abilities to offer support and "emotional re-regulation after difficult encounters" is the fourth core competency (NCTSN, 2018, n.d., p. 2). After a particularly stressful or exhausting patient interaction, the nurse's experience of STS may be mitigated by the supervisor's targeted support. The supervisor should consider educating the nurse about the dynamics of self-regulation, assessing the nurse's well-being and internal thoughts they may be having about their performance. Last, the supervisor should support the nurse by reframing their role in the encounter and providing strategies to help the nurse, allowing for the nurse's choice of best-fit strategies (NCTSN, 2018).

> Jenna listens closely, without making assumptions about what Kristen is feeling and processing. Jenna purposely educates Kristen about strategies she can use to reframe her interactions with patients. Jenna begins by disclosing how she still witnesses Kristen's compassion, evidenced by the positive patient and peer responses she has directly observed and received. Jenna offers Kristen alternatives to the critical voice that reinforces Kristen's feelings of inadequacy by reframing Kristen's actual performance. Jenna offers Kristen several options moving forward, allowing Kristen to commit to consuming fewer social media sites and news during her time off. She also selects resources from various national nursing and healthcare organizations, such as meditation apps, to help her be more mindful.

The fifth core competency for supervisors surrounds knowledge of approaches such as Psychological First Aid (PFA) to support individuals in the aftermath of disasters, emergencies, and crisis events (Brymer et al., 2006). Specific to supervisors, nurses should be contacted to offer compassionate help without assumptions of what the nurse is experiencing. Acting as a role model, the supervisor should present calmly and ensure their own emotional regulation (NCTSN, 2018).

> Kristen continues to share how she has been struggling since the pandemic and wonders at times what's wrong with her and why she just can't forget about it all. Jenna reflects on what is being shared and views it as sacred; she conveys that Kristen lost the normalcy of nursing care during the pandemic. Kristen practiced during a natural disaster when staff, supplies, and other resources were scarce, even rationed. She encourages Kristen to allow herself to grieve.

The sixth competency for supervisor trauma-informed care enlarges the lens from individual to service delivery. This competency helps infuse the organization into becoming trauma-informed. For example, nurses are instructed to deliver care with the knowledge that patients' behaviors may be influenced by their past traumas. Reconceptualizing the questions posed encourages nurses to think about what happened to the patient versus what is wrong with the patient (NCTSN, 2018). In this way, viewing the patient as an object, a room number, or a diagnosis is discouraged.

> Jenna understands that many of her staff were nurses during the pandemic. Those who were not still take care of patients in times of crisis, making them vulnerable to STS. She plans to enlist the hospital's director of education/onboarding, the clinical nurse specialist, and employee assistance staff to design online modules related to trauma-informed care for both patients and nursing staff.

Next, the supervisor should take a resiliency-building, strengths-based approach as one strategy to promote nurse resiliency. Compassion with the self, teams, and patients and avoiding isolation through team support promote nurses' recovery from traumatic stress and events (NCTSN, 2018). The eighth core competency requires observation and is related to the supervisor's ability to differentiate between expected attitudes and behaviors and those related to STS. Being attuned to staffs' attitudes and typical stress reactions versus those that reflect a distorted worldview is critical (NCTSN, 2018).

Jenna listens for Kristen's descriptions of her nursing care and nursing outcomes. At one point, Kristen states, "It seems every case ends badly." Then, she corrects herself and adds, "No, that's not true, but at times it feels that way." Jenna affirms that such a perception is natural to think periodically but reinforces that some cases have positive outcomes. Jenna then assesses Kristen's peer support, and Kristen reports that she would be lost without her "nursing peeps."

The final, ninth, core competency is about the supervisor's honesty, transparency, and vulnerability in self-disclosures of personal STS. Although characterized by the supervisor's sharing, this competency is for the benefit of the nurse who is supervised (NCTSN, 2018). Such disclosures should align with the American Nurses Association's (ANA, 2015) ethical standards. In Provision 2.4, professional boundaries are outlined (ANA, 2015). In this context, nurses are advised to maintain professional boundaries; however, in Provision 1.5: relationships with colleagues and others (ANA, 2015), nurse leaders' therapeutic use of self to support nurses experiencing STS is reflected in creating an environment of respect and dignity.

As mentioned, Jenna disclosed her own struggle with STS; however, when further questioned by Kristen, Jenna also shares that she is part of a support group facilitated by a mental health professional to work through her own experiences during the pandemic. By doing so, Jenna indirectly minimizes stigma related to mental health assistance and working through past trauma. Jenna maintains confidentiality by not disclosing other nurses in the group. The dialogue between Jenna and Kristen ends, but Jenna follows up with Kristen to ensure she is processing and recovering from past and present STS.

# A HEALING ORGANIZATION

A trauma-informed organization is also a healing organization. *Healing* is defined as actions that enable relationships to restore an employee's interpersonal connections (Powley, 2012, 2013). Healing moves the organization from a disabled state to a place of renewed energy (Powley, 2012). Organizational healing requires attention to employees' well-being, as employees are also transformed by being healed. Employees' well-being can be measured by factors such as mental and physical health, psychological functioning, and demonstrated behaviors (Gallego-Toledo, 2015).

A healing organization is one that values and sustains the attitudes and behaviors that facilitate recovery, repair, and wholeness (Marquitz et al., 2016). A healing culture values behaviors that enhance healing. Trust, communication, compassion, service, and a commitment to active learning are the core components of organizational change needed to create a healing culture (Ananth, 2009, p. 59). Healing is not resilience, hardiness, or adaptation. The actions and interactions of the people in the organization should become compassionate, caring, and supportive.

# BECOMING WHOLE

Caring Science is a lens by which to reframe and revitalize an organization. The use of caring consciousness and action serves as a foundation for transforming and healing an organization that has been traumatized (Messina, 2019). Becoming whole requires a leader that embeds patterns of compassion, caring, mutual support, courage, and faith. Employees need supportive actions to heal the organization's social fabric, sense of continuity, expectations, culture, and identity. The leader will need to utilize language that signals an end of former processes and practices. Language creates our experience of reality, and how we choose to name things influences how we experience them and how we value them. The language of business and commerce has resulted in many traumatized organizations. The language of caring, helping, healing, and a relational language of being is needed for healing to take place (Quinn, 2002). Leaders must bring about regrowth of group well-being, translating into their willingness to engage with the organization (Powley & Cameron, 2006).

# PRAXIS OF EMBRACING

Some actions can build a healing organization. Approaching the organization from a paradigm that embraces the whole person in relation to the environment where the transference of energy occurs (work) will bring about healing. As described by Jean Watson (2008), the Caritas Process will be discussed as a praxis of embracing the organization for healing.

**Embrace** a model of kindness and compassion in interactions with individuals within and outside the organization. Leaders who use honesty and kindness can help members see what is going on and regain the traction needed for an organization to progress forward. Displaying equanimity under challenging situations will help bring about a sense of stability that a traumatized organization needs. Leaders will need to demonstrate their humanity by being present, physically and emotionally. For an organization to heal, a leader should demonstrate through action and language that they care about what happens to them and will do whatever they can to help them in a time of need.

**Inspire** faith and hope in the mission of the organization. The leader must offer optimism, confidence, and energy to help employees reconnect with the mission. This will require setting priorities to move the organization forward and to bring about a regrowth in potential. Employees should hold reflection sessions to set a path to promote intentional human connection (Halldorsdottir, 1991). The more authentic a leader can be in guiding the other, the more likely healing will occur.

**Trust** must be cultivated. A wounded organization will be hesitant to trust. Employees will be guarded, unsure of what feelings and information to share. Leaders will need to be fully present as trustworthy. Institute structures and facilitate processes that set expectations for ethical and direct communication (Durant et al.,

2015). Listening and reflecting before actions will build trust through a stance of compassion. The compassion that results from the awareness of others' emotions, listening, reflection, and voicing are central to facilitating a transition toward healing (Lawrence, 2015). Being fully present at the moment with unconditional compassion and acceptance of others' potentially painful experiences from organizational trauma becomes a catalytic healing instrument to individuals' change transformation (De Klerk, 2019).

**Nurture** a nonjudgmental attitude within yourself as a leader. The process of caring for another promotes direct, constructive, and respectful communication. As a leader, meet the employees where they are along the trajectory to healing. This means engaging in proactive problem-solving, reframing a situation to see the potential or positive side. Many situations can be opportunities if perceived in an approach that does not feed pessimism. For example, one can show respect for things that have meaning to others, such as rituals, service delivery practices, learning, and desires. A leader must promote, support, and enhance an environment that fosters healthy growth. Examining an employee's strengths and helping to ensure that the person is in the proper position to grow and positively impact the organization is a skill that requires authentic communication.

**Forgive** the past. This will require allowing individuals the opportunity to share their stories, reflect on their feelings and experiences. Bring a forward-vision approach instead of one that is always looking back. Employees will need to have a leader authentically listen. *Forgiveness* is the release of anger and resentment (Vanzant, 2013). Releasing the negative energy that has trapped an individual will enhance optimism and empower the person to move forward. Forgiveness can improve anxiety and depression. The inability to forgive will result in toxicity within the person and impact the environment in which they find themselves. Forgiveness encourages compassion (Kanov et al., 2004).

**Deepen** ways of knowing/being/doing/becoming and committing to creatively problem solve. The leader must create a healing environment by a positive outward affect such as smiling and displaying positive gestures. Celebrate victories regardless of size, and give positive reinforcement (Kirkpatrick, 2006). Reinforcing productive communication and interpersonal exchanges can bring about organizational change (Smollan, 2014). Employees will see the approach of rewarding the norm. Develop new rituals that bring a positive feeling. Create greater autonomy of work for all employees, including clinicians, reduce excessive bureaucracy, recognize and celebrate employees, and respect employees for their engagement and contributions (Ananth, 2009, p. 59).

**Balance** is equalizing and knowing when to step in and step back. Caring leadership is about what leaders can grasp and sense from the other. Leaders bring balance to an organization through learning and knowing whether and how to remove authority from or grant power to others, and bearing responsibility for what emerges through empathic and tacit modes of knowing (Watson & Disser, 2005). Leaders need strategies to balance decisiveness vs. flexibility, certainty vs. ambiguity, and control vs. complexity (Watson & Disser, 2005). An organization needs to provide its employees with a clear and vital vision. Using creativity to uncover the imagination of employees as you move toward a rebirth of the traumatized organization will bring about a readiness to learn (Zell, 2003).

**Co-create** a healing environment by engaging employees with dignity and respect. Employees need a supportive and protective environment. Leaders must look for ways to reduce stress. Bring nature and natural light into space. The physical environment impacts moods, spirit, and energy. Healing environments should be beautiful and stimulate positive awareness, encourage relaxation, and balance constancy and flexibility. The density of individuals in space can impact individuals' psychological health, such as anxiety and depression (Schaller, 2012). Leaders need to change the environment to be a healing space, which may require leaders to renovate a place. Employees will feel valued regardless of the scale of a change, including painting walls or placing new light fixtures.

**Minister** to the body-mind-spirit of the employee (Watson, 2018). The leader must have continual attention to the emotional life of the organization and its members. Coaching employees requires communication skills that provide feedback for growth and reassurance. For example, leaders help employees navigate during difficult times and support decision-making processes aligning with organizations' values. It is crucial for leaders to know individual employees and find out what is important to them. When employees feel cared for, they are rejuvenated. Building strength, resolve, and courage for daily life will help employees thrive in their work environment. For example, sacred spaces in some units are quiet spaces to recharge or a place for teams that respond compassionately when a death occurs in an employee's life.

**Openness** to different (infinite) possibilities is a characteristic of a leader suitable for a traumatized organization. The leader is suggestive, enabling, and facilitating in a complex environment. Operating in the realm of multiplicity, a leader can bring about healing by creating a community of support, accountability, and inspiration (Swengros et al., 2014). Being open allows you to challenge ideas about how things should work. If you quickly decide how things should be, you limit your ability to consider other approaches. Leaders should not judge other people, as you could be closing off unique possibilities. Being intellectually curious, creative, and imaginative means that you have the openness needed to work with a traumatized organization for healing emergence.

While the Caritas Process can inform leaders in healing an organization, many strategies are needed to heal an organization. For example, one must treat employees with respect, adopt greater flexibility to collaborate with employees, appreciate good work, embrace diversity, teach instead of reproach, and create a culture of relationships to enhance performance (Cameron, 2003).

# TRANSFORMING ORGANIZATIONS

Organizational transformation is needed to help organizations sustain healing when they are faced with trauma. Such a transformation creates a new culture, a unified mission to be a trauma-informed organization. This transformation is multifaceted and reflects staff education and training, assessment, and revision of policies and procedures. It is a systematic approach to creating a new organization with a focus on internal and external practices and ensuring those who make up the organization are trauma aware.

Trauma-informed care training and education are a wellness framework that improves employee satisfaction and engagement while reducing burnout and turnover. In addition, conducting an organizational assessment can help the leader understand how well individuals function in their work. The Substance Abuse and Mental Health Services Administration (SAMHSA) National Center for Trauma Informed Care has developed a self-assessment tool. This tool can provide the leader with information to share with employees to co-create a trauma-informed organization.

Embracing a trauma-informed system aims to reduce the negative consequences of trauma (Hodas, 2006) by integrating trauma-informed values into policies, procedures, and practices (SAMHSA, 2015; Woll, 2013). Employees will need to reengage and be open to receiving training about trauma-informed practices for system change. The training provides information about the prevalence and effects and the tenets of trauma-informed practice to increase staff knowledge, improve attitudes, and change behavior. Reviewing the SAMHSA (2014a) Treatment Improvement Protocol for Trauma-Informed Care can provide the leader and employees with an approach for moving an organization forward. The protocol provides 16 non-training components that can be integrated into trauma-informed organizational interventions.

SAMHSA (2014a) also provides a framework for organizations and systems to address trauma. Organizational leaders should role model these practices, purposefully educating themselves to be competent as trauma-informed leaders through the four "Rs." The first "R" is the **realization** of trauma's impact on individuals, groups, communities, and organizations. An awareness of how trauma is threaded into the world of healthcare means that the culture changes. The realization of trauma changes into **recognition** of trauma by changing how assessments are conducted, interventions are carried out, and patients and staff are approached. Sensitive racial, ethnic, cultural, gender, and age approaches guide how recognition translates into practices. The third "R" is the systemic organizational **response**, transforming the organization's culture to be trauma sensitive. Organizational missions are revised, and a new discourse reflects this awakening. Each member of an organization is called to become trauma-aware and informed. Last, the organization's policies and procedures are structured to **resist retraumatization** for staff and clients (SAMHSA, 2014a). It is an organization's goal to bring healing rather than a toxic environment to its employees and clients and avoid retraumatization.

The implementation of informed organizational response and collective energies to avoid retraumatization require cultural and systematic change. Changing organizations and moving its people toward healing and committing to the principles of trauma-informed care isn't easy—but the rewards are great. Leaders need to be passionate about nurse well-being and build sustainable resilience. The Sanctuary Model is an approach to enact institutional change toward transforming organizations to be trauma-informed (Bloom, 2000; Bloom & Sreedhar, 2008).

The Sanctuary Model is founded in trauma theory, constructivist self-development theory, burnout theory, and systems theory (Esaki et al., 2013). Thus, this approach situates the individuals and the organizations that have experienced traumatic events, as characterized by mutual interactions (Esaki et al., 2013). Labeled as an *organizational intervention*, the Sanctuary Model calls for shared values, which rely on leadership to model these values, use emotional intelligence, ensure "social immunity" to violence, and employ open communication (Bloom, 2017, p. 6; Esaki et al., 2013). Recalling how important feeling physically and psychologically safe is to processing and healing from trauma, the Sanctuary Model uses the acronym "SELF" to structure a common language within organizations: Safety, Emotions, Loss, and Future (Bloom, 2000, 2017). Identifying which of these concepts is present in a problem faced by the organization can forward solutions to addressing the difficulty (Bloom & Sreedhar, 2008).

Assessment of safety is structured in four dimensions: physical, psychological, so-cial, and moral safety (Bloom, 2017). Nurse leaders are called upon to overtly ask nurses how safe they feel. Aspects of workplace violence (both internal and exter-nal) and moral distress are folded into these dimensions. Debriefing after adverse events, conducting root cause analysis of the event, and acknowledging the poten-tial trauma experienced are ways of increasing safety. Emotions and the regulation of emotions is also a component of SELF (Bloom, 2017). When faced with crisis and disagreement, nurses and patients express their emotional feelings. Being able to respect and manage these emotions is a goal of those within the organization. Setting expectations of how to process and express emotions can be a successful strategy for nurse leaders (Bloom, 2017).

Loss is also a part of SELF (Bloom, 2017) and is inherent in psychological trauma. Recognizing loss, processing what is no longer present, and honoring what is gone are woven into healing (Bloom, 2017). Again, both individual- and system-level losses are to be recognized. Last, looking to the future can be helpful when ad-dressing a problem of an impending loss, lack of safety, and potential dysregulat-ed emotions (Bloom & Sreedhar, 2008, 2017). Nurse leaders envision a positive future where individuals and the organization share common trauma-informed values and address current and future problems.

In sum, trauma-informed transformation toward care competence is vital for a healthy organization. Community Connections (http://www.communityconnec-tionsdc.org), a private, not-for-profit mental health and substance abuse agency, managed to help change the culture of an entire agency through a trauma-in-formed approach. In a trauma-informed approach, the emphasis is on understand-ing the whole individual and appreciating the context in which they live their lives. Another resource for managers or leaders to use is Partner for Healing (http://part-nerforhealing.org), which has exercises that can be conducted at staff meetings.

# ORGANIZATIONAL POST-TRAUMATIC GROWTH

As trauma-informed practices become cultural norms, organizational post-traumatic growth becomes possible. In a parallel manner to individuals who achieve transcendence and post-traumatic growth, a new organization emerges with collective awareness and insights. A trauma-transformed organization may occur through an Appreciative Inquiry (AI) approach and the four cornerstone ideas behind AI: Discovery, Dream, Design, and Destiny (Cooperrider & Whitney, 1999; Fry et al., 2002; Grieten et al., 2018; see Figure 7.1). *Appreciative Inquiry* is a strengths-based method of organizational change that has been used as a framework in healthcare organizations (Hung et al., 2018). In the context of this discussion, it is a conduit for organizational growth due to what has been gained by operationalizing trauma-informed organizational strategies. Assuming that trauma-informed practices are infused within the organization, especially within individual staff members, it's time for leaders to move the organization to a new level of functioning where psychological safety is a given; voices are heard; and trust, forgiveness, and compassion are cultural norms. In essence, nurse leaders need to move the nursing staff toward new possibilities of existing in the present and envisioning a new future. Of note: Trauma-informed practices are the catalysts for this positive growth and the freedom to explore possibilities.

As an organization is newly transformed, nurse leaders take on the process of **Discovery** (Cooperrider & Whitney, 1999; Fry et al., 2002). In Discovery, nurses are encouraged to identify what works well in the present, including trauma-informed practices. Leaders inquire about what excites nursing staff, what changes have been effective, what keeps them working at the organization. This record of Discovery is critical; nurse leaders want to retain what has a positive impact and sustain the efforts of achieving a trauma-informed organization. Employees resist change when they fear losing something that is valuable to them.

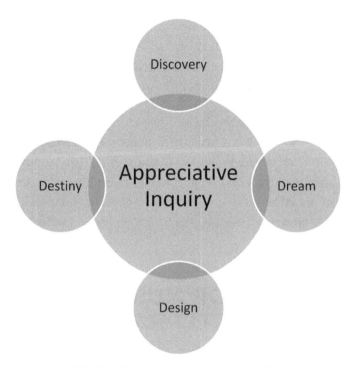

**FIGURE 7.1** Appreciative Inquiry (AI).

As narratives of Discovery are compiled, patterns emerge, which forms a foundation for future-oriented thinking. Nurses are called upon to **Dream** (Cooperrider & Whitney, 1999; Fry et al., 2002). Nurses are innovators and have the most sophisticated and pragmatic knowledge of healthcare systems' weaknesses and strengths. While "workarounds" are notoriously invented and used by bedside nurses, these point-of-service providers are rich sources of information. Leaders need to not only allow but encourage nurses to Dream of what could be now that trauma is mitigated in their organizations. Toxic energy has been channeled into an inspired focus of what the future could look like.

By dreaming, nurses are then encouraged to **Design** the future through shaping innovation, piloting ideas, and drafting processes (Cooperrider & Whitney, 1999;

Fry et al., 2002). Nurses co-create and operationalize the concepts through **Destiny** (Cooperrider & Whitney, 1999; Fry et al., 2002). Innovations are solidified and tested, and the cycle continues as results are compared to what was uncovered during the Discovery and Dream phases.

Nurse leaders pose purposeful questions to their staff throughout these steps: What is valuable and what must we ensure is retained (Discover)? What is possible, and what should our future look like (Dream)? What can be done and how (Design)? And what initiatives realize our Dreams (Destiny)? (Cooperrider, 2012). The ability for an organization to grow into an innovative, adaptable, co-created entity is stabilized and strengthened by the trauma-informed work nurse leaders have accomplished.

# IMPLICATIONS FOR NURSING: INTEGRATING INTO PRAXIS

The nurse leader's influence in mitigating—and contributing to—organizational trauma should be recognized. The leader needs to consider what traumas affecting nurses are integrated into the nurse's role and which are avoidable (Foli et al., 2020). For example, secondary traumatic stress can be viewed as inherent in the role of the comforting, compassionate, caring nurse. Secondary traumatic stress is then seen as unavoidable. In contrast, to provide safe and quality patient care, the nurse needs sufficient staffing levels, supplies, access to interdisciplinary team members, and other resources. The adequate level of resources and staffing is under the control of organizational and nursing leadership (ANA, 2020). Therefore, insufficient resource trauma is avoidable, given a vigilant leader who can successfully advocate for the nursing professionals in the organization and ensure nurses have the resources they need (Foli et al., 2020).

Whether the organization is a school of nursing or a healthcare organization, the ability to understand the risks associated with a traumatized organization and strategies for healing are imperative. Recently, the importance of well-being for nursing students has received increased visibility due to the recent resolution by the American Association of Colleges of Nursing (AACN, 2020) to enhance resilience among nursing students and faculty. The American College Health Association reports that 45% of college students stated they felt so depressed it was difficult to function, 66% reported overwhelming anxiety, and 13.3% seriously considered suicide in the last 12 months (AACN, 2020).

According to the ANA (2019), 70% of nurses report putting the health, safety, and wellness of their patients before their own. Stress in the workplace impacts patient outcomes. This stress comes about due to the nurse staffing crisis. Typically nursing represents 40% of operating costs, and decreased staffing levels can increase the overall bottom line of an organization. However, research has shown that appropriate staffing levels reduce errors, mortality rates, and length of patient stays (ANA, 2020). Creating a healthy workplace culture is a critical principle identified by the ANA.

Whether you are considering an individual nurse or an organization made up of nurses, taking the healthy nurse, healthy nation challenge should be one of the first commitments to improving oneself and the organization. The ANA has a toolkit designed to provide organizations with exemplars of practices to enhance wellness (2021). For example, every organization should have a wellness committee to develop interventions that best fit the organization. Financial resources should be committed to ensuring that employees have avenues to relieve stress and enhance well-being. The Virginia Nurses Association has the "Take Five Challenge." Nurses commit to taking five minutes a day for 21 days to improve their health by focusing on physical activity, nutrition, rest, quality of life, or safety. Adding sleep to this list has been suggested by other organizations as a way to improve health (Virginia Nurses Association, 2021).

# SUMMARY

Organizational compassion positively affects employee satisfaction, retention, and productivity, and employees will reward companies that treat them humanely. Typically, it has been found that units with the highest employee satisfaction scores tend to have the highest patient satisfaction, best clinical outcomes, and successfully comply with their budgets (Ananth, 2009). As individuals step up to be a leader in an organization, especially in traumatized organizations that require healing, they should consider the use of Jean Watson's theory as a framework.

Leaders should ask themselves if they place people first and show concern for others. They must design opportunities for employees to build trusting relationships (Bragg, 2001) and strategies for creating healthy work environments. Caring is the foundation for healing organizations.

Within a trauma-informed context, the nurse leader's goals include advocating for nurses experiencing STS, and policies and practices that transform an organization toward a healing institution. Cultural shifts in system-wide practices should be designed to understand what happened to people and the organization versus blaming people or events that occurred. Ultimately, organizational post-traumatic growth allows for new possibilities for both nurses and patients as the environment becomes safe, adaptable, innovative, and nurturing.

# REFLECTIVE QUESTIONS

1. Consider an experience that made you feel traumatized at your workplace. What was the situation? What happened to you? How would you describe (a) the *event*, (b) the *experience*, (c) the *effects* of the workplace trauma?

2. Could you describe the strategies that leaders can use to help you heal from that trauma?

3. How do you as a nurse leader impact the organization and help it heal and remain a healing organization?

4. What are your suggestions for organizational leadership teams to promote a caring-healing environment?

5. Describe ways to enhance organizational post-traumatic growth.

---

# NARRATIVE

Jameson Hospital is a 530-bed acute care hospital. The critical care unit has 12 beds and is typically 90% occupied. Typically, there are six nurses on each shift. On a Thursday night, the unit had 12 patients and one of the night shift nurses had called in, leaving five nurses on duty to work 7pm to 7am. During the shift, Nancy grabbed some medication and cross checked it with Sarah. Nancy went into room 12 and administered the medication; within minutes the patient went into V-fib. A code was called and during the middle of resuscitation, Nancy realized she had pulled the wrong dosage of the medication resulting in the patient arresting. Nancy immediately told the physician running the code hoping that the information would help save the patient. The patient died. The family was informed of the death. However, no one informed the family of the cause of the death. The organization reported both Nancy and Sarah to the Board of Nursing, resulting in Nancy losing her license and Sarah being placed on probation. The nursing staff slowing became aware of what had happened as both nurses were friends with other nurses in the unit and everyone was heartsick over the loss of two critical care nurses, and the short staffing that everyone felt played into the outcome. The hospital administration held a staff meeting telling everyone to not discuss the case. Each week that passed, the nursing staff sunk deeper into depression. The nurse who had called out sick that night ended up resigning after four weeks, unable to take the side glances; it seemed everyone was wondering if she had worked her shift, would this have happened? Even those nurses who worked on the night shift eventually resigned over the course of four months.

---

# RESPONSE TO THE NARRATIVE

1. Describe how organizational trauma evolved in this case.

2. Discuss the cumulative impacts of organizational trauma in this scenario.

3. Describe ways of using caring consciousness and actions to promote organizational caring-healing when trauma occurs.

4. Explain how the Sanctuary Model could be utilized as a viable approach in this case.

# AUTHOR BIOGRAPHIES

**Sonya R. Hardin, PhD, CCRN, NP-C, FAAN,** is Dean and Professor at the University of Louisville. She oversees over 100 FTEs, delivering education to over 1,100 students. Her work history includes hospital and academic management. Hardin has a PhD in nursing from the University of Colorado and master's degrees in business and health administration from Pfeiffer University in North Carolina. She earned master's and bachelor's degrees in nursing from the University of North Carolina at Charlotte. She also completed post-doctoral fellowships at Stanford University and the University of North Carolina at Chapel Hill. She has conducted research in academic-service partnerships, nursing theory, and heart failure.

**Karen J. Foli, PhD, RN, FAAN,** is an Associate Professor at Purdue University School of Nursing whose work is bound together by the lens of psychological trauma. She is an expert in nurse-specific psychological trauma and co-author of the award-winning book, *The Influence of Psychological Trauma in Nursing* (2019, Sigma). Her middle-range theory of nurses' psychological trauma has been applied to emergency nursing as a model toward healing. With this trauma-informed lens, Foli has an active research program surrounding nurses' substance use, with funding from the Substance Abuse and Mental Health Services Administration (SAMHSA), and the National Council of State Boards of Nursing: Center for Regulatory Excellence, among others. Foli is a Fellow in the American Academy of Nursing. She was inducted into the Purdue University Book of Great Teachers in 2018. She also received the Sigma Theta Tau Honorary Society of Nursing, Delta Omicron Chapter Award for Outstanding Mentoring in 2017.

# REFERENCES

American Association Colleges of Nursing. (2020). *Resolution: A call to action for academic nurse leaders to promote practices to enhance optimal wellbeing, resilience, and suicide prevention in US schools of nursing.* https://www.aacnnursing.org/Portals/42/Downloads/Meetings/2020/ANLC/7-2020-Resolution-For-AACN-Nurse-Wellness-Suicide-Prevention.pdf

American Nurses Association. (2015). *Code of ethics for nurses with interpretive statements.* Author. https://www.nursingworld.org/practice-policy/nursing-excellence/ethics/code-of-ethics-for-nurses/coe-view-only/

American Nurses Association. (2019). Healthy nurse healthy nation: Year two highlights 2018-2019. *American Nurse Today.* https://www.nursingworld.org/~4a6d20/globalassets/docs/ana/practice/hnhn18-19highlights.pdf

American Nurses Association. (2020). *ANA's principles for nursing staffing* (3rd ed.). Author.

American Nurses Association Enterprise. (2021). *Well-being initiative.* https://www.nursingworld.org/practice-policy/work-environment/health-safety/disaster-preparedness/coronavirus/what-you-need-to-know/the-well-being-initiative

Ananth, S. (2009) Creating healing organization. *Explore, 5*(1), 59–60.

Arnold, T. C. (2020). An evolutionary concept analysis of secondary traumatic stress in nurses. *Nursing Forum, 55,* 149–156.

Berquist, R., St-Pierre, I., & Holmes, D. (2017). Uncaring nurses: An exploration of faculty-to-faculty violence in nursing academia. *International Journal for Human Caring, 21*(3), 112–119.

Bloom, S. L. (2000). Creating sanctuary: Healing from systematic abuses of power. Therapeutic communities. *The International Journal for Therapeutic and Supportive Organizations, 21*(2), 67–91.

Bloom, S. L. (2017). Some guidelines for surfing the edge of chaos, while riding dangerously close to the black hole of trauma. *Psychotherapy and Politics International.* doi: 10.1002/ppi.1409

Bloom, S. L., & Sreedhar, S. Y. (2008). The Sanctuary Model® of trauma-informed organizational change. *Reclaiming Children and Youth, 17*(3), 48–53.

Bragg, T. (2001). Healing betrayal: Work relationships. *Industrial Management, 43*(3), 29–31.

Brymer, M., Jacobs, A., Layne, C., Pynoos, R., Ruzek, J., Steinberg, A., Vernberg, E., & Watson, P. (National Child Traumatic Stress Network and National Center for PTSD). (2006). *Psychological first aid: Field operations guide* (2nd ed.). https://www.nctsn.org/sites/default/files/resources//pfa_field_operations_guide.pdf

Cameron, K. (2003). Organizational virtuousness and performance. In K. S. Cameron, J. E. Dutton, & R. E. Quinn, *Positive organizational scholarship* (pp. 48–65). Berrett-Koehler.

Cooperrider, D. L. (2012). The concentration effect of strengths. *Organizational Dynamics, 41*, 106–117.

Cooperrider, D. L., & Whitney, D. (1999). *Appreciative inquiry.* Berrett-Koehler.

De Klerk, J. J. (2019). Leading transitions in traumatically experienced change-a question of doing or being? *Journal of Organizational Change Management, 32*(3), 340–355.

Durant, A. F., McDermott, S., Kinney, G., & Triner, T. (2015). Caring Science: Transforming the ethic of caring-healing practice, environment, and culture within an integrated care delivery system. *The Permanente Journal, 19*(4), e136–e142.

Esaki, N., Benamati, J., Yanosy, S., Middleton, J. S., Hopson, L. M., Hummer, V. L., & Bloom, S. L. (2018). The Sanctuary Model: Theoretical framework. *Families in Society: The Journal of Contemporary Social Sciences, 94*(2). doi: 10.1606/1044-3894.4287

Foli, K. J., Reddick, B., Zhang, L., & Krcelich, K. (2020). Nurses' psychological trauma: "They leave me lying awake at night." *Archives of Psychiatric Nursing, 34*(3), 86–95. http://doi.org/10.1016/j.apnu.2020.04.011

Fry, R., Barrett, F., Seiling, J., & Whitney, D. (2002). *Appreciative inquiry and organizational transformation: Reports from the field.* Quorum Books.

Gallego-Toledo, J. M. (2015). *The relationship between perceived frequency of change and the wellbeing of telecom professionals* [Doctoral dissertation]. The University of the Rockies.

Grieten, S., Lambrechts, F., Bouwen, R., Huybrechts, J., Fry, R., & Cooperrider, D. (2018). Inquiring into Appreciative Inquiry: A conversation with David Cooperrider and Ronald Fry. *Journal of Management Inquiry, 27*(1), 101–114. doi: 10.1177/1056492616688087

Griffith, D. M., Mason, M., Yonas, M., Eng, E., Jefferies, V., Plihcik, S. & Parks, B. (2007). Dismantling institutional racism: Theory and action. *Am J Community Psychology, 39*, 381–392.

Halldorsdottir, S. (1991). Five basic modes of being with another. In D. A. Gaut and M. M. Leininger (Eds.), *Caring: The compassionate healer* (pp. 37–49). National League for Nursing.

Hodas, G. R. (2006). *Responding to childhood trauma: The promise and practice of trauma informed care.* http://www.childrescuebill.org/VictimsOfAbuse/RespondingHodas.pdf

Hung, L., Phinney, A., Chaudhury, H., Rodney, P., Tabamo, J., & Bohl, D. (2018). Appreciative inquiry: Bridging research and practice in a hospital setting. *International Journal of Qualitative Research Methods, 17*, 1–10. doi: 10.1177/1609406918769444

Kanov, J. M., Maitlis, S., Worline, M. C., Dutton, J. E., Frost, P. J., & Lilius, J. M. (2004). Compassion in organizational life. *The American Behavioral Scientist, 47*(6), 808–827. https://doi.org/10.1177/0002764203260211

Kirkpatrick, M. K. (2006). Social action for a healing/caring healthcare system through the arts. *International Journal for Human Caring, 10*(2), 42.

Lawrence, P. (2015). Leading change – insights into how leaders actually approach the challenge of Complexity. *Journal of Change Management, 15*(3), 231–252.

Marquitz, M., Badding, S. & Chermack, T. J. (2016). The effects of scenario planning on perceptions of grief in organisational change. *International Journal of Technology Intelligence and Planning, 11*(1), 1–19.

Messina, M. J. (2019). *Failed dependency: Leadership strategies to prevent, mitigate and heal organizational trauma in behavioral health systems* [Doctoral dissertation]. Ashford University.

National Child Traumatic Stress Network. (2018), *Using the secondary traumatic stress core competencies in trauma-informed supervision.* https://www.nctsn.org/sites/default/files/resources/fact_sheet/using_the_secondary_traumatic_stress_core_competencies_in_trauma-informed_supervision.pdf

National Child Traumatic Stress Network. (2020). *Trauma-informed organizational assessment (TIOA) information packet.* https://www.nctsn.org/sites/default/files/resources/special-resource/trauma_informed_organizational_assessment_information_packet.pdf

Norman, V., Rossillo, K., & Skelton, K. (2016). Creating healing environments through the theory of caring: The official voice of perioperative nursing the official voice of perioperative nursing. *AORN Journal, 104*(5), 401–409.

Powley, E. H. (2012). Organizational healing: A relational process to handle major disruption. In G. M. Spreitzer & K. S. Cameron (Eds.), *The Oxford handbook of positive organizational scholarship* (pp. 855–866). Oxford University Press.

Powley, E. H. (2013). The process and mechanisms of organizational healing. *The Journal of Applied Behavioral Science, 49*(1), 42–68.

Powley, E. H., & Cameron, K. S. (2006). Organizational healing: Lived virtuousness amidst organizational crisis, *Journal of Management, Spirituality & Religion, 3*(1–2), 13–33.

Quinn, J. F. (2002). Revisioning the nursing shortage: A call to caring for healing the healthcare system. *Frontiers of Health Services Management, 19*(2), 3–21. https://search.proquest.com/docview/203892978?accountid=10639

Schaller, B. (2012). *Architectural healing environments.* Architecture Senior Theses, Paper 62. http://surface.syr.edu/architecture_theses/62

Smollan, R.K. (2014). Control and the emotional rollercoaster of organizational change. *International Journal of Organizational Analysis, 22*(3), 399–419.

Substance Abuse and Mental Health Services Administration. (2014a). *Treatment improvement protocol for trauma-informed care.* TIP 57. https://store.samhsa.gov/shin/content/SMA14-4816/SMA14-4816.pdf

Substance Abuse and Mental Health Services Administration. (2014b). *SAMHSA's concept of trauma and guidance for a trauma-informed approach.* HHS Publication No. (SMA) 14-4884. https://ncsacw.samhsa.gov/userfiles/files/SAMHSA_Trauma.pdf

Substance Abuse and Mental Health Services Administration. (2015). *Trauma-informed approach and trauma-specific interventions.* http://www.samhsa.gov/nctic/trauma-interventions

Swengros, D., Herbst, A. M., Friesen, M. A., Mangione, L. & Anderson, J. G. (2014). Promoting caring-healing relationships: Bringing healing touch to the bedside in a multihospital health system. *Holistic Nursing Practice, 28*, 370–375.

Tafoya, D. W. (2018). Trauma in organizations: Triggering organizational trauma and the trauma model. In *Managing organizational crisis and brand trauma* (pp. 39–70). Palgrave Macmillan, Cham.

Vanzant, I. (2013). *Forgiveness: 21 days to forgive everyone for everything* (1st ed.).Smiley Books.

Virginia Nurses Association. (2021). *Champion spotlight.* https://engage.healthynursehealthynation.org/blogs/24/1556

Vivian, P., & Hormann, S. (2013). *Organizational trauma and healing*. CreateSpace.

Watson, J. (2008). *Nursing: The philosophy and science of caring* (rev. ed.). University Press of Colorado.

Watson, J. (2018). *Unitary Caring Science*. University Press of Colorado.

Watson, J., & Disser, A. (2005). Continuing the dialogue: Promoting harmony in caring-healing environments by balancing economic costs, management, and technological system demands with informed, leadership actions to assure professional practices of compassionate human caring. *International Journal for Human Caring, 9*(2), 128.

Woll, P. (2013). *Safety, strength, resilience, and recovery: Trauma-informed systems and communities*. Department of Behavioral Health and Intellectual Disability Services.

Zell, D. (2003). Organizational change as a process of death, dying and rebirth. *The Journal of Applied Behavioral Science, 39*(1), 73–96.

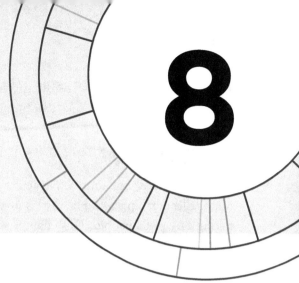

# HEALTHCARE LEADERSHIP IN PLANETARY AND ENVIRONMENTAL HEALTH

Barbara Sattler, DrPH, RN, FAAN

---

## LEARNING OBJECTIVES

After completing this chapter, the learner will be able to:

- Appreciate the integral connection between a healthy planet and healthy people

- Describe key attributes and gifts that nature provides for creating healthier and more grounded leaders

- Explore how nurse leaders can move beyond institutional walls to address social determinants of health and healing

- Catalyze conversations and actions for nursing leadership to create and lead from a more expansive vision for health

---

# OVERVIEW

If the adage that we cannot have healthy people on a sick planet is true, then our nursing leadership should be just as invested in taking care of the earth as it is in taking care of its people. This chapter will explore what it might mean to take care of the earth and how our investment in the earth and all of her creatures will help us heal the planet and heal ourselves.

# CARING FOR MOTHER EARTH AS AN EXTENSION OF OURSELVES

What if we asked the trees to help guide our leadership? What might we discover about the world and ourselves if we seek counsel from new sources of wisdom? Mother Nature can teach us different things depending on our goals. And sometimes, she can suggest new goals.

In our haste to find solutions, we sometimes don't take the time to really investigate the problems. Sitting with our problems in nature can create opportunities for our imagination to be unleashed in a way that sitting in a conference room and brainstorming with others cannot. One exercise is not intended to replace the other, but both can create insights into better defining our problems and their solutions.

Simard (2021) spent years in nature as a forest scientist resulting in remarkable discoveries about how trees in the forest are interdependent, communicative, and generous. Her book, *Finding the Mother Tree: Discovering the Wisdom of the Forest*, describes her personal journey and her scientific inquiries. Trees, she notes, are networked by underground mycelium, fungal threads that occasionally poke their heads up in the form of mushrooms. Mycelia create a network that helps trees communicate with each other about their needs and then allows them to respond to each other's needs by sending healing gifts in the form of water, carbon, nutrients, alarm signals, and hormones. Within forest networks, trees don't just communicate with their own species but rather communicate with diverse populations of trees. Perhaps the trees have healing gifts for us, as well.

Mertins (n.d.), who engages in "nature mentoring," has compiled a list of the attributes and gifts that nature provides when we spend time in her presence (see Table 8.1). This practice of sitting in nature and nature's associated gifts can make us better, healthier, and more grounded leaders.

## TABLE 8.1  Nature's Gifts

| | |
|---|---|
| Naturalist Intelligence | Being able to see patterns and develop empathy for all living beings. |
| Presence and Awareness | Opening a quiet space in which to both leave our worrying and painful thoughts behind and focus on the beauty and healing presence of the natural world. |
| Using Your Senses | Being in nature allows us to increase our sensory awareness—our sight, hearing, feeling, and observational skills. |
| Unstoppable Focus | Our focus is increased by quieting our minds and then being captivated by a cloud, tree, and bird's song. |
| Stillness and Meditation | This gift of stillness creates the conditions for a natural state of meditation. Our breathing slows, our mind quiets. |
| Authenticity | Listening to ourselves without judgment or the interference of the many outside influences and seeing our true path in life. |
| Awe and Wonder | Immersing in nature unveils a world of magic, majesty, and mystery. |
| Gratitude and Appreciation | Nature helps renew our sense of gratitude and allows us to slow down among positive things in life. |

*continues*

**TABLE 8.1**  Nature's Gifts (cont.)

| | |
|---|---|
| Emotional Freedom | Nature teaches us that we do not have to be a slave to our feelings or be entrenched in how we experience or see our situations or challenging problems. We have the choice to be free. |
| Pleasure in Simple Things | Nature is so generous, yet she helps us realize what "things" we really need and what we don't. |
| Relationships and Emotional Intelligence | We learn to be present and interact with people in a deeper and more authentic way. |
| Self-Acceptance and Healing | Nature promotes mental and emotional spaciousness and self-reflection—critical to the healing process. |
| Unconditional Love | Nature allows us to exist without judgment and encourages us to do the same—expanding our capacity to love ourselves and others. |
| Spiritual Connection | Nature instills a feeling of faith in the truth that we are all connected. No one is alone. We are all loved. |

*Based on "Nature Mentoring: What Does Nature Teach Us? 14 Lessons from the Natural World"*
*(Mertins, n.d.)*

Today is a time when we need all of the attributes and gifts that we can receive freely in nature to address the complex problems and existential threats that we face.

Trees recognize and utilize the power of community not just to survive but to flourish. They send out stress hormones to each other in times of scarcity, and other trees respond. The oldest trees, known as "Mother Trees" (or hubs) especially support the vulnerable young trees and share their wisdom with other trees through a wide array of chemical signals.

# WHAT AILS US

Perhaps, if we sit with a tree, she will sense our vulnerability, our stress and share her wisdom and healing. She might ask us, "What ails us?" This simple question would require a thoughtful and complex answer. While we might answer what ails us as an individual, we might also address the question more broadly as nursing leaders.

What does ail us? When we look at the etiologies of our collective ailments, here are some of the things that might come up. Between 30%–55% of our diseases are attributed to the social determinants of health (World Health Organization, n.d.). These determinants include how we educate, house, feed, and care for each other's basic needs. And yet, our healthcare systems do very little to address these needs. Forests give us oxygen, food, shelter, medicines, fuel, and furniture.

There is nothing wasteful in nature—nature runs like an efficient circular economy. Humans are extremely wasteful and increasingly to the detriment of Mother Nature. While we humans manage to waste about 30% of all the food we produce in the US and globally, we still manage to have significant numbers of food insecure populations and even larger numbers of nutrition insecure populations. Nutrition insecurity is another thing that ails us. We know that poor nutrition is a risk factor for cancer, diabetes, cardiovascular diseases, and other chronic diseases (Centers for Disease Control and Prevention, 2021), yet our healthcare systems do virtually nothing about nutrition insecurity. In fact, we don't include a screen for food insecurity, not to mention nutrition insecurity, when we see patients in our hospitals or clinics. We don't ask.

Vivek Murthy, the US Surgeon General during the Obama Administration, observes that we are suffering from an epidemic of loneliness that is ailing us in the US. According to Murthy, the experience of loneliness is more strongly associated with increased mortality than smoking or obesity (2020). Unlike the social support networks that mycelium provides for trees, our internet-based social networks are not really supporting us.

In his book, *Bowling Alone: The Collapse and Revival of American Community*, Putnam (2000) comprehensively explored how we are increasingly disconnected from each other and the damaging effects that this has on our *social capital*—the networks of relationships among people who live and work together which serve to create a common societal purpose. Some of the structures that support these efforts are faith-based organizations, voluntary organizations, local clubs (garden clubs, civic clubs), and so on. But they also include bowling alleys, roller skating rinks, bingo halls, and other places where people gather socially. Putnam provides empirical evidence demonstrating that we now belong to fewer organizations that meet, know little about our neighbors, meet with friends less often, and even get together with our families less often. The simple act of joining and participating in groups is associated with increased longevity.

Forest resources generally flow from the older, stronger trees to the youngest and smallest. When a Mother Tree senses that a younger tree needs additional nutrition, she sends it to the younger tree via the biological lifelines that mycelium networks create. Seedlings cut off from the underground networks are more likely to die than those in the network. In a Cigna study on loneliness (Cigna, 2018), they specifically called attention to the fact that more teens, our social network champions, feel lonelier and more socially isolated than ever before, unrelated to their social media use. Our teens and young adults are experiencing high rates of suicide, depression, and anxiety.

Louv (2005) coined a new diagnosis in his book *Last Child in the Woods: Saving Our Children from Nature-Deficit Disorder*. Louv documents how modern American culture has sanitized children's experience with nature and how children's closely managed and orchestrated time is often denuded of unstructured time in nature. This deficit has meaningful effects on children, robbing them of time in which nature is a teacher of many things—pattern recognition, system awareness, and using multiple senses at once. Pilot studies addressing the benefits of children's wilderness experiences suggest that nature immersion experiences could address the risk of "nature-deficit disorder," improve health, and prepare future environmental leaders (Warber et al. 2015).

The average American child spends 44 hours a week at some kind of electronic screen (Kaiser Family Foundation, 2005). Increased screen time is associated with obesity, violence, and lower intelligence scores. Louv offered recommendations to address nature-deficit disorder, and there was a wholehearted response to Louv's suggestions. The National Wildlife Association developed a program that supports a "Green Hour" in every child's day. The US Forest Service has an initiative called More Kids in the Woods, and there is a new organization called the Children's Nature Network. During COVID-19, experimentation with outdoor education flourished, including those that were part of the *National COVID-19 Outdoor Learning Initiative*, a Green Schoolyards America project (https://www.green-schoolyards.org).

In a final act of generosity, as older trees are dying, they send their carbon to their neighbors. In the Cigna study, the social nature of humans and the importance of having communities were shown to be critical. "People who are less lonely are more likely to have regular, meaningful, in-person interactions; are in good overall physical and mental health; have achieved balance in daily activities; and are employed and have good relationships with their coworkers" (Cigna, 2018, para. 5).

Our healthcare system offers very little to address the social isolation and loneliness that is causing health and mental health challenges for a wide swath of people in our communities. It does little to nothing to increase the social capital in communities or to address the stress-inducing issues that many children, teens, and young adults are experiencing.

# TRANSFORMING OUR HEALTHCARE SYSTEM

If our healthcare system is not designed to address the social determinants of health, the quality of social capital in our communities, the loneliness and isolation so many are experiencing, and the quality of nutrition that is contributing to significant health risks in our communities, then how can we apply our nursing leadership beyond the walls of our hospitals and healthcare systems to address these issues?

In her provocative TEDMED talk, Robin Guenther (2015), an architect whose award-winning nature-informed Restorative Designs of hospitals, asks, "How do we move from a system that delivers health care to one that creates actual health?" She suggests that our healthcare system has been stuck in a "massive industrial paradigm that actually has very little to do with health" and is rather a "sick care system that is focused on advanced stages of the disease and largely irrelevant to the health needs of most people." Guenther compares our hospitals to other industries, like chemical manufacturing and fossil fuels, which include stressful unhealthy workplaces, and create waste and other negative external impacts. Our hospitals contribute to the problems they ostensibly intend to solve.

In the healthcare system's efforts to address disease, we concurrently contribute to the contamination of rivers and lakes with pharmaceuticals, to the massive accumulation of plastic waste, and greenhouse gases responsible for climate change. What might a reimagined healthcare system look like? Tweaking our existing healthcare system without addressing the crushing blow that we are having on Mother Nature will not bring us health. One that prevents people from getting sick, heals those who are sick, and takes care of Mother Earth simultaneously will bring us all health.

How do we create those conditions? For us to survive, we must change. For things to change, we need nursing leaders who believe that change is necessary. We need to foster our sense of hope in the future to bring this spirit to our work. Mother Nature is waiting to help us with this—we need only ask.

An essential component of our leadership role is fostering new leaders and creating a powerful cadre of responsible citizens and changemakers. We need to be radically inclusive so that our choirs sing brightly. Simply, we are all the better off when we are all better off. Moreover, let's make sure that along the way, we create opportunities for joy. No one wants to be in the doom and gloom club. Invite the art community to join us—their creative proclivities should be welcome. Some of today's truths are incredibly hard to face, yet we must find our buoyancy in their presence. Joy and hope come with responsibility, and as leaders and together, we can build our response-ability.

As we are experiencing the truths about loneliness, food insecurity, and other human conditions, we are also in the period of the sixth-largest extinction of species on earth. If we are authentic as a Mother Tree would compel us to be, we must be present with the pain and suffering in the world, but we must also recognize that of our healthcare system is not designed to address any of these issues. Perhaps, the Mother Tree would have something to say similar to Albert Einstein's oft-quoted phrase, "We can't solve problems by using the same kind of thinking we used to create them." Our relationship with and dominion over nature and dominion over disease must be re-envisioned and reinvented.

# THE RIGHT QUESTIONS

There are many ways to lead. This book explores many of them. While there are certainly dozens of ways to be a leader, the question any leader might want to start with is "What is the change I wish to see in the world?" or (more precisely), "What is the change that I want to help make happen in the world?"

Nursing leadership is focused on nursing education, nursing's roles in healthcare delivery, and the healthcare system, all for obvious and good reasons. If these are the foci of much of our leadership, what will it take to pivot and address the things we know are making people unwell and vulnerable. For instance, can we effectively advocate for excellent K–12 education for all children and a school nurse in every school? Should we also be visible advocates for affordable housing and nutritious food for everyone? Furthermore, how about access to safe drinking water or making sure that the pollinators that are required for the plants that feed us don't go extinct? Can we organize our collective voices more effectively? Perhaps visibly advocating for a wider range of health-related issues would bring more nurses into our nursing organizations—nursing organizations that many nurses perhaps currently consider irrelevant to them.

# RIGHTS OF NATURE

The "rights of nature" is a concept first codified by Bolivia when their national government created the Law of the Rights of Mother Nature. A national office was created to defend the rights of Mother Earth. The binding principles of this law are:

- Harmony
- Collective good
- Guarantee of the regeneration of Mother Nature
- Respect and defend the rights of Mother Earth
- No commercialization [of living systems]
- Multiculturalism

Moreover, the rights that are imbued to Mother Nature are the following rights:

- To life
- To the diversity of life
- To water
- To clean air
- To equilibrium
- To restoration
- To pollution-free living

What if Mother Nature wrote a law for the Rights of Humans to Health and Well-Being? How different would the principles and rights be from the ones listed above? We might even want to think about the Rights of Future Generations. Even imagining what might be included in such a paradigm-shifting idea helps us to break with our old thinking and see anew. Our current extractive economic system relies on exploitation and unbridled growth. What would a caring economy look like? What (r)evolutionary changes might we explore to create the world that we all want to live in?

If we were to listen, what would our rainforests ask of us? They are the "lungs of the earth," providing us with 20% of the world's oxygen, yet they are under violent attack. What is our role as nursing leaders and as healers worldwide to call out the emergency that this particular violence is causing? What happens when we run out of oxygen? Perhaps, the forests would ask that we help protect them through policy and advocacy and even suggest that we plant more trees, especially in our urban areas where we know that co-benefits of the presence of trees lower community violence rates and improve mental health metrics.

# INDIGENOUS WISDOM

Indigenous voices are telling us "what we yearn to know again: that as kin to the animals and plants, rocks and winds of this sacred world, we can tap its power, take part in its healing" (Macy & Brown, 2014).

In *Braiding Sweetgrass: Indigenous Wisdom, Scientific Knowledge, and the Teachings of Plants*, Kimmerer (2013) explains that in some Indigenous cultures, there is no word for waste. Yet in our culture, we have whole throwaway communities that live in "sacrifice zones" breathing toxic air and drinking contaminated water. Others of us can have energy and products without a thought about the harm that has been caused. We have chosen not to know this—and yet we do. Our work starts with seeing our whole community, human and non-human. Our role is to amplify our most vulnerable communities' needs, not necessarily to lead them, but also to listen and support them.

Kimmerer recognizes that science as a way of knowing is too narrow and quotes a fellow Native scholar Greg Cajete, who shares that "in indigenous ways of knowing, we understand a thing only when we understand it with all four aspects of our being: mind, body, emotion, and spirit." Kimmerer goes on to say that "it is the whole human being that finds the beautiful path." She reminds us that when connecting through ceremony, we "marry the mundane to the sacred" and "it is a vehicle for belonging—to family, to a people, and to the land." Finding and building our communities are a path to health. This work is calling us.

There is a tenet in Native American lore that our decisions today should be considered in the context of their effect on the seventh generation forward. This longer view would certainly change many of today's policy-making processes and outcomes. In Native terms, we need to be in "right" relations now, and that will foster our healing.

Willoya (1962), in his book about Native warriors, describes an ancient prophecy: "When the Earth is sick and dying, all over the world people will rise up as Warriors of the Rainbow to save the planet." An Inuit offers a modern addition to this prophecy quoted in Willoya's book: "Great are the tasks ahead, terrifying are the mountains of ignorance and hate and prejudice, but the Warriors of the Rainbow shall rise as on the wings of the eagle to surmount all difficulties. They will be happy to find that there are now millions of people all over the earth ready and eager to rise and join them in conquering all barriers that bar the way to a new and glorious world! We have had enough now of talk. Let there be deeds."

The words of Black Elk, a native elder, guides our challenging work ahead:

*"Heal me, four quarters of the world, a relative I am!*

*Give me the strength to walk the soft earth, a relative to all of us!*

*Give me the eyes to see and the strength to understand, that I may be like you.*

*With your power only can I face the winds."*

–Black Elk

# ACKNOWLEDGING THE CATASTROPHES: A FIRST STEP

Our environmental catastrophes are of a scale that we can no longer merely amass good deeds at the individual level and expect to come out of this alive. We cannot recycle our way out of these cataclysms. This requires urgent collaborative leadership at the local, state, national, and global levels.

In 2019, the American Public Health Association declared climate change a health emergency, recognizing that its trajectory is placing humankind in harm's way (APHA, 2019). And, as with all health harms, there will be many populations that will be more vulnerable to its effects.

What are the skills that we need to lead today? We need to be armed with science, of course, and we need to identify who holds power and authority to make the changes we want to see. When operating with a broader lens, we will see more and different organizations and agencies that we will need to work with. There will be a learning curve. Power mapping is a way to visually display who has power within a community, or when developing a campaign for change, and where there are potential levers for influencing change. Power mapping is a tool often used by community organizers but is not typically part of our nursing leadership repertoire. Creating a power map can be a useful exercise as we expand the scope of our change-making and advocacy.

In 2015, the Rockefeller Foundation-Lancet Commission on Planetary Health issued a report and concurrently coined the frame of "planetary health" (Whitmee et al., 2015). This new frame recognizes that humans exist both in human systems and have a place within natural systems. In light of the litany of planetary threats, including massive species extinctions and deforestation, the report calls for "urgent collective action." Nurses must be part of this collectivity.

An expanded definition of "health policy" will be necessary. For the most part, nurses' policy leadership has been applied to the system in which we care for people when they are sick. We have spent much less time preventing illness. While we acknowledge the criticality of the social determinants of health, we have not significantly applied our policy acumen to addressing education, housing, or economic stability. We spend even less time addressing clean air and water, food and nutrition security, or other essentials that are absolutely critical to human health. In part, this latter lack of attention stems from the fact that we have not been teaching nurses about air, water, agriculture, or even climate change, whose cascading effects are presenting an existential threat to life on earth.

We do pick up the pieces when our air pollution causes childhood asthma and worsens chronic lungs diseases. We do take care of families whose children have been lead poisoned from their drinking water. Furthermore, we do take care of our communities after being ravaged by climate change–related fires, floods, and extreme weather events. However, to date, we have not substantially connected the dots to environmental health advocacy as a role for nursing leaders. If nurses are the most trusted voices regarding health, then we have tremendous potential to influence policies that will lead to environmental and planetary health.

An expanded understanding of the forces at play in environmental and planetary health policy is important. Anyone who has done tobacco/smoking policy over the last 50 years fully understands the tobacco industry's role in first denying the science regarding health risks, then fighting any and all anti-smoking policies. We will have similar experiences moving forward with other industries. We will have barriers to overcome.

While incrementalism is often the path we take in the policy arena, we need significant, audacious actions now. Moreover, leaders that will help propose them. We are regrettably behind schedule to save the planet. There is no time for baby steps. Physicist and systems thinker Fritjof Capra reminds us that on a limited planet, we cannot have unlimited growth (Capra & Henderson, 2009).

As nurses, we can continue to make changes within the healthcare system. However, if that limited scope is contextualized in a society that is perpetuating a runaway train economy, we will have dramatically failed to keep people healthy. No tweaks to our healthcare system, large or small, will prevent a massive, predicted health crisis. Our challenge will be to find a path to sustainable communities, in our countries and globally, which will no longer outpace nature's ability to regenerate and sustain life.

The path to solutions will require systems thinking well beyond the healthcare system to economic, political, and ecological systems. Nevertheless, we are reminded that sometimes small changes can generate great ones. And so, we are being called into territories, relationships, and actions that may be unfamiliar to nurses and nurse leaders—to join hands and hearts with new brothers and sisters, and new organizations. Big change is going to be necessary, and a big tent will be required.

# IMPLICATIONS FOR NURSING: IMAGINING A NEW STORY

If the earth were our patient, all of the alarms would be sounding right now. Our life support systems are imperiled. The causes of climate change and the resulting environmental degradation—increased duration of extreme heat, drought, flooding, and famines—are unthinkable to most people.

Nobel Prize winner Wangari Maathai was recognized for her phenomenal work in planting trees in Africa and healing whole communities in the process. Her wisdom was born in the earth.

> Trees are living symbols of peace and hope. A tree has roots in the soil yet reaches to the sky. It tells us that in order to aspire we need to be grounded, , , , Today we are faced with a challenge that calls for a shift in our thinking, so that humanity stops threatening its own life support system. We are called to assist Earth to heal her wounds, and in the process, heal our own. (Maathai, 2004, para. 25)

As nurses, we can see a landscape of incredible pain and suffering, and we are being called to action. We need to be the translators of science to the broader citizenry. Nevertheless, merely engaging in the criticality of the science debate will not be sufficient. We need to develop a new story to tell. While the story must be steeped in the scientific evidence, it must also help to bring a vision of what "might be"—a positive vision, one of hope and possibilities. A story with an expansive vision of health.

The story must contain a more seductive message than the current ones offered by the industries that are exhausting the Earth's resources and health. It is difficult for most people to imagine how we can escape the morass. The current mode of activism is more often than not reactive and negative. We are often "against" policies or practices (no fracking, no development, etc.), but we have not offered a grand picture of what we are for. And yet, people are craving a positive vision to counter-balance the daily evidence of climate change's catastrophic trajectory. What could our communities look like in the near and far future, and what is the path we must take to get there? If we don't know what it looks like, if we do not take the time to dream and co-imagine, we will never be able to co-create, and we will never get there. Our challenge is to invigorate our imagination.

# SUMMARY

As leaders, we can gather the broadest array of communities to explore what it would look like if we reimagined the future and tell that story forward and tell the story about how to get there. This is a BIG story, but it's a story that no one is telling. There is a need to create it, tell it, and use a more expansive "language." Bringing artists into the mix allows us to think visually and aurally in a different way—to bring new fertility to the landscape of exploration. We can consult the Mother Tree. We can drill deeper than words to find a place that is not dependent on words but is nevertheless more powerful. There we can find hope and grace and the courage to lead where we need to go. And then we must go.

*"The best way to predict the future is to design it."*

–Buckminster Fuller

# REFLECTIVE QUESTIONS

1.  Why might it be helpful to seek out nature when considering an important work challenge, life question, or career choice?

2.  As nurse leaders, why is it important to consider how we, as a society, address the social determinants of health?

3.  How did we become a society so fraught with loneliness and anxiety and how is that contributing to health risks? What can we do about this?

4.  How might national nursing organizations begin to advocate for positive changes regarding the social determinants of health and why does that really require collective action?

5.  What DOES the more beautiful world our hearts know is possible look like? Think expansively. Paint it as clearly as possible.

---

# NARRATIVE

## FACILITATED GROUP EXERCISE

Cover large tables with craft paper, give each student a marker, and have the students stand around the table. Ten students per table works well.

Ask the students to take turns identifying the "systems" that make up our communities and have them describe what works and doesn't work regarding these systems and what are sometimes the unintended consequences of the systems. Start them with the transportation system and ask them to draw the elements (e.g., roads/highways, public transportation, sidewalks, biking paths, airports, ferries, etc.). Ask them what the positive and negative effects are of this system. What are the health-promoting aspects of this system and what are not?

---

# AUTHOR BIOGRAPHIES

**Barbara Sattler, DrPH, RN, FAAN,** is a Professor Emerita at the University of San Francisco and an international leader in environmental health and nursing. She is a board member of the Alliance of Nurses for Healthy Environments, which is integrating environmental health into nursing education, practice, research, and policy/advocacy. She integrated environmental health as a core competency into the population DNP program. While at the University of Maryland, she directed the Maryland Hospitals for Healthy Environments, a 10-year statewide initiative that helped hospitals develop sustainable policies and practices to achieve the triple bottom line of employee health, patient health, and ecological health. She has been an advisor to the US EPA's Office of Child Health and the Principal Investigator on a host of grants from NIEHS, USDA, HUD, and the EPA. She helped to found Health Care Without Harm, a national organization focused on greening the healthcare sector.

# REFERENCES

American Public Health Association. (2019). *A declaration on climate change and health.* https://www.apha.org/-/media/files/pdf/topics/climate/190429_declaration_climate_health.ashx

Capra, F., & Henderson, H. (2009, September 14). Qualitative Growth: A conceptual framework for finding solutions to our current crisis that are economically sound, ecologically sustainable, and socially just. https://www.fritjofcapra.net/qualitative-growth/

Centers for Disease Control and Prevention. (2021). *Poor nutrition.* https://www.cdc.gov/chronicdisease/resources/publications/factsheets/nutrition.htm

Cigna. (2018). *New Cigna study reveals loneliness at epidemic levels in America.* https://www.multivu.com/players/English/8294451-cigna-us-loneliness-survey/

Guenther, R. (2015). *TEDMED Talk: Why hospitals are making us sick.* https://www.youtube.com/watch?v=HsOiDw2iDjA

Kaiser Family Foundation. (2005). *The effects of electronic media on children ages zero–six: A history of research — issue brief.* https://www.kff.org/other/issue-brief/the-effects-of-electronic-media-on-children/

Kimmerer, R. W. (2015). *Braiding sweetgrass: Indigenous wisdom, scientific knowledge, and the teachings of plants.* Milkweed Editions.

Louv, R. (2005). *Last child in the woods, saving our children from nature-deficit disorder.* Workman Publishing Company.

Maathai, W. (2004, December 10). *Nobel lecture.* https://www.nobelprize.org/prizes/peace/2004/maathai/26050-wangari-maathai-nobel-lecture-2004/

Macy, J., & Brown, M. (2014). *Coming back to life.* New Society Publishers.

Mertins, B. (n.d.). *Nature mentoring: What does nature teach us? 14 lessons from the natural world.* https://nature-mentor.com/nature-lessons/

Murthy, V. (2020). *Together: The healing power of connection in the sometimes lonely world.* Harper-Collins.

Putnam, R. D. (2000). *Bowling alone: The collapse and revival of the American community.* Simon and Schuster.

Simard, S. (2021). *Finding the mother tree: Discovering the wisdom of the forest.* Alfred A. Knopf of Penguin Random House.

Warber, S. L., DeHudy, A. A., Bialko, M. F., Marselle, M. R., & Irvine, K. N. (2015). Addressing "nature-deficit disorder": A mixed methods pilot study of young adults attending a wilderness camp. *Evidence-Based Complementary and Alternative Medicine, 2015,* Article ID 651827. https://doi.org/10.1155/2015/651827

Whitmee, S., Haines, A., Beyrer, C., Boltz, F., & Capon, A. G. (2015). Safeguarding human health in the Anthropocene epoch: Report of the Rockefeller Foundation. *Lancet, 386*(100007), 1973–2028.

Willoya, W. (1962). *Warriors of the rainbow: Strange and prophetic dreams of the Indians.* Naturegraph Publishers.

World Health Organization. (n.d.). *Health topics: Social determinants of health.* https://www.who.int/health-topics/social-determinants-of-health#tab=tab_1

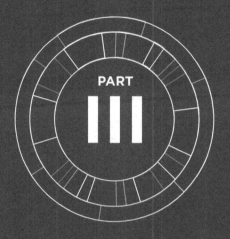

PART

# III

# APPLYING NOVEL LEADERSHIP THEORIES INTO PRACTICE

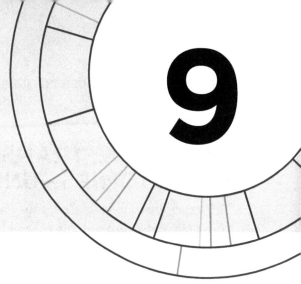

# 9

# QUANTUM CARING LEADERSHIP: A NEW ONTOLOGY INTO PRACTICE

Jean Watson, PhD, RN, AHN-BC, HSGAHN, FAAN, LL (AAN)
Tim Porter-O'Grady, DM, EdD, ScD(h), APRN, FAAN, FACCWS
Sara Horton-Deutsch, PhD, RN, PMHCNS, FAAN, ANEF
Kathy Malloch, PhD, MBA, RN, FAAN
Jim D'Alfonso, DNP,  PhD(h), RN, NEA-BC, FNAP, FAAN

## LEARNING OBJECTIVES

After the completion of this chapter, you will be able to:

- Distinguish the unitary principles of wholeness in nursing from the separatist principles of healthcare leadership

- Define the intersecting principles of Caring Science and Quantum Leadership

- Describe Quantum Caring Healthcare Leadership and its principles

- Critique the theory for leading in a quantum unitary reality to sustain humanity

# OVERVIEW: TRANSCENDING DICHOTOMIES—UNITARY THINKING

This paper draws upon and expands the previously published Watson, Porter-O'Grady, Horton-Deutsch, and Malloch works published in 2018. Unitary nursing has been evolving in nursing scholarship and theories over the past few decades to clarify and articulate its disciplinary foundation. Contemporary nursing discourse challenges nursing to engage in disciplinary-specific knowledge development through extant nursing theory and unifying philosophical worldviews. Prominent nursing leaders raise questions about the survivability of nursing without a shared ontological, philosophical, and ethical disciplinary worldview (Barrett, 2017; Grace et al., 2016; Newman, 2003; Newman et al. 1991; Phillips 2017). Without clarity of the disciplinary foundation for theory, knowledge, and practice, the nursing profession can easily lose its way. The profession will otherwise continue to be guided by pressures from institutional cultures to adhere to practices of distancing and objectifying humans and health, conforming to control dynamics, and the dominant conventional medical clinical paradigm.

Nursing's long-standing focus on the whole person and environment, in relation to universal human-environment health, has been acknowledged as unitary (Cowling, 1999; Newman, 2003; Newman et al., 1991; Rogers, 1970; Watson & Smith, 2002). The continuing disciplinary discourse of paradigms evolved from Rogers' (1970) original Science of Unitary Human Beings to current theories and scholarship, making a case for unitary thinking as the highest level of consciousness, congruent with the nursing phenomena (Cowling et al., 2008; Newman, 2003; Newman et al., 1991; Phillips, 2017).

Likewise, nursing scholars have acknowledged that caring is the fourth metaparadigm concept, replacing the concept of nursing (Conway, 1985; Cowling et al., 2008; Watson & Smith, 2002). Nursing is the study of the human environment, health, and healing through caring—or caring in the human health experience (Newman et al., 1991; Smith, 1999). These definitions reflect the disciplinary focus on wholeness, along with nursing's ethical-moral covenant to sustain human caring-healing and health, requiring an evolved consciousness of oneness and connection.

Within the unitary paradigm, everything is connected at the energetic, quantum level, and small acts have a ripple effect in the field. Human beings are viewed as whole. Caring moments within the unitary paradigm have been perceived as "mutuality" of human-to-human patterning (Newman et al., 1991). Watson refers to these human caring moments as *transpersonal moments*, whereby a caring moment transcends time, space, and physical presence (Watson, 1999, 2005) and creates a new field of possibilities.

This awareness transcends differences through a human-to-human authentic connection; unitary consciousness seeks to avoid dualism of "either/or" thinking, embracing "both/and" reality. This unitary oneness experience is transformative, resisting dichotomies and transcending differences, resulting in an evolution of consciousness (Watson, 1999, 2005, 2008, 2017). Awareness of the unitary consciousness arises when disparate ontologies about caring and the human-universe relationship are uncovered, depending upon paradigmatic perspectives. For example, three nursing paradigms are identified: Particulate-Deterministic; Interactive-Integrative; and Unitary-Transformative (Newman et al., 1991). We can see the first two levels are located within a separatist, parts-focused worldview or ontology; parts versus wholeness—meaning the human is separate from the environment and wider universe, the mind is separate from the body, and so on. That is, within the first two paradigms, the relations and processes in the human environment field are separate entities we seek to control or at least interact with to manage our body, physical field, and environmental reality (Newman et al., 1991).

The unitary paradigm awakens nursing to its timeless phenomena, of wholeness, to the human-universe reality of oneness, and connection of all. This evolved consciousness within Caring Science can be framed as a relational unitary worldview (Watson, 2005, 2008). It is when we locate nursing's phenomena of wholeness, healing-health, and caring within the unitary field that we have ontological disciplinary congruence for a relational-unitary ontology, versus a separatist, ontological worldview (Watson, 2008, 2017).

# QUANTUM REVOLUTION—HEALTHCARE LEADERSHIP

While nursing's disciplinary discourse and theories have evolved to the unitary principles of wholeness, caring, and health (Cowling et al., 2008; Newman et al., 1991; Watson & Smith, 2002), healthcare leadership is still primarily embedded in Newtonian separatist outdated principles versus the unitary principles of our human-environment-universe (Porter-O'Grady & Malloch, 2011; see Table 9.1).

**TABLE 9.1** Newtonian Characteristics of Leadership (Porter-O'Grady, 2016, p. 19)

- Hierarchical structures
- Focus on control
- Vertical orientation
- Reductionist scientific processes
- Top-down decision-making
- Mechanistic models of design
- Process-driven action

Meanwhile, in the field of quantum physics, the world has been experiencing a "second quantum revolution," even metaphorically. It takes the field beyond the first revolution of Newtonian physics of particles-parts-matter, motion, and movement into the larger field of quantum from micro to macro levels—i.e., everything in the universe is connected. This second revolution is shared by research and scholarship of notable common familiar names of physicists, such as Planck, Bohr, Schrödinger, Heisenberg, Bohm, Bell, and others.

The movement of *quantum* thinking is uncovering that everything is connected at the micro-level of the physical world. This thinking is now more than just a theory. While not all physics theorists agree that quantum is more than just a theory, there is increasing agreement that quantum principles work in the larger micro-macro world, if not the universe. Quantum theory and Quantum Leadership principles emphasize integration, synthesis, and relatedness and recognize that change is not a thing or an event but rather a dynamic that is constitutive of the universe (Porter-O'Grady & Malloch, 2010). This quantum worldview parallels the growing commitment of nursing scholars to unitary thinking for nursing phenomena.

New quantum breakthroughs have led to more mainstream images of quantum as a reality. For example, among the general public, *quantum,* even as a metaphor *for the unitary oneness of the mystery of the universe,* takes on new meanings, exemplified by the 70s movement, with popular books such as Gary Zukav's *The Dancing Wu I Masters* and Capra's *The Tao of Physics.* Currently, we see the "quantum world" of oneness evident at the environmental-planetary level, with common discourse among the public about climate change, global warming, and threats to the survival of all species, including the human species.

Indeed, the second quantum physics revolution has engaged the general public to the extent that folks are informed of such phenomena as wave-particle theory of light and matter. This awakening has led to medical science theory and research in phenomena of "non-locality" and "non-local consciousness": Consciousness is not confined to the brain (Phillips, 2017; Watson, 2005). Moreover, Rogers' Science of Unitary Human Beings posited energy as the fundamental unit of living, including indivisible fields within fields, beyond the physical plane (Rogers, 1992). This

Rogerian view of quantum indicates that everything is energetically connected and co-extensive with the entire universe.

These unitary quantum principles were most recently summarized by Phillips (2017), the prominent Rogerian unitary scientist scholar. Phillips highlighted selected views of science to include the following (p. 223):

- Everything in the universe manifests wave frequencies, vibrations, resonances of patterns, and fields.

- The universe is unitary, integral, and alive.

- Spirit and soul are of the universe and are integral.

- The universe manifests conscious awareness.

- The universe manifests thought, information, and knowledge.

- The universe and communication …can be non-local.

- Humans have a mind that is not confined to the brain (non-local consciousness).

This view of unitary science declares it is a holographic universe—the whole is in the part, and the part is in the whole.

# QUANTUM LEADERSHIP—UNITARY PRINCIPLES

The scholarship in Quantum Leadership has been underway for a couple of decades, offering a new level of unitary consciousness in nursing and healthcare leadership education and practices (Porter-O'Grady & Malloch, 2010, 2013, 2015, 2016, 2017). These unitary, quantum converging themes can be found in Quantum Leadership science, in contrast to non-unitary Newtonian paradigm approaches. Porter-O'Grady & Malloch (2016) identified characteristics of Quantum

Leadership. These characteristics are congruent with the unitary field of thinking and the "second quantum revolution" (Balents, 2016; see Table 9.2).

These characteristics reveal principles of both unitary and quantum emergence and convergence. These characteristics directly contrast to conventional, parts-focused healthcare leadership principles; those embedded in the Newtonian physics worldview are more aligned with the particulate deterministic medical science worldview. As Porter-O'Grady and Malloch's (2010, 2015, 2017) quantum scholarship evolved, they identified the different worldviews and how each level reflects different paradigms. For example, the Newtonian approaches reflect the particulate-deterministic paradigm; their work then evolved from the transactional parts-model (Interactive paradigm) to the quantum level, consistent with a Unitary Caring Science worldview.

**TABLE 9.2**  Quantum Healthcare Leadership–Unitary Principles (Porter-O'Grady & Malloch, 2016, p. 21):

- Non-linear structures
- Focus on connections—relatedness
- Value-driven actions
- Complexity-based models of design
- Multi-focal processes
- Multi-systems within systems
- Everything is connected

# CARING SCIENCE

Caring Science is an extant, evolved model of science grounded in a moral-ethical ontological framework of relations and unity that promotes and sustains human dignity, caring, healing, and health for all (Watson, 1999, 2005, 2008, 2017). For more than 40 years, Caring Science scholarships and the Theory of Transpersonal Caring have transformed nursing from the inside out by an expanded discipline-specific unitary worldview, acknowledging nursing's covenantal relationship with global humanity and Transpersonal Caring moments (Watson, 2017). This Caring Science Theory seeks to sustain human caring-healing and love through knowledgeable, compassionate service to humankind.

The 10 Caritas Processes (Watson, 2008) of Caring Science Theory identify universals of human caring and love that guide the caring-healing practitioner-leadership principles for patients, nurses, and healthcare systems around the world (see Table 9.3).

## TABLE 9.3   10 Caritas Processes

1. Embrace: Sustaining humanistic-altruistic values—Practice of loving-kindness, compassion, and equanimity for self/other.

2. Inspire: Being authentically present—Enabling faith/hope; Honoring subjective inner, life-world of self/other.

3. Trust: Being sensitive to self/others by cultivating own spiritual practices; beyond ego-self to transpersonal presence.

4. Nurture: Developing and sustaining loving, trusting, and caring relationships.

5. Forgive: Allowing for expression of positive and negative feelings—Authentically listening to another person's story.

6. Deepen: Creatively problem-solving, solution-seeking through caring processes; full use of self and artistry of caring-healing practices.

7. Balance: Engaging in transpersonal teaching-learning caring relationship; Staying within other's frame of reference—shift toward coaching model for health/wellness.

8. Co-create: Creating a healing environment at all levels—subtle environment for energetic, authentic caring presence.

9.    Minister: Reverentially assisting with basic needs as sacred acts; touching the spirit of others; sustaining human dignity.

10.   Open: Opening to existential-spiritual, mystery, unknowns—allowing for miracles.

# CARING SCIENCE AND UNITARY PRINCIPLES

Watson's Theory of Transpersonal Caring is guided by unitary philosophical-ethical principles of unity of all; healing is transformative through evolving transcendent consciousness. Indeed, Caring Science is based upon the Ethic of Belonging and the Ethics of Face from Emmanuel Levinas, the French philosopher who posited the Ethic of Belonging as the first principle of science (Levinas, 1969; Watson, 2005). The Ethic of Belonging is consistent with the unitary paradigm that we all "belong to the infinite field of the universe" (Levinas, 1969) and are connected and belong to one whole. In his philosophy of Ethics of Face, Levinas noted the "face" of others we encounter is irreducible and without bounds, whereby one person's level of humanity reflects on the other—we are all connected (Watson, 2005).

Watson's Caring Science, drawing upon Levinas, posits that the field of nursing resides within the infinite sacred circle of life-death—all connected with and belonging to a universal, infinite Source (Watson, 2005, 2008). The notion of Source is close to what Phillips refers to as an "*Energyspirit*—the indivisible and invisible soul of the universe" (Phillips, 2017, p. 223). According to Levinas's work *Totality and Infinity* (1969), humanity will either evolve to a higher level of consciousness or humans will objectify, totalize, and destroy humanity.

Transpersonal Caring Theory posits a caring moment as transcending time, space, and physicality, connecting with an infinite field of possibilities (Watson, 1999). Transpersonal Caring consciousness affirms an evolution of human consciousness. This consciousness leads to our ability to affirm ethically and morally that we all belong to the infinite field of universal love energy. This is the great mystery and sacred nature of our being in the physical world yet connected with infinity—a universal field of the oneness of all (Phillips, 2017; Rogers, 1992; Watson, 1999, 2005).

# UNITARY CONVERGENCE: QUANTUM LEADERSHIP SCIENCE AND TRANSPERSONAL CARING SCIENCE

While Quantum Leadership theory and science have evolved in scholarship and practices, the scholarly work has not been explicitly located within a distinct disciplinary, nursing-specific theoretical foundation. In the meantime, Caring Science has evolved separately from Quantum Leadership science yet resides within the shared quantum unitary worldview. However, Caring Science has not been linked directly to Quantum Leadership scholarship, even though Caring Science scholarship is consistent with quantum thinking. By transposing Caring Science and Quantum Leadership into a disciplinary matrix context, we find congruence. This congruence is at the philosophical-ethical, ontological, theoretical level. The new integration unites quantum and caring leadership toward a distinct disciplinary foundation for new leadership practices and principles.

Drawing upon the core unitary, quantum aspects of Quantum Leadership (QL), and Caring Science (CS), we can identify Unitary Disciplinary-Specific Commonalities. These comprise shared, nursing ethic, ontological, philosophical, epistemology, and praxis convergence for Quantum Caring HealthCare Leadership (QCL).

Guided by these evolved shared, unitary quantum disciplinary commonalities, the following principles for Quantum Caring HealthCare Leadership are offered.

# IMPLICATIONS FOR PRACTICE

Contemporary nursing discourse challenges nurses to engage in disciplinary-specific knowledge development through extant nursing theory and unifying philosophical worldviews. Prominent nursing leaders raise questions about the survivability of nursing without a shared ontological, philosophical, and ethical disciplinary worldview (Barrett, 2017; Grace et al., 2016; Newman et al., 1991; Phillips 2017).

Two divergent areas, Caring Science and Quantum Leadership scholarship, have evolved separately. However, by using a disciplinary ontological-ethical matrix analysis, convergence and synergy were uncovered between quantum knowledge, unitary thinking, Caring Science, and Quantum Leadership: *Quantum Caring Healthcare Leadership Model.*

## QUANTUM LEADERSHIP AND CARING SCIENCE COMMONALITIES

- **Ethic:** Both QL and CS share Ethic of Belonging (to infinity) as foundation starting point for unitary science worldview; this ethic serves as a basis for QCL principles and practices to honor social mandate to sustain human dignity and human-organizational, dynamic evolution.

- **Ontology:** QL and CS both embrace a unitary ontology and quantum worldview thinking, honoring oneness and infinite connections, thus generating QCL constructs of caring community and relational accountability as healthcare leadership principles.

- **Philosophical—Values:** Both QL and CS honor the unity of the whole person mind-body-spirit, shared human-valued connections across time, extending into infinity; thus, generating QCL healthcare principles that explicitly embrace the diversity of human spirit, creativity, awe, wonder, infinite possibilities unfolding.

- **Theoretical:** Both QL and CS share unitary perspectives related to human caring and the 10 Caritas Processes whereby Transpersonal Caring moments potentiate new human-environment field patterning; dynamics of human expression of love and caring create sustainable healthcare leadership principles and lead to complexity-based, ontologically designed models of organizational structure.

- **Epistemology:** Both QL and CS share the principles of transcendent consciousness whereby the leadership values, philosophy, and ontological worldview affect the entire field of knowledge and what counts as knowledge. The expanding Quantum Caring Leadership epistemology adheres to new models of knowing and research, including non-physical Quantum Leadership models—for example, the concept of presence; of consciousness; intuition; and authenticity and similar human phenomena. Embracing all ways of knowing—artistic, personal, relational, intuitive, empirical, ethical, spiritual, and so on, along with co-creative, exploratory methodologies; expanded epistemology has the potential to generate new theories, knowledge, and new forms of Unitary healthcare caring leadership inquiry.

- **Praxis:** Both QL and CS celebrate praxis as an informed moral practice of new forms of healthcare. QCL science, guided by a unitary, quantum worldview of infinite creative unknowns and emergence QCL principles, seeks evidentiary, community building, creating space for authentic emergence of human-caring community structures, allowing for expressions of love and human caring. Quantum Caring Leadership Praxis invites an evolution of human consciousness, opening to spirit, mystery, wonder, the awe of nature, and the infinite universe.

- **Together:** QL and CS provide and affirm a shared ethical, ontological, philosophical disciplinary worldview to inform, if not transform, nursing and healthcare leadership: *Quantum Caring Healthcare Leadership Model.*

New healthcare, nursing-specific leadership models will be required to participate in a quantum-unitary reality to sustain humanity. In response, in 2021, the Watson Caring Science Institute has developed the Caritas Leadership Program. Uniquely, this leadership program is a spiritual journey to discover and honor each individual's experience in a safe space built on mutual respect, embracing differences, non-judgment, self-care, and love. Once the nurse leader's experience is honored and voiced, they expand their leadership contribution by radiating trust, care, and compassion to others. Being open to feedback, expressing appreciation, being responsive, recognizing others' contributions, demonstrating humility, and treating others with dignity and respect are core unitary/quantum components. Upon self-discovery through the Leadership Circles, participants articulate and translate a Caritas Leadership ontology into human caring/Caring Science organizational leadership practices. As nurse leaders broaden their focus from a medical-care system to a caring, healing healthcare system, they collectively co-create caring-healing cultures.

## QUANTUM CARING HEALTHCARE LEADERSHIP PRINCIPLES

- Quantum Caring Healthcare Leadership principles involve the universality of human caring community as a quantum unitary phenomenon.

- Quantum Caring Healthcare Leadership principles build upon the 10 Caritas Processes of Caring Science and Transpersonal Caring as a theoretical guide for expanding nursing disciplinary foundation for new models of universal, caring-healing healthcare.

- Quantum Caring Healthcare Leadership builds upon Quantum Leadership principles of non-linear structures; relational-ethical accountability and complexity quantum-based models of design—allowing for ontological-infinite emergence of caring-healing health communities.

- The universals of Quantum Caring Healthcare Leadership integrate with Caritas Processes of Transpersonal Caring Science theory, creating a language and structure for substantive human leadership models as quantum acts of love and caring (Porter-O'Grady & Malloch, 2010; Watson, 2008, 2017).

- Quantum Caring Healthcare Leadership principles build upon the Unitary Caring Science "Ethic of Belonging and Love" as a nursing, discipline-specific, and unitary ethical view of science—allowing for concepts such as non-local consciousness, non-physical phenomena, human caring transpersonal field, and human health (healing) experiences as mystery, infinite unknowns.

- The discipline of nursing and Quantum Caring Healthcare Leadership principles are grounded in a unitary view of science and nursing phenomena distinctly evolved beyond the conventional Western, separate-parts paradigm, and Newtonian worldview of science.

- The unifying framework of Quantum Caring Healthcare Leadership grounds the discipline within an expanding view of science, adhering to nursing's moral-ethical imperative as the starting point to sustain humanity itself and, specifically, human caring-healing and health practices for our world.

- New patterns of Quantum Caring Leadership principles offer directions for the whole person-whole system, caring-healing, and global healthcare organizations.

Quantum Leadership science has long held a shared unitary nursing caring disciplinary perspective, although not made explicit. This chapter uncovered and made explicit ontological-philosophical disciplinary congruence between Caring Science and Quantum Leadership. An evolved Quantum Caring Healthcare Leadership model invites new provocative thinking and critique, both for the discipline and an informed new unitary, quantum caring consciousness for all healthcare leadership.

# SUMMARY

Nursing leadership continues to evolve from transformative, transactional leadership principles to a unitary quantum caring worldview of the infinity of relationships-universe. Caring Science has evolved more explicitly, underpinned by "second quantum revolution" science and Quantum Leadership principles. By integrating the ethics and unitary ontology of Caring Science with energetic Quantum Leadership principles, both Quantum Leadership and Caring Science are transformed and metamorphosed into a new discipline-specific entity: the *Quantum Caring Healthcare Leadership Model*.

# REFLECTIVE QUESTIONS

1. How do you integrate the Caritas Processes into practice including care for self, others, and your organization/community?

2. How is unitary consciousness visible in your role as a nurse leader? What more can you do?

3. What does Quantum Caring Leadership mean to you?

4. How can the principles of Quantum Caring Leadership be utilized to sustain humanity?

5. Why does embracing a unitary quantum caring worldview matter?

# NARRATIVE

An invitation to present to the regional quality council of a large healthcare system was extended to a Chief Nurse Executive (CNE), the direct result of notable and sustained improvements in quality outcomes, operational performance, and service metrics over two years.

In sharing the team's story, the CNE identified that despite dutifully implementing the same system-wide initiatives and best practices supported by detailed playbooks, checklists, and service scripts, their hospital's scorecard remained among the lowest in the region. Following extended leadership gaps and turnover, the new and current nurse executive assessed the landscape, identified a unique and disruptive opportunity, and proposed a different approach to address performance gaps that involved integrating established Caring Science Theory and emerging Quantum Leadership principles. The leadership and clinical teams were engaged and subsequently espoused their support during open leader forums, enthusiastically embracing the vision to transform their culture through Quantum Caring Leadership (QCL) principles, evidence, and informed moral action.

The leadership message and commitment were that this hospital or community of leaders and care teams would begin a journey to consciously lead and act through human connections and authentic caring relationships. Conventional leadership approaches had previously focused on controlling processes, competency, metrics, and compliance. Fostering trust and shifting the culture required education, mentoring, coaching, and role modeling that were both ubiquitous and aligned with QCL. Teams had to discover new ways of being and becoming together, unlearn divisive or separatist thinking, and develop evolved practices that were more congruent with quantum caring leadership. The focus was on supporting the ongoing development of confident, caring clinicians and leaders committed to establishing an authentic, caring, compassionate, and healing culture. Learning forums were conducted regularly to model appreciative dialogue and discover the shared meaning behind new or emerging initiatives. The change was no longer something to fear or resist but increasingly perceived as an opportunity to learn, grow, adapt, and improve care together. Clinicians were engaged every step of the way and soon adopted a credo, "Nothing about us, without us!" to represent their commitment to full engagement. In addition to authentic dialogue and intentional inclusion, decisions were no longer made in an office. Instead, they encouraged and supported them, being made as close to the point of care as possible. Experiential learning events on QCL, Caring Science integration, and the 10 Caritas Processes helped guide leader and care team commitments to self-care, resilience, connectedness, caring moments, and healing environments. Growing evidence of intentionality, presence, connectedness, and authentic caring connections was best reflected in narratives. Inviting and celebrating caring moments before meetings and in shift huddles/cuddles helped infuse a steady sense of joy and meaning in their collective work.

In closure, the CNE reinforced that hospital leaders have continually evolved and come to value their role as navigators, translators, and champions of a harmonizing QCL message that unites teams under a shared vision in order to achieve uncommon results. Their commitment to relationships and connectedness helped engender trust. Through consistent QCL practices, they have nurtured ongoing growth, quality, success, and the ability for patients, individuals, teams, and the organization to flourish together. Empowered through QCL practices, care teams are increasingly aware, fully engaged, and owning their practice, which we have observed to be a liberating, organic, transformative, renewable, and indispensable source of continued success and sustained performance as a caring community.

Discuss the potential impact of sustained congruence between theory and leadership practices (QCL) on patient care, the nursing workforce, and organizational performance. In pairs or small groups, create a list of QCL characteristics identified in the narrative. The list of QCL characteristics invites participants to share a leadership experience where QCL characteristics were either clearly evident or notably absent.

# AUTHOR BIOGRAPHIES

**Jean Watson, PhD, RN, AHN-BC, HSGAHN, FAAN, LL (AAN),** is Distinguished Professor and Dean Emerita, University of Colorado College of Nursing Anschutz Medical Center, USA; founder of the original Center for Human Caring in Colorado; a Fellow of the American Academy of Nursing (FAAN); Founder and Director of nonprofit organization, Watson Caring Science Institute; past President of the National League for Nursing; founding member of International Association in Human Caring and International Caritas Consortium. She held the nation's first endowed chair in Caring Science for 16 years; holds 15 Honorary Doctoral Degrees, including 12 International Honorary Doctorates. Her work is studied and implemented around the world. She is a widely published author and recipient of many awards and honors, has authored or co-authored over 30 books on caring, and is designated as a *Living Legend* by the American Academy of Nursing, its highest honor, and an Honorary Scholar for the Global Academy of Holistic Nursing.

**Tim Porter-O'Grady, DM, EdD, ScD(h), APRN, FAAN, FACCWS,** Senior Partner for Tim Porter-O'Grady Associates LLC & Clinical Professor, Emory University School of Nursing, is an advanced practice nurse in geriatrics/wound specialties and holds two doctorates. He has served as Clinical Professor, Leadership Scholar at The Ohio State University, College of Nursing, and Professor of Practice and Leadership Scholar at Arizona State University, College of Nursing and Health Innovation for 10 years, and is currently a Clinical Professor at Emory University, School of Nursing. He is nationally/internationally recognized as an expert/futurist in clinical health systems, leadership, professional governance, and health systems innovation. He has consulted with over 600 clinical systems worldwide and has lectured at over 1,000 settings globally. He has authored/co-authored 28 books and over 200 journal publications and is a nine-time winner of the AJN Book of the Year Award.

**Sara Horton-Deutsch, PhD, RN, PMHCNS, FAAN, ANEF,** is a Caritas Coach and a Professor and the Director of the Kaiser Permanente/USF Partnership at the University of San Francisco, where she mentors the next generation of nursing leaders through the lens of Caring Science and values-based leadership. She also serves as a Faculty Associate with the Watson Caring Science Institute. In 2021, she co-created and initiated the Caritas Leadership Program, a uniquely customized six-month program guiding participants through executive Caring Science leader dialogues, interactive circles, and participant transformation projects. She is also a founding partner of Better Together Healing, LLC, a holistic practice partnership specializing in an integrative approach to heal the self, build collaborations, and create healthy and bounded communities. As a therapeutic practitioner and Caritas leadership coach, she collaborates with healthcare professionals and organizations seeking balance and growth who are open to engaging in innovative approaches to healing. Her comprehensive approach includes certifications in professional coaching and training through the Leadership Circle and Working with Resilience, providing comprehensive profiles and assessments to raise the conscious practice of leadership and build regenerative success at work.

**Kathy Malloch, PhD, MBA, RN, FAAN,** Clinical Professor, The Ohio State University, is a nationally known writer and speaker and has been a registered nurse for over 50 years. Malloch has published extensively in proctored health journals and co-authored 15 textbooks on leadership and innovation with Tim Porter-O'Grady. She is a frequent presenter and author on leadership topics, healthcare innovation, professional nursing practice, and patient classification systems. Malloch served as the first program director for the Arizona State University, College of Nursing and Health Innovation, Master's in Healthcare Innovation program. This innovative, multidisciplinary program is the first of its kind in the country. Most recently, Malloch and Porter-O'Grady created the Executive DNP Program at OSU College of Nursing, Columbus, Ohio. Currently, she consults with The Ohio State University, College of Nursing Master's in Healthcare Innovation program and serves as the Associate Director of Education and Evidence-Based Practice at the Arizona Board of Nursing.

**Jim D'Alfonso, DNP, PhD(h), RN, NEA-BC, FNAP, FAAN,** Executive Director, Professional Excellence and the KP Scholars Academy & Adjunct Faculty University of San Francisco, served as a Chief Nurse Executive/COO and Associate Vice President prior to joining Kaiser Permanente (KP) in 2011. As Executive Director for the KP Scholars Academy, he leads programs to advance research, professional development, continuing education, and health systems transformation. D'Alfonso received his Doctor of Nursing Practice (DNP) with a focus in executive leadership from the University of San Francisco (USF), where he serves as Adjunct Faculty. In 2015, he received an honorary doctorate in Caring Science for his career-long contributions. He is a board-certified nurse executive (NEA-BC), Certified Caritas Coach, Master HeartMath Executive Trainer (HMET), a Distinguished Fellow of the Nursing Academies of Practice (FNAP) and Fellow of the American Academy of Nursing (FAAN). He has published extensively and lectured across the US and internationally. A text he co-authored: "Kaiser Foundation School of Nursing, A Legacy of Disruptive Innovation," was published in June 2020.

# REFERENCES

Barrett, E. (2017). Again. What is nursing science? *Nursing Science Quarterly, 30*(2), 129–133.

Conway, M. E. (1985). Toward a greater specificity in defining nursing's metaparadigm. *Advances in Nursing Science, 7*(4), 73–81.

Cowling, W. R. III. (1999). A unitary-transformative nursing science: Potentials for transcending dichotomies. *Nursing Science Quarterly, 12*(2), 132–137.

Cowling, W. R., Smith, M., & Watson, J. (2008). The power of wholeness, consciousness and caring. A dialogue on nursing science, art and healing. *Advances in Nursing Science, 31*, E41–E51.

Grace, P. J., Willis, D. G., Roy, C., & Jones, D. A. (2016). Profession at the crossroads: A dialog concerning the preparation of nursing scholars and leaders. *Nursing Outlook, 64*, 61–70.

Levinas, E. (1969). *Totality and infinity*. Duquesne University Press.

Newman, M. A. (2003). A world of no boundaries. *Advances in Nursing Science, 26*(4), 240–245.

Newman, M., Sime, A., & Corcoran-Perry, S. (1991). The focus of the discipline of nursing. *Advances in Nursing Science, 14*(1),1–6.

Phillips, J. (2017). New Rogerian theoretical thinking about unitary science. *Nursing Science Quarterly, 30*(3), 223–226.

Porter-O'Grady, T., & Malloch, K. (2010, 2013, 2015, 2017). *Quantum leadership*. Jones and Bartlett.

Porter-O'Grady, T., & Malloch, K. (2016). *Leadership in nursing practice: Changing the landscape of health care*. Jones and Bartlett Learning.

Rogers, M. E. (1970). *An introduction to the theoretical basis of nursing*. F. A. Davis.

Rogers, M. E. (1992). Nursing science and the space age. *Nursing Science Quarterly, 5*, 27–34.

Smith, M. (1992). Caring and the science of unitary human beings. *Advances in Nursing Science, 21*(4), 14–28.

Smith, M. (1999). Caring and science of UHB. *Advances in Nursing Science, 21*, 14–28.

Watson, J. (1999). *Postmodern nursing and beyond*. Churchill-Livingstone.

Watson, J. (2005). *Caring Science as sacred science*. F. A. Davis.

Watson, J. (2008). *Nursing: The philosophy and science of caring*. University Press of Colorado.

Watson, J. (2017). Global caritas literacy. In S. Lee, P. Palmieri, & J. Watson (Eds.), *Global caring literacy* (pp. 3–11). Springer.

Watson, J., Porter-O'Grady, T., Horton-Deutsch, S., & Malloch, K. (2018). Quantum caring healthcare leadership. Integrating quantum leadership with Caring Science. *Nursing Science Quarterly, 31*(3), 253–258.

Watson, J., & Smith, M. (2002). Caring Science and the science of unitary human beings: A trans-theoretical discourse for nursing knowledge development. *Journal of Advanced Nursing, 37*(5), 452–461.

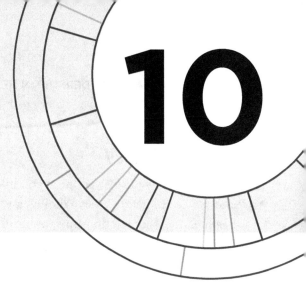

# 10

# CARING SCIENCE–INFORMED LEADERSHIP

Grissel Hernandez, PhD, RN, MPH, HNB-BC, NPD-BC, SGAHN
Marcia Hills, PhD, RN, FAAN, FCAN
Chantal Cara, PhD, RN, FAAN, FCAN
Jean Watson, PhD, RN, AHN-BC, HSGAHN, FAAN, LL (AAN)

## LEARNING OBJECTIVES/SUBJECTIVES

After completing this chapter, you will be able to:

- Describe the underlying ethic, philosophy, and unitary worldview of Caring Science

- Critique dominant leadership separatist worldview in contrast to unitary caring worldview

- Examine one's own worldview and institutional patterns

- Review Caritas ontological leadership literacy/illiteracy (*dyspraxis*) toward self/other

- Translate Caritas Process language into Caritas ontological leadership guide for informed moral leadership practice/praxis (*eupraxis*)

- Explore national/international exemplars of Caritas ontological leadership in academic and clinical administrations, resulting in what may be framed as a form of sacred activism

# OVERVIEW

This moment: yes, *this* very moment, in our work and our world, we are invited and required to enter an expanding, awakening worldview of science, of life, of healing, of caring relationships, of health, of hospitals, of medicine, of education, of communities, of civilization, and of course of Caritas or Watson Caring Science–informed leadership—the focus of this chapter.

BUT the problem is: We can't get *'There'* from *'Here.'* Where is *'Here'*? Where is *'There'*?

*'Here* is where we as nurses, educators, and leaders largely are situated still; lost, unconsciously or consciously, trapped in the outer world of fear, institutional constraints, biocidic (life-destroying), oppressive cultures and practices; succumbing to conformity; or trying valiantly to advance in the dominant separatist worldview of fear, ego, control, institutional power—a dominating system culture.

*'Here'* is where still, we seek to find our way in a worldview and in systems that are turned inside out and upside down and have gone astray from their core values, missions, and commitment to humans and humanity, sustaining dignity and oneness of ALL. That is why we can't get to *'There'* unless we unravel, constructively critique, creatively and intellectually disrupt, and transcend the *'Here,'* wakening to a unitary transformative worldview and cosmology of the universe to which we all Belong.

So, how are we to proceed in such a tumultuous turning point for our world, our work, our Being/Becoming more evolved, more conscious, more intentional, a more engaged professional as nurses, always searching for ways to sustain human caring and preserve humanity? How are we to humanize ourselves, institutions, or our practices to find meaning and purpose when all seemingly is dissolving or has already dissolved in front of our eyes?

Where and What is *'THERE'* then? How do we get *'THERE'*? When the controlling energy, 'HERE' is focused on staying *'HERE'*? *'HERE,' in our sickness unto death,* remaining in an outdated worldview of separation and physical material—matter (i.e., economics) at all costs, generating stagnation and poverty of spirit, and destruction of human-planet-earth existence.

# CARING SCIENCE-INFORMED LEADERSHIP—A PATH TO THE *'THERE'*

This new *'There'* is where Caring Science and Caritas Nursing Leadership has always been—but on the margin. *There* now is where nursing steps into the center, with voice, language, and informed moral action; more advanced in its disciplinary foundation, awakening the human spirit, widening our unitary, relational worldview, returning to the heart of our humanity and the heart of nursing education and healthcare, our universe.

In Caring Science, we enlarge our universe of nursing, of education, of practice, of caring, of humanity, of global civilization, of Mother Earth, guiding our professional-disciplinary responsibility. More specifically, Watson Caring Science calls and guides us toward informed moral (*eupraxis*) practice, honoring circle of life/death care as a sacred science, and toward Caritas informed leadership as a form of sacred activism (Watson, 2018, 2019).

Thus, Watson Caring Science is informed by a unitary worldview of connectedness; it holds a reverence for the sacred circle of life-death, via the explicit "Ethic of Belonging"—before our separate Being. Our belonging to each other and the infinite field of Universal Cosmic Love opens the human heart and science for a transcendent and transformative worldview of ONENESS; whereby we all Belong to this energy of Cosmic Love for life, for renewal, for mystery, healing, wonder, for awe; for a return to the sacred art in our science and our lifeworld.

In this new *'There'* to which we seek, we now reside in a unitary field of quantum proportions, whereby everything in the universe is energetically connected to everything else. This Caring Science–informed leadership introduces and disrupts the dominant *'Here'* reality by offering a new starting point and unitary foundation platform. This new *'There'* invites and uncovers another way from our no-longer-working, *Here*.

Watson Caring Science–informed leadership includes:

- Ethic of *Belonging* as the first principle of (Caring) Science—comes before our separate Being

- Language of 10 Caritas Processes to articulate, teach, practice, research, and lead by uncovering and living out the invisible, yet universal phenomenon of human caring for self/system/society

- New Ontological Ways of Being as Caritas Literate guide to be in the right relation at all levels

- Expanded epistemology: critique of knowledge; questioning what counts as knowledge; honoring all ways of knowing for practice, research, education, leadership, and policy

- Disruption of conventional thinking about science, about knowledge, about consciousness, about life, and about death and human-universe

- Caritas leadership *eupraxis* (*good* practice) as a guide to *'There'* for informed moral justice

Thus, Caring Science offers an awakened Human-Universe Consciousness, Ethic, Unitary Ontology, Epistemology, for Caritas literacy for (*eupraxis*) *good* (ontologically literate) leadership Praxis. Caritas literacy has been acknowledged as ultimately an ontology of being/becoming that comes from within the subjective, inner lifeworld of each person, morally aroused for reflective and contemplative self-growth. These self-caring practices contribute to the whole of humanity (Watson, 2017, p. 7).

This new '*There*' is underpinned by deep personal/professional values, purpose, high vibrational language; an open worldview that disrupts and transcends; constructively deconstructs the dominant ontological, illiterate '*Here*' (*dyspraxis*, bad practice) in current, conventional, institutional structures, practices, policies, and culture.

## CARITAS ONTOLOGICAL LEADERSHIP LITERACY

What is Caritas Ontological Leadership Literacy?

Simply put, the ontology of Caritas leadership literacy begins with self, in the beginning, and the end: being present and open to compassion, mercy, gentleness, gratitude, loving-kindness, humility and equanimity toward and with self, and higher self/Source. This Caritas (loving self-relational ontology) literacy forms (versus deforms) and guides the human creative spirit, away from *outer* patterned system-cultures, of non-relational (*dyspraxis*), toward reconstructing that draws upon *inner* subjective, creative life force of self/other in relation—co-creating Caritas ontological *eupraxis* as foundation for Caring Science leadership.

Caritas ontological literacy invites an evolved level of ontological leadership. Such literacy involves intentional consciousness of a love of humanity and all living things; the immanent, subtle, radiant, shadow, and light vicissitudes of experiences of our humanity—honoring with reverence the mystery, unknowns, higher deeper dimensions of a unitary universe of Oneness (Watson, 2008). This unitary caring, relational consciousness influences all levels of nursing: clinical care, education, research, practice, management, politics, and policy.

## ONTOLOGICAL LEADERSHIP *ILLITERACY*

The counterpoint to Caritas (relational-loving-ontological literacy for leadership) is Ontological *illiteracy*—that is inhumane, task-conscious foci, stifled emotions, and repressed expressions and feelings; authoritative mindset, insensitive, dehu-manizing, punitive-distrusting atmosphere, and dividing-separating actions. This (often unconscious) cultural-institutional pattern becomes a dysfunctional, yet somehow subtly acceptable, normative leadership style—a power-over style of leadership, perpetuating illiterate practices, standards, and policies (e.g., fixation with adhering to "compliance" demands, versus co-creating a culture of compas-sion for *eupraxis* leadership)

Ontological *illiteracy* leads to a controlling, harsh culture—impersonal institu-tions, corporate mindsets, that discriminate with the use of distancing objective criteria and language that labels, divides, and often incites fear and distrust as a means of control. Caritas *ontological literacy* is the opposite of Caritas *ontological illiteracy*. Caritas ontological *literacy* invites liberating, compassionate learning, trusting, and supporting, co-creative emergence from within the whole. This form of literacy honors diversity, equity, a mix of talents, and constructive, humane critique, committed to shared humanity to serve the whole.

# CARING SCIENCE LEADERSHIP PRAXIS

The next section of this chapter will explore, uncover, and invite some other ways of implementing ontological Caritas (i.e., Caring Science) leadership—in acute care and academy/education with clinical-administrative leadership responsibili-ties. As such, these acute care and wonderful academic-clinical exemplars highlight *eupraxis* models; they move us closer to '*There*'—guided by Caring Science and Caritas Ontological Literacy for new forms of caring-loving leadership of Caritas/ LOVE. Through Caritas ontological leadership processes and practices, nursing is humanizing previously ontologically illiterate leadership systems toward heart-cen-tered, authentic, lasting, timeless leadership for self/system/society—our world.

# CARITAS LEADERSHIP IN ACUTE CARE: CREATING A CARING, HEALING ENVIRONMENT

This section describes lessons learned from Caritas Leadership within acute care settings; we explore experiences of nurse leaders in the roles of nurse manager, nurse director, chief nursing officer, or administrators creating a caring, healing environment. After introducing Caritas Leadership in acute care nursing administration, we describe three elements that facilitate Caring Science–informed leaders to create a caring, healing environment for staff and identify six Caritas Processes that serve as building blocks for Caritas Leadership practice.

Leadership is an expression of love and caring. Our leadership matters. Nurse leaders are central to creating caring, healing environments in acute care settings and have an ethical and moral obligation to articulate their contributions as caring practitioners in their organizations. Nurse leaders can create caring, healing environments by grounding their leadership practice within a conceptual framework and solid foundational knowledge of caring in nursing.

Caring Leadership entails embodied, situational, relational, and action-driven practices or interventions (a way of being, knowing, and doing) that facilitate human flourishing for leaders, staff, students, and organizations (Hernandez, 2015). Leaders who practice Caring Leadership find meaning in their work by engaging in self-leadership and loved-based actions, role model by leading the way, developing and empowering others, and demonstrating a deep commitment to creating a humanistic caring culture within their organizations. As a result, these leaders make their staff feel valued, supported, and cared for, positively influencing job enjoyment, satisfaction, and retention. Caring is imperative for highly effective organizations to reach their true potential and inspire leaders to lead with heart, soul, integrity, kindness, and vision, focusing on love and caring as the leading force and economic resource (Hoyle, 2002; Ray, 1987; Watson, 2018).

And yet, our fast-paced, complex, and fragmented healthcare organizations lack humanistic caring, adding an extra layer of complexity and providing new challenges for nurse leaders. The *'Here,'*—that is, the absence of caring, healing environments—are experienced by nurse leaders as "the disconnected, illiterate unconscious actions and practices from a dehumanizing organization hindering the creation of a caring, healing environment" (Hernandez, 2020, pp. 167-168). In these dehumanizing organizations, particularly during intense financial pressures or pandemics emergencies, love and caring are unconsciously and perhaps even unintentionally neglected, overshadowed by attention to "one-size-fits-all," quick solutions, and task-oriented aspects of the business, including leadership practices for the sake of public safety. Leaders practicing in these dehumanizing organizations feel isolated, disconnected from themselves and others, suffer from extreme burnout, and cannot engage deeper in their work, much less contribute to creating caring, healing environments. This neglect gives rise to individuals and organizations losing meaning, purpose, joy, and enthusiasm with their work, and they might stop caring for the people they serve (Hernandez, 2020).

This dehumanization requires a reimagining of conventional organizational structures and a bolder, more intentional approach to nursing administration leadership to meet new challenges (Cara et al., 2011; Spitzer & Kingman, 2011). Bringing a caring, humanistic approach to organizational culture requires a new caring consciousness of nurse leaders in administrative roles who embrace leadership practices supporting their ability to listen to their inner wisdom and acknowledge their interconnectedness by becoming more thoughtful, mindful, intentional, and purposeful in their actions. These Caritas leaders would inspire, strategize, mobilize, nurture, and usher a new era of meaningful healthcare transformation in their organizations, our *'There,'* by fostering deep-rooted "caring, healing" internal and external environments. These caring, healing environments, the *'There,'* are steeped in mutual respect, value for the caregiver, employees' sense of self-fulfillment and well-being, inclusivity of thoughts and ideas, creativity in the workplace, and the commitment to celebrate and develop the potential in every individual

(Hernandez, 2020; Meanger, 2014; Uusiautti, 2013; Williams et al., 2011). Nurse leaders practicing from a Watson Caring Science framework (e.g., Caritas Coaches) might be this new caring and conscious leader positioned to hear the *'There'* call to transform and create caring, healing environments at all levels of their organizations and beyond. Caritas Coach nurse leaders are advanced Caring Science practitioners who live and embody Watson Caring Science and Caritas in healthcare and focus on people in a transpersonal relationship—coach and person being coached (Anderson, 2014).

Watson Caring Science provides a road map for reclaiming the art and science of caring and the healing power of love, compassion, authentic presence, reflection, intentionality, and gratitude in human-to-human encounters (Watson, 2018). Watson Caring Science reconnects nurse leaders with the moral and ethical dimensions of caring in nursing, reminding us of our continued social covenant with the public to advocate for patients and staff alike while preserving their dignity and humanity. Watson Caring Science's humanistic philosophy provides nurse leaders a framework for creating a caring, healing environment in healthcare organizations and focuses on the transpersonal relationship between leaders and others (Watson, 2008, 2012, 2018). Watson's (2008) 10 Caritas Processes offer a framework for nurse leaders' artistic creation of a caring, healing environment and provide the language and ontological literacy for what we do, our way of being, and the environment we choose to create.

**Caritas Process #8** speaks to "creating a healing environment at all levels; subtle environment" (Watson, 2008, p. 129). And in her revised Unitary Caring Science (Caritas-Veritas), "appreciating patterns; re-patterning; radiating energetic heart presence; 'being' the Caritas field" (Watson, 2018, p. 140). In Caritas Process #8, Watson (2008) defines three levels of the healing environment: physical environment, repatterning environment, and nurse as the environment. The first level describes the physical environment, including comfort, privacy, safety, cleanliness, and aesthetic surroundings. The second level serves as an invitation for nurse leaders to use theory as a guide to support the repatterning of the environment by promoting healing, harmony, and the use of caring, healing modalities (i.e., imagery, visualization, relaxation, music-sound, intentional touch, art, etc.) to assist in creating a more caring, healing environment (Watson, 2007, 2008). Lastly, the third level is an expanded view of the environment influenced by Quinn's (1992) "nurse as the environment." This evolved healing environment considers the nurse and their evolved caring consciousness, presence, and intentionality as the crucial ingredients in the environment (Watson, 2002, 2005, 2008, 2018). In the third level of environment, the nurse self is viewed as an energetic, vibrational field, integral with the patient, staff, and external environment. In this evolved caring, healing environment, we move beyond the physical environment (first level) and bring our attention to the nurse leader and their caring consciousness affecting the entire field (Watson, 2007). The nurse leader as the environment, as an evolved environment, is congruent with Quantum Caring Leadership with the energy of Caring and Love as a source for leadership (Watson et al., 2018). So how can Caring Science–informed leaders like Caritas Coaches create a caring, healing environment for their staff? Moreover, what might a model of Caring Science–informed leadership look like?

# CARITAS LEADERSHIP: ENGAGING HEART, HEAD, AND HANDS

Caring Science–informed leaders (Caritas nurse leaders) create a caring, healing environment by engaging the heart, head, and hands as *"the embodied, caring-loving consciousness engaged in informed, moral actions and practices"* (Hernandez, 2020, p. 163). This section describes three elements that Caritas leaders use to create caring, healing environments.

# HEART: NURSE LEADER AS THE ENVIRONMENT

Caring Science–informed nurse leaders engage their hearts by being *the environment.* Caring Science–informed nurse leaders embody and live the Caritas Processes while interacting with the staff and engaged with themselves as individuals. These Caritas nurse leaders are deeply aware of how their energy affects their environment and conduct themselves in ways that elevated the energy field of their environment. Creating a caring, healing environment is about how nurse leaders make their staff feel by engaging in self-caring micropractices, authentic presence, and mindful listening, demonstrating loving attention to themselves and staff (Hernandez, 2020). Watson Caring Science emphasizes caring for the caregiver, permitting nurse leaders to slow down, engage in mindful and intentional self-caring practices, thus becoming better versions of ourselves as we engage with others in our daily interactions. Some self-caring practice interventions include intentional pause, breathing awareness, centering by engaging in prayer or repetition of a sacred phrase or mantra, movement, mindful eating, and gratitude journals. Watson Caring Science allows nurse leaders to love and care for others and, as significantly, allow others to love and care for them. A Caring Science–informed nurse leader recognizes that taking care of themself makes them a more effective and efficient nurse leader in supporting and engaging others to co-create caring, healing environments.

Caring Science–informed leadership practices that create caring, healing environments are a "way of being," encouraging a practice of heart-centered leading to influence change within the organization (Turkel, 2014; Watson, 2009). Caritas nurse leaders are the environment by providing loving attention to the staff by their authentic presence and mindful listening. These nurse leaders demonstrate loving attention by sitting with staff during difficult moments, making themselves available, and engaging in mindful, authentic listening when staff share their stories. A Caring Science–informed leader becomes a mindful listener by listening differently, engaging in purposeful silence, and inviting staff to engage in storytelling. This loving attention allows the nurse leaders to go beyond the surface and become a vessel of love, caring, and healing for the staff. In turn, they allow staff to feel safe; show vulnerability; and be seen, heard, and nonjudged (Hernandez, 2020). Caritas nurse leaders embody caring consciousness by "radiating energetic heart presence and 'being' the Caritas field" (Watson, 2018, p. 140).

## HEAD: INTEGRATION OF THEORY-GUIDED PRACTICES TO REPATTERN THE ENVIRONMENT

Caring Science–informed nurse leaders engage their heads by integrating their in-depth knowledge and understanding of Watson Caring Science to ground their leadership practice in theory to repattern the environment (Hernandez, 2020). Caring Science–informed nurse leaders are open to loving-kindness, compassion, and new creative knowledge inspired by personal, unknown, empirical, ethical, aesthetic, spiritual, sociopolitical, and emancipatory ways of knowing. Caring Science theory-informed practices become the foundation and roadmap for developing, implementing, and evaluating organizational caring hiring practices, annual performance evaluations, self-caring practice interventions, coaching and mentoring relationships, and strategic goal integration (Hernandez, 2020). An example of using Caring Science as a framework to repattern and reimagine the environment is using Caring Science language in job descriptions to articulate expectations of caring behaviors or caring literacy. Nurse leaders design caring hiring practices, including pre-interview coaching and preparation that enhances self-awareness, empowerment, and self-management for potential candidates. In addition, it is essential to employ a holistic approach to the interview experience by being authentically present, inviting deep breathing before the interview begins, and rearranging the interview space to create a more intimate and welcoming environment. Another aspect of creating caring hiring practices includes engaging in holistic interviewing, focusing on questions that provide a whole-person view of the candidate, and noticing how they show up and their way of being. For existing staff, the annual performance evaluation process is transformed into an opportunity to share caring moments that can influence employees' practice quality, establish caring behavioral expectations, and reflect their commitment to creating a caring culture in their units, departments, and organizations (Hernandez, 2020).

Another way Caritas nurse leaders repattern the environment using Caring Science theory-guided practice is by developing self-caring practice interventions or inservices infused with Caring Science for staff. For example, nurse leaders use the 10 Caritas Processes as a template to introduce Watson Caring Science, creating course materials with practical exercises and tools, making Caring Science practice actionable and attainable. Caring Science informs nurse leaders' evolving relationships with staff and colleagues as coaches and mentors by demonstrating authentic presence and authentic listening, and meeting staff where they are to create lasting, caring relationships. Finally, Caritas nurse leaders use Watson Caring Science as a framework to translate caring language and practices in developing and implementing an intentional Caring Science integration plan that incorporates critical strategies in praxis, education, research, and enculturation that aligns with the mission, vision, values, and strategic priorities of their organization. This strategic Caring Science integration plan cascades to all levels of nursing from the boardroom to the bedside. Caritas nurse leaders articulate and advocate for an intentional and mindful pathway for Caring Science and integration of Caring Science into the fabric of their organization, particularly at the executive nursing leadership level, as pivotal to the successful integration and creation of a sustainable caring, healing environment.

## SELF-CARING MICROPRACTICES

- **Authentic presence** can be achieved by engaging in Intentional pause and Breathing awareness—slowing down, bringing focused attention to our breathing, and pausing—this can be done when we wash our hands, before starting a meeting or answering a call, at the beginning and end of any human interaction, before answering emails.

- **Centering**: engaging in ways to remain calm by relaxing, renewing, and refreshing to adjust your environment. The goal of centering is to be in touch with your inner self so that you can cope with the daily stresses that occur at work and at home. You can center by engaging in prayer or repeating a sacred phrase/mantra or reading an inspirational quote.

- **Nurturing Self**: You nurture self by remembering you must pay attention to mind-body-spirit. You can do this my engaging in movement—taking the stairs, taking frequent breaks during the day, going outside, or engaging in Mindful eating (schedule your lunch breaks and do not cancel, do not eat at your desk, have a "no shop talk" rule during lunch).

- **Gratitude journals**: Using journals as a tool for reflection and appreciation for the day allows us to shift our focus to look for the positive in our lives. Journaling can be done as a narrative of the day, writing one or two examples of what we were grateful for, drawing how our day went, or writing a poem. A gratitude journal allows us to use multiple ways of knowing and engage in creative/aesthetic expressions.

# HANDS: CREATING PHYSICAL OR EXTERNAL CARING, HEALING ENVIRONMENTS

Caring Science–informed nurse leaders engage their hands by *creating physical or external caring, healing environments* providing comfort measures that support and protect staff in their areas of work, psychological safety, privacy, and aesthetic surroundings (Hernandez, 2020). For example, nurse leaders promote comfort measures by encouraging the creation of renewal room and proactively promoting staff self-caring practices. These renewal rooms allow the staff to take their breaks uninterrupted while enjoying soothing music, massage chairs, or simple relaxation techniques. Offering designated spaces for staff to take their breaks and re-focus during their shift can help reduce staff daily stressors and support self-caring practices (Andrus, 2016; Crewe, 2016; Hernandez, 2020; Shanahan et al., 2016).

Another way Caritas nurse leaders create a physical/external caring, healing environment is by promoting psychological safety and privacy; building trusting relationships for staff in their units and departments; and supporting their well-being and protecting human dignity. Some examples include "re-arranging the physical environment to provide dedicated space to mourn, promoting team cohesion and a work-family atmosphere" (Hernandez, 2020, p. 143). Caring Science–informed nurse leaders engage in the creative use of self and multiple ways of knowing to mobilize resources to provide shift coverage for staff needing to go home and providing in-person or virtual check-ins as part of their daily leadership practice (Hernandez, 2020). Psychological safety and building trusting, caring relationships are achieved by creating team cohesion and a home-like atmosphere at work, encouraging milestone celebrations and team-inspired events at work and outside work. Caritas nurse leaders used their direct report meetings, inservices, nursing forums, and rounding with staff as opportunities to engage them in "meaningful, authentic, caring conversations" (Hernandez, 2020, p. 148) and role model this behavior as an expectation of how to engage with the staff and others in their daily interactions. Lastly, Caritas nurse leaders can promote shared governance by engaging staff in designing new hospital buildings and finding creative ways to reaffirm their commitment to Caring Science and humanistic care by placing life-affirming and inspirational messages in inpatient rooms, nursing stations, or handwashing stations, fostering group identification and empowerment.

Caring Science nurse leaders are open, accessible, and take advantage of their routine check-ins and daily huddles with staff to get to know them personally and build trusting relationships, thus identifying basic staff needs like when staff need to go home to attend to a sick child or parent or are too distraught to care for another patient after a death event. This level of personal insight and awareness from nurse leaders creates an environment where staff feel safe sharing their feelings without judgment and feel supported by leadership and the rest of the team (Hernandez, 2020). This inclusive leadership can help reduce psychological distress for staff by creating a psychologically safe environment, encouraging belonging, and valuing their uniqueness (Carmeli et al., 2010; Hirak et al., 2012; Randel et al., 2018; Zhao et al., 2020).

# 10 CARITAS PROCESSES: ESSENTIAL BUILDING BLOCKS FOR CARITAS LEADERSHIP PRACTICE

Hernandez (2020) identified six Caritas Processes as essential building blocks for Caring Science–informed leaders to create caring, healing environments for staff (Watson, n.d.):

1. **Embrace** (Practice of Loving-Kindness)

2. **Inspire** (Faith-Hope, being authentically present)

3. **Trust** (Transpersonal presence; cultivating own spiritual practices)

4. **Nurture** (Trusting, caring relationships)

5. **Forgive** (Authentically listening to another person's story)

6. **Deepen** (Creatively problem-solving, "solution-seeking"; creative use of self and all ways of knowing/being/doing/becoming)

These Caritas-in-action practices allow nurse leaders to reflect on their actions and make decisions as they move from the dominant '*Here*' to '*There,*' engaging deeply in the work of elevating caring consciousness to their practice and organizational structure and processes. Caring Science–informed nurse leaders communicate heart-centered vision and exhibit loved-filled, theory-guided actions and behaviors that promote an environment of mutual connection for leaders and staff alike (Hernandez, 2020). They do this by engaging in practices to get to know the staff as unique individuals, identifying their gifts and inspiring them to use their skills and talents to achieve personal and organizational goals. The embodiment of Caring Science–informed leadership reflects an evolved caring, healing environment framework that considers the nurse leader and their evolved caring consciousness, presence, and intentionality as vital ingredients in the environment (Watson, 2008). Moreover, the Caring Science journey extends beyond our professional nursing leadership practice into personal experiences, transforming the way we view our world. A leadership practice rooted in Watson Caring Science helps reframe and make sense of commitment and passion, and it transforms our lives.

The next section will focus on Caring Science leadership within another domain of nursing practice: the academy embracing both education and research.

# ACADEMIC CARITAS LEADERSHIP: LESSONS LEARNED FROM NURSING EDUCATION AND RESEARCH

This section describes lessons learned from Caritas Leadership within the academy; we explore experiences within both nursing education and research. Being an academic requires that nursing professors contribute to the development of nursing's disciplinary knowledge (research and scholarship) and teach in post-secondary education that disseminates our disciplinary knowledge in a way that encourages students and developing scholars to find their understandings, their perspectives, and their voice. After introducing academic Caritas Leadership, we describe some lessons learned, followed by an exemplar of the lesson—an experience one of us (Dr. Hills) has had while facilitating learning or engaging in nursing education and nursing research. We then link those lessons to Watson's Caritas Processes. We describe three lessons: 1) Have an unyielding trust that "people are able," 2) Develop allies and collaboration, 3) Seize the opportunity, push the door open and step in.

# ACADEMIC CARITAS LEADERSHIP

Leadership is often considered a process to influence others toward a common goal. Literature pertaining to "caring leadership" has been primarily discussed in relation to clinical healthcare and organizations (Boykin et al., 2014; Brousseau et al., 2017; Levay & Andersson Bäck, 2021; Saks, 2021; Solbakken et al., 2018; Watson et al., 2018). For example, in their meta-ethnography, Solbakken et al. (2018) concluded that "caring in nursing leadership means nurturing and growing relationships to safeguard the best nursing" (p. E1). Moreover, they explain that a caring leader must inspire, motivate, dialogue, guide, and teach their staff to foster quality patient care (Solbakken et al., 2018). In her work, Boykin (2012, p. 1) describes caring-based leadership as "a commitment by nurse leaders to use caring to guide all decisions that he or she makes with the intention to create, maintain and sustain environments where nurses can truly nurse. In these environments, nurses feel nurtured and can respond to the calls for nursing in their unique way." Overall, Brousseau et al. (2017) consider caring favorable to nursing leadership because underlining management practices from a humanistic perspective fosters professional growth and development. In fact, according to Watson et al. (2018, p. 256), a caring leadership aims "to honor social mandates to sustain human dignity and human-organizational, dynamic evolution." Nonetheless, to our knowledge, little literature has addressed Caritas Leadership in the academic realm of nursing.

What does it mean to be a Caritas leader in the academy? We believe that academic Caritas leaders lead with kindness, passion, humility, and engagement; they listen to, value, and trust people to enable educational and organizational humanization for all—students, staff members, nurse educators, faculty, and faculty managers. They are also invited to develop a sophisticated caring and critical consciousness to "read" the situation in its full illumination. Understanding the status quo and what supports it is essential in Caritas Leadership.

Being and becoming informed by reflective practice and critical consciousness, Caritas Leadership in the academy is founded on an understanding of "caring as a moral imperative to act ethically and justly" (Hills et al., 2021, p. 133). Although we believe that caring is the ethical, ontological, and epistemological foundation of nursing, we are concerned that, as a discipline, nursing continues to be embedded in a behaviorist, biomedical, positivist reductionist paradigm. Unfortunately, this seems to be true in all aspects of nursing—practice, education, administration, and research. As Watson (2012) declares,

> It is critical for nursing … to be clear about sustaining a meaningful ethical, philosophical foundation … lest we lose our way in this chaotic, post-modern era of change … Nurses now are invited to become visionary leaders … [and] shape international transformative worldview change, rather than conform to outdated modes that no longer work. (p. 3)

Caritas Leadership in the academy is grounded on a relational ontology, especially in educational, research, and sociopolitical domains, crucial to advance nursing as both a discipline and a profession. In other words, Caritas leaders are authentic and congruent in their words and actions. They need to be social activists, inspiring, collaborating, sojourning with others—students, nurse educators, professors, administrators, community, government, and decision-makers—in their co-created transformative learning journey. As Brousseau and Cara (2021, p. 179) uphold, "political skills and emancipatory power of influence rooted in humanism can only contribute to creating a better environment for the future of nursing education as well as the global nursing profession."

In this section, we describe three lessons that we have learned from our experiences with Caritas Leadership.

## LESSON 1: HAVE AN UNYIELDING TRUST THAT "PEOPLE ARE ABLE"

Being an effective Caritas leader requires that we hold, maintain, and sustain a deep commitment to the belief that *people are able*. So often in nursing leadership, we, as nurses, want to control the situation by telling others what steps we are going to take to meet our goals. Creating a process that honors and encourages people's capacities to be empathic, respectful, caring, compassionate, authentic, and willing and able to express their positive and negative feelings and speak to inequities and inequalities, requires a complex integration of Caritas literacy and capacities.

Caritas leaders have a deep belief that people know what is best for them. Because nurses have a comprehensive understanding of health, diseases, illness, and healing, it is often difficult for them to step back or step forward to "allow" patients/clients to make decisions about their health and healthcare options/decisions. This is also true in the academy for nurse educators/researchers. Therefore, Caritas leaders advocate for this liberation for people. They understand that when people have engaged in decision-making about their own health/education, they are more likely to adhere to the goals they set for themselves.

For instance, in a Canadian federally funded project, "In From the Margins: A Collaborative Action to Improve Access to Appropriate Health Services for Indigenous People Living with HIV, AIDS and Substance Misuse," the research team was committed to truly "hear" the story of Indigenous community members. The team held a focus group (research language) or "firepit" (Indigenous language) at the new Primary Health Care (PHC) facility that was developed and funded by the government to support access to healthcare for Indigenous community members. The research team discovered that only 30% of the community accessing this facility were Indigenous. The team pursued the issue and discovered that Indigenous people did not feel welcomed or safe at the PHC center. The community members reported that no one greeted them; no one offered them coffee, tea, or water; no one guided them. They weren't sure what to do or when their appointment actually was. The research team learned so much from one meeting and made changes immediately because of the methodology used, Collaborative Action Research and Evaluation (CARE). Being interested in people's ideas acknowledges that they are able and know what is best for themselves. As a result, the PHC management hired an Indigenous greeter; put coffee, tea, and water in the waiting room; and removed the plexiglass that shielded the nursing station from the clients.

A key strategy in this collaborative research design is to act, make changes, and monitor the impact of the change strategies. In other words, you do not wait to do a post-test, as in orthodox research. You make changes as soon as you understand the "challenge" as a team. An unexpected outcome when the plexiglass was removed was that all the nurses quit! Of course, initially, this was shocking, but we soon realized this was an opportunity. These nurses were uncomfortable working with Indigenous people without what they perceived as the protection of the plexiglass. The management team hired new nurses, and employment criteria ensured that these nurses were comfortable in an open, inviting, and welcoming environment.

From this exemplar, we are reminded notably of **Caritas Process #8**, "Creating a healing environment at all levels; subtle environment for energic authentic caring presence" (Watson, n.d.). By paying attention to the environment, the research team not only demonstrated their concern for the community's safety, health promotion, and accessibility to healthcare but also engaged in social action as they encouraged the management team to greet clients at the door into a more welcoming and open environment and transform their staff's nursing practice in the community. In other words, nurse educators/researchers, as Caritas leaders, assist managers in their journey from '*Here*' to '*There*' to transform the healthcare delivery system.

Informed by this Caritas Process, nurses from the PHC center participating in this research project, while engaging in an "authentic caring presence" (Watson, n.d.), encouraged clients to feel safe, comfortable, and reassured within the healthcare environment. Such an authentic caring presence invites nurses to consider their clients as *being able* and respect, support, and protect their clients' human dignity.

Lastly, all research team members acknowledged that they were all part of this physical environment. As Watson (2008) explains,

> Holding authentic, heartfelt, positive thoughts such as loving-kindness, caring, healing, forgiveness, and so forth, vibrates at a higher level than

having lower thoughts, such as competition, fear, greed, anxiety, hostility … the entire field can be and is being repatterned by the nurse's consciousness… the *Caritas Nurse … Becomes* the environment, affecting the entire field. (p. 140)

## LESSON 2: DEVELOP ALLIES AND COLLABORATION (IN PRACTICE, IN POLICY, IN RESEARCH, IN EDUCATION)

Developing relationships with others is a critical component of Caritas Leadership in the academy. Of course, this takes time, but there are strategies that Caritas leaders use to ensure that leadership is relationship-based—for example, purposely discussing what ideas and values team members can be counted on to hold throughout a collaborative effort. Creating a shared vision based on the group's values is an effective strategy in articulating a futuristic perspective of where you want to go together—getting from '*Here*' to '*There*.' For nursing education, we can ask, "How do nurses need *to be* in order to practice nursing in" 10 years? "What do nurses need *to know* to practice nursing in" 10 years? "What do nurses need to be able *to do* to practice nursing" in 10 years? (Hills et al., 2021, p. 160; italics by authors). These futuristic reflective questions serve as a strategy to create the structure and design of Caring Science nursing programs.

Another critical aspect of developing allies and collaboration is that Caritas leaders are aware of their strengths and surround themselves with others with complementary capacities. For example, some nurse educators/researchers think, read, and understand "the big picture" first; others automatically see and focus on a situation or development details. Hence, Caritas leaders who surround themselves with people who have different and complementary capacities are better able to explore many perspectives.

Caritas leaders in the academy embrace collaboration. Historically, the following definition was created by one of the authors when she was involved in a deeply collaborative Caring Science nursing curriculum development project that required a more nuanced understanding of collaboration beyond the traditional definitions. Historically, as Hills (1992) explains,

> Collaboration is the creation of a synergistic alliance that honours and utilizes each person's contribution in order to create collective wisdom and collective action. Collaboration is not synonymous with co-operation, partnership, participation, or compromise. Those words do not convey the fundamental importance of being 'in relationship' nor the depth of caring and commitment that is needed to create the kind of reciprocity that is collaboration. Collaborators are committed to, care about and trust in each other. They recognize that, despite their differences, each has unique and valuable knowledge, perspectives, and experiences to contribute to the collaboration. (p. 14)

This definition has been used extensively and is meaningful in all forms of Caritas Leadership (Cara et al., 2021; Hills, 2016; Hills & Watson, 2011; Hills et al., 2021).

One of the first activities that Caritas leaders engage their team in is the co-creation of a shared vision. Know where you want to go together—from '*Here*' to '*There*.' Seeing into the future requires a caring commitment to others and a deep trust in the collaborative process as a shared caring journey (Hills et al., 2021). This means working from a perspective of love, not fear. Caritas leaders are not ego involved, and they know how to engage every member of the team as they work and arrive together at the top of a plateau—a flat surface where there is room for everyone. It is not about one person—the leader—arriving at the top of the mountain and being revered. We conceptualize this process as "leading from beside" (Hills, 2016).

For this exemplar, many of the Caritas Processes come to mind. The one that we wish to highlight in this chapter is **Caritas Process #7**: "Engaging in transpersonal teaching and learning within the context of a caring relationship; staying within other's frame of reference—shift toward coaching model for expanded health/wellness" (Watson, n.d.).

For example, to develop this Collaborative Caring Curriculum, Caritas leaders needed to consider all actors' perceptions and past experiences and their meanings to collaboratively engage and commit to a shared vision regarding the transformation's insight for their nursing undergraduate programs. Moreover, Caritas leaders were required to be sensitive and conscious of each college's "frame of reference" to assist them in revolutionizing their academic practice from 'Here' to 'There.' Without this approach, some colleges might have been less likely to engage in the Caring Science Curriculum transformation throughout the province (Hills et al., 1994).

Naturally, to be successful in such a transformative academic journey, **Caritas Process #4**, "Developing and sustaining loving, trusting-caring relationships" (Watson, n.d.), is primordial. Being informed by this fourth Caritas Process reminds us that nursing is a fundamentally relational discipline and profession (Cara et al., 2021; Hills et al., 2021; Létourneau et al., 2017; Watson, 2018). Additionally, all members of the collaborative team "can come to realize that they share each other's journey, toward learning, development, transformation, and empowerment" (Cara et al., 2021, p. 118). As McDowell et al. (2013) explain, relying on Watson's fourth Caritas Process, "cultivating these caring-helping-trusting relationships with self and others is an integral part of caring leadership and is vital in encouraging the heart of those for whom ...we are privileged to lead" (p. 50).

## LESSON 3: SEIZE THE OPPORTUNITY, PUSH THE DOOR OPEN AND STEP IN...

Caritas leaders in academia can "see" opportunities. Although many systems and organizations have rigid rules and regulations, often there is a "crack" where the light pours in. In a sense, Caritas leaders recognize "cracks" as opportunities, and they step in. They embrace equity, facilitate and advocate for others to develop their voice. Caritas leaders encourage others to speak their truth, creating opportunities for others to claim their power. They can engage in critical dialogue because they have developed a critical caring consciousness that allows them to see the hegemony and create counter-hegemony (Hills et al., 2021). Understanding hegemony requires Caritas leaders to understand power relations. To understand that there is always a choice about how to use your power. Caritas leaders always choose "power with" relationships and speak out when they encounter inequities, "power over," uncaring or disrespectful situations. As Shor and Freire (1987) explain, to be silent is not a neutral position. It actually endorses this hegemony: "Washing one's hands of the conflict of the powerful and the powerless means to side with the powerful, not to be neutral" (p. x). This is a precious mantra that Caritas leaders live by.

In 2019, three of the authors were engaged in the development of the 6th International Caring Conference. We engaged the local health authority who supported and sponsored the conference. We recognized very early that we did not want this initiative to be a "one-off" event. So, we decided to develop a "sustainable project" to maximize the impact of the conference on healthcare systems. After the conference, we initiated a Systems Change research project entitled *Reawakening a Culture of Caring in Healthcare Systems: Nurses Leading Health and Social Change*. We received funding and established a partnership research team consisting of faculty members and health authorities, leaders, administrators, clinical nurse leaders, and clinical nurse educators. We completed the pilot project by holding focus groups consisting of teams of clinical nurse leaders and educators. Each team outlined an action project that they thought would "reawaken the caring culture" in their unit. The research team created three modules on Caring Science and Collaborative Action Research and Evaluation (CARE), which develops research and caring capacities and literacy for nurses in practice. We are ready now to apply for a larger grant to expand the project.

To be an effective and successful academic Caritas leader, one needs to be able to see opportunities. Often people in authority open "a crack" in the door, and then

Caritas leaders can see the light that the "crack" lets in, and they step into that light. They have the confidence and courage to raise their voices in acts of advocacy and addressing inequities. Nurses for years have expressed concern about the lack of caring and compassion in healthcare systems. This project is designed for academics to collaborate with them so that nurses can lead the changes needed to reawaken a culture of caring in healthcare. Rather than continuing with our "sickness care" focus on diseases, academics collaborating with nurses in practice assist in putting "health" and "caring" back into "healthcare." This is another example of moving from 'Here' to 'There' by collaborating to develop Caritas Leadership within healthcare systems by moving outside the academy.

Pertaining to this exemplar, we are informed notably by **Caritas Process #6,** "creatively problem-solving 'solution-seeking' through the caring process; full use of self and artistry of caring-healing practices via the use of all ways of knowing/being/doing/becoming" (Watson, n.d.).

Guided by this Caritas Process, academic Caritas leaders were engaged to truly understand the situation, including its opportunities and challenges, using all "ways of knowing" to decide the best administrative, practice, political, and academic strategies as social activists in transforming healthcare systems. Caritas leaders were invited to know themselves and others as caring persons to "seek new solutions" to challenges, difficulties, and problems from a Caring Science perspective. They especially used a focus group strategy to collaborate and get to know each other's perspectives.

Needless to say, as Watson explains:

> The complexity of decision making and acting within *Caritas Processes* requires critical thinking, clarity of rationale, and use of scientific evidence; but it also demands ... creative, integrative, critical thinking necessary for engaging in a systematic, synthesized problem-solving focus for an individualized [project]... (Watson, 2008, p. 114).

All 10 Caritas Processes have been guiding the Caritas team in their leadership journey by offering them a philosophical-theoretical-ethical-epistemological-ontological to guide their academic praxis.

# IMPLICATIONS FOR PRACTICE

Although we believe that caring is the ethical foundation of nursing, we are concerned that, as a discipline, nursing continues to be embedded in a behaviorist, biomedical, positivist, reductionist paradigm. Unfortunately, this seems to be true in all aspects of nursing—practice, education, administration, and research. As Watson (2012) declares,

> It is critical for nursing ...to be clear about sustaining a meaningful, ethical, philosophical foundation...lest we lose our way in this post-modern era of change...Nurses now are invited to become visionary leaders...[and] shape international transformative worldview change rather than conform to outdated modes that no longer work. (p. 3)

For significant change to occur, for us to get from 'Here' to 'There,' we need to mentor our Caritas leaders to work together and with others to embrace this type of leadership. Nurses can no longer sit on the sidelines. They are invited to seize the opportunity to lead and change these conventional, outdated systems and structures.

We believe that once you have committed, everything else follows. So many times, we are told that things won't work. We need more money, resources, or people involved. This keeps us stuck in the 'Here.' From our experiences, commitment comes first. As Johann Wolfgang Von Goethe, a famous German poet, and writer, once explained:

> Until one is committed, there is hesitancy, the chance to draw back, always ineffectiveness, concerning all acts of initiative (and creation).

There is one elementary truth, the ignorance of which kills countless ideas and splendid plans: that the moment that one definitely commits oneself, then Providence moves too. All sorts of things occur in one's favour that would never otherwise have occurred. A whole stream of events issues from the decision, raising in one's favour all manner of unforeseen incidents and meetings and material assistance which no man could have dreamed would come his way. Whatever you can do or dream, you can begin it. Boldness has genius, power, and magic in it. Begin it now!

# SUMMARY

We invite all nurses to develop their Caritas Leadership to move from '*Here*' to '*There*,' to engage in a worldview shift from an organization focused on bureaucracy to one dedicated to moving all nursing domains to embrace a Caring Science philosophy, ethic, ontology, and epistemology—to move nursing practice, administration, sociopolitical action, education, and research from reductionist, biomedical perspectives to a holistic Caring Science way of being, knowing, and doing that emancipates nurses to Become the way nurses long to be.

# REFLECTIVE QUESTIONS

1.  How is Caritas Leadership visible in your practice? What more can you do?

2.  What distinguishes Caritas/Caring Science–informed leadership from conventional patterns of leadership?

3.  How do Caritas leaders create a caring, healing environment?

4.  Why is it essential for an academic Caritas leader to trust that *people are able?*

5.  How would you describe Caritas leaders in the academy?

## NARRATIVE

### GROUP CIRCLE/GUIDED DIALOGUE ACTIVITY

Create a healing space for a group to gather in person or virtually. Engage in a centering exercise such as lighting a candle/flameless candle and intentional breathing awareness. Engage in any micropractice that can create a safe space for participants (e.g., inspirational reading).

In a group circle format of two or more, reflect on your individual, current nursing leadership experiences and invite participants to share how they are integrating and/or how they can begin to integrate Caring Science–informed leadership practices.

### ADDITIONAL SUGGESTIONS

Group facilitators are invited to use the reflective questions provided above to guide the dialogue.

Create a word cloud with the practices identified and share with each participant as a visual reminder of their commitment to Caring Leadership.

# AUTHOR BIOGRAPHIES

**Grissel Hernandez, PhD, RN, MPH, HNB-BC, NPD-BC, SGAHN,** is Executive Director, Center for Education and Professional Development, Stanford Health Care, and Faculty Associate, Watson Caring Science Institute. She coordinates the integration plan of Watson's Caring Science theory into practice, education, leadership, and research initiatives. She has over 20 years of Nursing Professional Development experience in ANCC Magnet and the Malcolm Baldrige National Quality Award designated organizations. Her qualitative research study aimed to describe and understand the lived experience of nurse leaders practicing within Watson Caring Science framework (Caritas Coaches), creating a caring, healing environment for staff. Hernandez is board-certified in Holistic Nursing by AHNCC, board-certified Nursing Professional Development by ANCC, Watson Caring Science Caritas Coach, and a Global Academy of Holistic Nursing Scholar. In addition, she is a board member of the International Association of Human Caring (IAHC), Watson Caring Science Institute, American Holistic Nursing Credentialing Corporation (AHNCC), and member of the AHNCC Committee on Equity, Diversity, Inclusion, and Social Justice (EIDSJ). Hernandez is currently completing her post-doctoral studies with Jean Watson.

**Marcia Hills, PhD, RN, FAAN, CFAN,** Professor and Associate Director, Research & Scholarship, School of Nursing, University of Victoria, British Columbia (BC), Canada, is an international scholar in Caring Science nursing education, curriculum and pedagogy, health promotion, and Collaborative Action Research & Evaluation (CARE). She was inducted into the American Academy of Nursing in 2012 and the Canadian Academy of Nursing in 2020. Hills has distinguished herself as: BC Collaborative Nursing Program Founding Director—the first Caring Science nursing program in Canada; Canadian Consortium for Health Promotion Research (CCHPR) President; Watson Caring Science Institute Distinguished Scholar of Caring Science, Faculty Associate, and Doctoral Program Academic Lead; and Global Alliance for Human Caring Education Founder/President. She has published three books on Caring Science nursing education and consulted extensively in the USA, the UK, New Zealand, Australia, Trinidad and Tobago, Kenya, Brazil, Chile, and Canada in the areas of: health promotion, primary healthcare, emancipatory caring curriculum and pedagogy, and CARE.

**Chantal Cara, PhD, RN, FAAN, FCAN,** Full professor, Université de Montréal, Distinguished Caring Science Scholar, Watson Caring Science Institute, invited professor/caring scholar, University of Colorado, USA, invited professor, Institut et Haute École La Source, Suisse Researcher, RRISIQ and CRIR, is a renowned bilingual expert in the field of Human Caring and a Visiting Caring Science Scholar/Professor at the University of Colorado and at the Haute École LaSource in Switzerland. For 30 years, Cara has been actively involved in the advancement of Human Caring in both French and English communities. Her numerous publications and conferences reflect her disciplinary commitment and leadership to advance humanization in both nursing education and healthcare. Moreover, she has co-authored, under Springer, two books on Caring Science and nursing education. Recently, she was a awarded the honorific titles of Distinguished Caring Science Scholar by the Watson Caring Science Institute, Fellow of the American Academy of Nursing, as well as Fellow of the Canadian Academy of Nursing.

**Jean Watson, PhD, RN, AHN-BC, HSGAHN, FAAN, LL (AAN),** is Distinguished Professor and Dean Emerita, University of Colorado College of Nursing Anschutz Medical Center, USA; founder of the original Center for Human Caring in Colorado; a Fellow of the American Academy of Nursing (FAAN); Founder and Director of nonprofit organization, Watson Caring Science Institute; past President of the National League for Nursing; founding member of International Association in Human Caring and International Caritas Consortium. She held the nation's first endowed chair in Caring Science for 16 years and holds 15 Honorary Doctoral Degrees, including 12 International Honorary Doctorates. Her work is studied and implemented around the world. A recipient of many awards and honors, she has authored or co-authored over 30 books on caring. Watson is designated as a *Living Legend* by the American Academy of Nursing, its highest honor, and an Honorary Scholar for the Global Academy of Holistic Nursing.

# REFERENCES

Anderson J. (2014). *Exploring application of the caritas coach role in nursing practice* [Unpublished dissertation]. Nova Southeastern University.

Andrus, V. (2016). *Cultivating mindfulness in nursing practice and self-care*. https://learn.ana-nursingknowledge.org/products/Cultivating-Mindfulness

Boykin, A. (2012). *Caring-based nursing leadership*. https://www.emergingrnleader.com/caringnursingleadership/

Boykin, A., & Schoenhofer, A., & Valentine, K. (2014). *Health care system transformation for nursing and health care leaders: Implementing a culture of caring*. Springer Publishing Company.

Brousseau, S., & Cara, C. (2021). Nurse educators' Political Caring Literacy and power to promote caring relationships in nursing education. In C. Cara, M. Hills, & J. Watson, *An educator's guide to humanizing nursing education: Grounded in Caring Science* (pp. 161–182). Springer.

Brousseau, S., Cara, C., & Blais, R. (2017). A Humanistic Caring Quality of Work-Life Model in Nursing Administration Based on Watson's Philosophy. *International Journal for Human Caring, 21*(1), 2–8. Doi.org/10.20467/1091-5710-21.1.2

Cara, C., Hills, M., & Watson, J. (2021). *An Educator's Guide to Humanizing Nursing Education: Grounded in Caring Science*. Springer.

Cara, C. M., Nyberg, J. J., & Brousseau, S. (2011). Fostering the coexistence of caring philosophy and economics in today's health care system. *Nursing Administration Quarterly, 35*(1), 6–14. Doi: 10.1097/naq.0b013e3182048c10

Carmeli, A., Reiter-Palmon, R., & Ziv, E. (2010). Inclusive leadership and employee involvement in creative tasks in the workplace: The mediating role of psychological safety. *Creativity Research Journal, 22*(3), 250–260. doi.org/10.1080/10400419.2010.504654

Crewe, C. D. (2016). *The Watson room: Managing compassion fatigue in clinical nurses on the front line* [Doctoral dissertation]. Walden University.

Hernandez, G. (2015). *Meta-synthesis in caring leadership: Reclaiming humanistic caring in nursing leadership*. Unpublished publication. University of Colorado.

Hernandez, G. (2020). The Lived experience of nurse leaders practicing within Watson Caring Science framework creating a caring, healing environment for staff [Unpublished dissertation]. University of Colorado Anschutz Medical Campus. https://hdl.handle.net/10968/6024

Hills, M. (1992). *Collaborative nursing program of BC: Development of a generic integrated nursing curriculum with four partner colleges*. Report to the Ministry of Advanced Education. Centre for Curriculum and Professional Development.

Hills, M. (2016). Emancipatory and collaborative: Leading from beside. In W. Rosa (Ed.), *Nurses as leaders: Evolutionary visions of leadership* (pp. 293–309). Springer Publishing Company.

Hills, M., Lindsey, E., Chisamore, M., Basset-Smith, J., Abbott, K., & Fournier-Chalmers, J. (1994). University-college collaboration: Rethinking curriculum development in nursing education. *The Journal of Nursing Education, 33*(5), 220–225. doi.org/10.3928/0148-4834-19940501-07

Hills, M., & Watson, J. (2011). *Creating a Caring Science curriculum: An emancipatory pedagogy for nursing*. Springer Publishing Company.

Hills, M., Watson, J., & Cara, C. (2021). *Creating a Caring Science Curriculum: A Relational Emancipatory Pedagogy for Nursing*. Springer.

Hirak, R., Peng, A. C., Carmeli, A., & Schaubroeck, J. M. (2012). Linking leader inclusiveness to work unit performance: The importance of psychological safety and learning from failures. *The Leadership Quarterly, 23*(1), 107–117. https://doi.org/10.1016/j.leaqua.2011.11.009

Hoyle, J. R. (2002). *Leadership and the force of love: Six keys to motivating with love*. Corwin Press.

Létourneau, D., Cara, C., & Goudreau, J. (2017). Humanizing Nursing Care: An Analysis of Caring Theories Through the Lens of Humanism. *International Journal for Human Caring, 21*(1), 32–40. doi: 10.20467/1091-5710-21.1.32

Levay, C., & Andersson Bäck, M. (2021). Caring Leader Identity Between Power and Powerlessness. *Organizations Studies, 00*(0), 1–20. doi.org/10.1177/01708406211006245

McDowell, J. B., Williams, R. L. II, Kautz, D. D. (2013). Teaching the core values of caring leadership. *International Journal for Human Caring, 17*(4), 43–51. https://iafhc.wildapricot.org/page-18066

Meanger, V. C. (2014). *Organizational climate and the theory of human caring in hospitals* (Doctoral dissertation, Walden University).

Quinn, J. F. (1992). Holding sacred space: The nurse as healing environment. *Holistic Nursing Practice* 6(4), 26–36. doi: 10.1097/00004650-199207000-00007

Randel, A. E., Galvin, B. M., Shore, L. M., Ehrhart, K. H., Chung, B. G., Dean, M. A., & Kedharnath, U. (2018). Inclusive leadership: Realizing positive outcomes through belongingness and being valued for uniqueness. *Human Resource Management Review, 28*(2), 190–203. Doi.org/10.1016/j.hrmr.2017.07.002

Ray, M. A. (1987). Health care economics and human caring in nursing: Why the moral conflict must be resolved. *Family Community Health, 10*(1), 35–43. doi: 10.1097/00003727-198705000-00007

Saks, A. M. (2021). A model of caring in organizations for human resource development. *Human Resource Development Review, 20*(3), 1–33. https://doi.org/10.1177/15344843211024035

Shanahan, M. M., Novack, G., & Andrus, V. L. (2016). *Fostering nurse renewal through compassion: A model for alleviating nurse workplace stress.* https://sigma.nursingrepository.org/handle/10755/621569

Shor, I., & Freire, P. (1987). *A pedagogy for liberation: Dialogues on transforming education.* Bergin & Garvey.

Solbakken, R., Bergdahl, E., Rudolfsson, G., & Bondas, T. (2018). International nursing caring in nursing leadership—A meta-ethnography from the nurse leader's perspective. *Nursing Administration Quarterly, 42*(4), E1–E19. doi: 10.1097/NAQ.0000000000000314

Spitzer, R., & Kingman, R. (2011). Caring and compassion, leadership essentials. *Nurse Leader, 9*(3), 6–7. doi: 10.1016/j.mnl/2011.03.009

Turkel, M. C. (2014). Leading from the heart: Caring, love, peace, and values guiding leadership. *Nursing Science Quarterly, 27*(2), 172–177. Doi.org/10.1177/0894318414522663

Uusiautti, S. (2013). An action-oriented perspective on caring leadership: A qualitative study of higher education administrators' positive leadership experiences. *International Journal of Leadership in Education, 16*(4), 482–496. Doi.org/10.1080/13603124.2013.770077

Watson, J. (n.d.). *10 Caritas Processes TM.* Watson Caring Science Institute. https://www.watsoncaringscience.org/jean-bio/caring-science-theory/10-caritas-processes/

Watson, J. (2002). Intentionality and caring, healing consciousness: A practice of transpersonal nursing. *Holistic Nursing Practice, 16*(4), 12–19. Doi: 10.1097/00004650-200207000-00005

Watson, J. (2005). *Caring Science as sacred science.* F.A. Davis Co.

Watson, J. (2007). Watson's theory of human caring and subjective living experiences: Carative factors/Caritas processes as a disciplinary guide to the professional nursing practice. *Texto & Contexto - Enfermagem, 16*, 129–135. doi.org/10.1590/S0104-07072007000100016

Watson, J. (2008). *Nursing: The philosophy and science of caring.* Revised new edition. University of Colorado Press.

Watson, J. (2009). Caring Science and human caring theory: Transforming personal and professional practices of nursing and health care. *Journal of Health and Human Services Administration, 31*(4), 466–482. PMID: 19385422.

Watson, J. (2012). *Human Caring Science. A theory of nursing.* Jones & Bartlett Learning.

Watson, J. (2017). Global advances in human caring literacy. In S. Lee, P. Palmieri, & J. Watson (Eds.), *Global advances in human caring literacy* (pp. 3–13). Springer.

Watson, J. (2018). *Unitary Caring Science. The philosophy and praxis of nursing.* University Press of Colorado.

Watson, J. (2019) Nursing's global covenant with humanity: Unitary Caring Science as sacred activism. *Journal of Advanced Nursing, 76*(2), 699–704. doi: 10.1111/JAN.13934

Watson, J., Porter-O'Grady, T., Horton-Deutsch, S., & Malloch, K. (2018). Quantum caring leadership: Integrating quantum leadership with Caring Science. *Nursing Science Quarterly, 31*(3), 253–258. doi: 10.1177/0894318418774893

Williams, R. L., McDowell, J. B., & Kautz, D. D. (2011). A caring leadership model for nursing's future. *International Journal for Human Caring, 15*(1), 31–35. https://iafhc.wildapricot.org/page-18066

Zhao, F., Ahmed, F., & Faraz, N. A. (2020). Caring for the caregiver during COVID-19 outbreak: Does inclusive leadership improve psychological safety and curb psychological distress? A cross-sectional study. *International Journal of Nursing Studies, 110*, 103725, 1–11. Doi.org/10.1016/j.ijnurstu.2020.103725

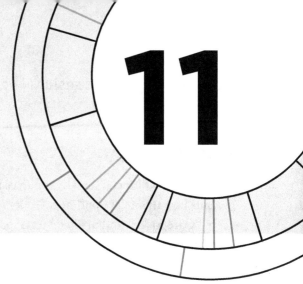

# 11

# PROMOTING EXCEPTIONAL PATIENT EXPERIENCE THROUGH COMPASSIONATE CONNECTED CARE

Mary Jo Assi, DNP, RN, NEA-BC, FAAN
Senem Guney, PhD

## LEARNING OBJECTIVES

After completing this chapter, readers will:

- Understand a data-driven model of human caring: the Compassionate Connected Care model

- Comprehend AI-enabled insights into human caring from patients' perspectives

- Explain leadership's roles in maximizing patients' voice through patients' experience

# OVERVIEW

This chapter will focus on why compassion, empathy, and caring are critical components of patient care and how leaders can leverage the Compassionate Connected Care model and artificial intelligence–generated insights to improve patient and caregiver outcomes. Before we go deeper into these topics, it is important to understand the difference between terms we commonly use in healthcare, such as sympathy, empathy, and compassion, as they are not interchangeable (Figure 11.1).

| SYMPATHY | EMPATHY | COMPASSION |
|---|---|---|
| The feeling of being sorry for someone | The ability to imagine and understand the thoughts, perspectives, and emotions of another person | A strong feeling of sympathy for people or animals who are suffering and a desire to help them |

*Oxford Learner's Dictionary, 2021*

**FIGURE 11.1** Sympathy, empathy, and compassion.

The two most relevant concepts for this chapter discussion are empathy and compassion. The ability to put oneself in another's shoes and to deeply understand what they are experiencing creates a strong human connection that can completely change the tone of any patient encounter. Empathy can foster compassion which includes the desire to do something to ease another person's suffering and is an action word in this context. As the chapter progresses, the reader will discover that the Compassionate Connected Care model is an action framework created to help healthcare organizations and leaders improve the experience of care for the patient and the caregiver.

# A DATA-DRIVEN MODEL OF HUMAN CARING: COMPASSIONATE CONNECTED CARE

*"It may seem a strange principle to enunciate as the very first requirement in a hospital that it should do the sick no harm."*

–Florence Nightingale

## BRENDA

Brenda's head was spinning as she hung up the phone with her urologist. "I'm sorry to have to tell you this, Brenda, but you have bladder cancer. We aren't sure how advanced it is, but test results indicate it has gone beyond the bladder wall. We have sent a referral to an oncologist who specializes in this type of cancer. Their office will be calling you to set up an appointment." And the office did call shortly after that and told Brenda that the oncologist would not be available for at least two weeks as he would be out of the country. Now panic was starting to set in. Brenda was a breast cancer survivor and had been down this road before. "Two weeks!!??" she thought, "How can I possibly wait two weeks to be evaluated and get my treatment plan underway?" She expressed this concern to the receptionist on the other end of the phone. "We'll get back to you," was the response.

Most if not all of us can relate to this scenario—whether it was personal or happened to a family member or friend, a conversation like this one turns our world upside down and stops us in our tracks. In this case, "Brenda" is a member of my family who told me about this experience shortly after it happened. "I waited for hours for the office to call back. When they finally did in the late afternoon, the provider's nurse told me she had met with the oncologist to lay out a comprehensive diagnostic evaluation plan that would start the next day and be completed by the time of my first scheduled visit two weeks later. "If they told me in the morning that they would be working on a plan throughout the day, it would have spared me much of the anxiety I experienced that day. I was pacing my kitchen floor all day long." The receptionist to whom she spoke in the morning did not intentionally mean to cause emotional suffering. She just didn't put herself in the patient's shoes. She was not tuned in to the anxiety and stress of the person on the other end of the phone. Brenda then shared that the oncologist called her later that evening and apologized that he wouldn't be able to see her for two weeks, understanding how anxious she must be. He then gave her his personal cellphone number and told her to call him at any time with questions or concerns she might have until they were able to meet in person at her first visit. "You know, I knew I would probably never call him—but the fact that he gave me that lifeline when I needed it most brought my stress level way down. I felt an immediate connection and knew I was in good hands."

In one day, at the very start of this journey, Brenda experienced a fairly common and often complained about healthcare scenario: an interaction with a healthcare team member who was probably well-meaning but through poor communication caused unnecessary anxiety and suffering; and another interaction with her oncologist who by his actions and acknowledging her deep anxiety and concern put her immediately at ease and established the start of a great provider-patient relationship that is still strong today four years later.

## LEADERSHIP, MISSION, AND VISION

Historically, Press Ganey was primarily a patient experience survey company. Their work was focused on creating robust survey tools yielding actionable data to healthcare organizations that could help them achieve their patient experience goals. With a change of leadership a decade ago came a change in perspective. It was time for leaders in the organization to reflect and refocus: What is most important to patients and caregivers? What is the best way to approach the work to achieve exemplary patient and caregiver experience and outcomes? In other words, we needed to go beyond just providing clients with data and partner with healthcare organizations to leverage their data to improve outcomes.

To that end, Press Ganey leaders revised the organizational mission to reflect a new paradigm emphasizing partnership and collaboration. Press Ganey's mission, to reduce patient and caregiver suffering, was adopted throughout the company. In considering the suffering construct, we know that patients may experience suffering related to their inherent diagnosis. They have concerns about how their diagnosis may impact their quality of life and disrupt their family and income. They experience fear about pain and anxiety related to short- or long-term mortality. And while we would eliminate all of these worries for our patients if we could, we can really only hope to mitigate those feelings—we can't eliminate them. Our patients and families also experience *avoidable suffering*—that is, the suffering caused by defects in care that are in our power to control. As our patients are already carrying the burden of unavoidable and inherent suffering, it is on us as caregivers to eliminate avoidable suffering to the greatest possible extent (Dempsey et al., 2014).

But how do we do that? What is it that patients really need from us? Those insights can be gleaned from the voice of the patient through patient experience survey data. Surveys provide us both quantitative data (through scaled questions) and qualitative data (through a patient comment). Both are important to understanding patient needs.

A frequent misperception is that the focus of patient experience work is to make the patient "happy." During a recent conversation with a colleague whose background is in hotels and hospitality, he mentioned that the goal of patient experience should be similar to the goal of hotel customers: "The patient should be happier leaving than when he arrived." However, we would challenge anyone to find a patient that is happy to be in a hospital bed, on a stretcher in the ED, or visiting a provider's office with influenza. Those patients are not happy to be there. Then, if the patient experience isn't about happiness, what is it about?

For the answer to that question, we need to turn to patient experience survey data. The Press Ganey national patient experience database is robust, with over 40 million patient responses annually. *Key drivers* are measures that are weighted most heavily with respect to global measures, such as likelihood to recommend and rating the hospital on a scale of 1 to 10. Key drivers are an important part of the data analysis report because they represent what is most important to patients when it comes to their experience of care. Key drivers help organizations better understand where they should focus their improvement efforts.

Reviewing both priority index national data and data at the organizational level, we see a consistent pattern: More than half of key patient experience drivers, regardless of the location of care, are predicated on caregiver ability to establish a human connection with the patient (Figure 11.2).

### Example: One Health Care Organization's Key Driver Report (Inpatient)

Key Driver Summary
Top Drivers: Rate Hospital 0-10 (CAHPS)                    → = Relies on Human Connection

| | Linear Correlation | Top-Box Ratio | Driver Index | Top-Box Score (Percentile Rank) |
|---|---|---|---|---|
| → Nurses treat with courtesy/respect (CAHPS) | 0.6 | 4.18 | 97 | 85.2 (33) |
| → Nurses listen carefully to you (CAHPS) | 0.61 | 2.63 | 69 | 75.3 (35) |
| → Staff provide care in safe manner | 0.62 | 2.52 | 69 | 70.5 (36) |
| → Nurses explain in way you understand (CAHPS) | 0.56 | 2.17 | 54 | 73.7 (32) |
| → Care and concern of the nurses | 0.6 | 2.5 | 66 | 70.8 (66) |
| → Doctors treat with courtesy/respect (CAHPS) | 0.46 | 2.23 | 41 | 84.0 (26) |
| → Good undertanding managing health (CAHPS) | 0.51 | 1.75 | 39 | 47.5 (26) |
| → Hosp. staff took pref. into account (CAHPS) | 0.52 | 1.72 | 41 | 42.7 (34) |
| → Doctors listen carefully to you (CAHPS) | 0.48 | 1.95 | 39 | 76.6 (32) |
| → Doctors explain in way you understand (CAHPS) | 0.46 | 1.86 | 35 | 73.4 (31) |

**FIGURE 11.2**

In analyzing HCAHPs data across multiple service lines, key drivers of high HCAHPS scores for hospitals included teamwork, room cleanliness, and caregiver listening and courteousness (Dempsey, 2017). What do these three things have in common? Safety. A great patient experience is not about making patients happy—

it is about making patients feel safe under our care. Not to *be* safe under our care by virtue of our licensure and training—patients expect to receive safe care from caregivers. Ensuring patients *feel* safe under our care is foundational to excellent patient care (Dempsey, 2017, p. 59).

## COMPASSIONATE CONNECTED CARE FOR THE PATIENT

Insights gained from key driver and priority index reports about what is most important to patients led to the creation of the Compassionate Connected Care model by Dr. Christy Dempsey, Press Ganey's Chief Nursing Officer Emerita, and a team of Press Ganey clinical leaders and research scientists (Dempsey & Assi, 2018). When organizations respond to survey results by responding to every question by itself, the impact can be overwhelming, which leads to "paralysis by analysis" and to the potential creation of many improvement initiatives based on individual questions. Dr. Dempsey took a different approach by grouping related patient experience survey questions into four categories: Clinical, Caring, Operational, and Cultural. Categorizing the questions in this way makes it more apparent to clinicians and caregivers what the area(s) of greatest need are from the patient's perspective (Figure 11.3). This enables the team to focus their efforts more narrowly on what matters most to the patient.

We know that quantitative data alone does not tell the whole story. Narratives based on personal experience and practice (in the case of clinicians) adds a richness to the model that cannot be derived from quantitative data alone. Dr. Dempsey and the Press Ganey team fielded a survey to hundreds of caregivers and patients to gather qualitative comments on what Compassionate Connected Care meant to them. The research team then used affinity diagramming to extract themes from the survey data. Six themes were identified:

1.   **Acknowledge suffering.** We should acknowledge that our patients are suffering and show them that we understand. Asking patients what they

are worried about provides an opportunity for caregivers and patients to connect on issues patients might be experiencing beyond their diagnosis. Anticipating their needs shows concern for their suffering.

2. **Body language matters.** Nonverbal communication skills are as important as the words we use. When caring for patients, caregivers should maintain an awareness of body position, facial expression, eye contact, and tone of voice.

3. **Anxiety is suffering.** Anxiety and uncertainty are adverse outcomes that must be addressed. Anxiety can negatively impact patients physically and emotionally, impairing sleep, rest, and healing. Caregivers must recognize and intervene to reduce anxiety to the greatest extent possible.

4. **Coordination of care.** We should show patients that their care is coordinated and continuous and that we, as caregivers, are always there for them. We need to convey that the relationship with the caregiver is present even when the caregiver is not providing direct care. Managing team members, bedside shift reports, thorough discharge teaching, and post-discharge follow-up calls are foundational to effective care coordination.

5. **Autonomy reduces suffering.** Autonomy helps preserve dignity for patients. We are not here to tell patients what to do. The patient must be a full participant in developing their plan of care.

6. **Caring transcends diagnosis.** Real caring goes beyond the delivery of medical interventions to the patient. Understanding what is important to a patient beyond their diagnosis or treatment plan creates the human connection necessary to establish trust. Trust is needed for patients to feel safe under our care (Dempsey, 2017).

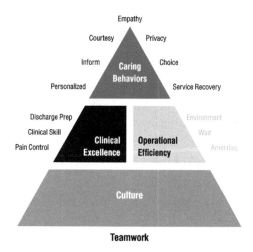

**FIGURE 11.3** Compassionate Connected Care for the patient.

No caregiver comes to work thinking, "I'm only going to do a mediocre job caring for my patients today." They want to take great care of their patients and know that compassion, empathy, and caring reduce patient suffering. Poor patient experience scores are demoralizing to caregivers working hard to manage patient care in a highly complex environment. So, what's getting in the way?

The healthcare landscape today is very different from what it was 20 years ago. Regulatory agencies and payors began focusing on patient care outcomes and attached financial penalties and bonuses to performance. There was a heavy emphasis on clinical processes of care. In 2003, for example, the Joint Commission and Centers for Medicare and Medicaid Services launched the first set of Core Measures (Joint Commission, 2021). While the intention to improve quality and safety outcomes is laudable, it can also de-emphasize the qualitative patient experience when the focus is heavily weighted on clinical tasks and processes by incentivizing success in implementing required care strategies reliably.

Academic and clinical preparation of caregivers has also changed over the past several decades. Nursing schools, for example, are challenged with the sheer amount of content they must deliver to prepare nursing students for entry into practice. There is an emphasis on clinical knowledge and skills, which are important to the provision of quality care. However, much of this work has now shifted to the simulation lab. Interaction with actual patients and families has decreased over time, so students are often less than prepared to respond with empathy and compassion to patients who are suffering. Dr. Dempsey shared the following anecdote. When she spoke about Compassionate Connected Care at a national Student Nurses Association event several years ago, there were over 1,000 people in attendance. She said that several dozen student nurses approached her afterward to say that they had not received any preparation of this kind during their coursework and wanted to learn more.

Other factors that can impede the ability of clinicians to provide compassionate and empathic care are related to the availability of adequate human and material resources. If staffing is critically low and/or material resources are inconsistently available, team members will expend their energy trying to cope with and manage care despite those deficiencies.

The primary role of leaders is to create a positive and healthy work environment in which teams can provide excellent patient care. As leaders, we must recognize, foster, and support the need to balance best practice clinical skills and Compassionate Connected Care. If we don't prioritize compassion and empathy as essential skills for practice, neither will our teams.

## COMPASSIONATE CONNECTED CARE FOR THE CAREGIVER

Concerns about caregivers' compassion fatigue, burnout, and turnover are not new. Clinician engagement has been declining over the past decade, with nurses and physicians consistently ranking at or near the bottom of engagement surveys in Press Ganey's national database year over year (Figure 11.4). During the worst period of the COVID-19 pandemic, the situation only worsened, with the negative impact on nurses being the most pronounced. Nurse engagement declined significantly in all measurement categories between March and December 2020 (Press Ganey, 2021).

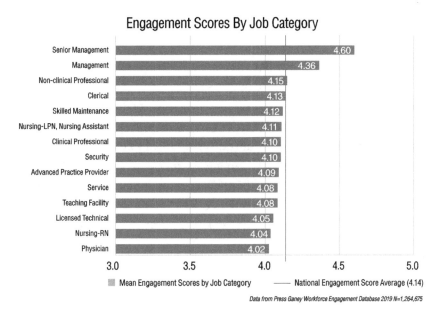

**FIGURE 11.4** Engagement scores by job category.

After the Compassionate Connected Care model for the patient was completed, the team began to consider the caregiver's experience. Many nurses, in particular, had been resonating strongly with the Compassionate Connected Care model for the patient as it helped them get back to why they had decided to enter the profession of nursing in the first place. In dialogue with many clinicians over the following year, they shared their stories and experiences. It became clear that in many ways, caregivers also suffer. And while as nurses, we have chosen a very challenging profession, it is critically important also to consider how best to support caregivers, keeping in mind that human connection is just as crucial to caregivers as it is to patients.

The team began to explore another dimension of the model, Compassionate Connected Care for the Caregiver, understanding that stress and fatigue were frequently repeated concerns of those caring for patients. Using the same methodological approach, the team reviewed the workforce engagement survey and categorized related questions into four categories: Connected, Clinical Excellence, Operational Efficiency, and Culture (Dempsey, 2017).

While similar in some ways to the patient version of the model, the constructs for caregivers are different as they encompass the role of the caregiver (see Figure 11.5). Connectedness is the connection of caregivers to the manager, team, and purpose. In this context, the engagement of caregivers is very much related to connectedness and the purpose of the organization. Clinical knowledge is an integral part of a nurse's professional identity. Caregiver experience also has an operational component that is strongly influenced by the environment in which patient care is provided. For caregivers to provide excellent care, they must have the appropriate human and material resources and management support to be successful. Lastly, caregiver experience is also influenced by organizational culture. Culture is a vital enabler (or detractor) of workforce engagement. Like patients, caregivers could have met or unmet needs in one or more of these domains.

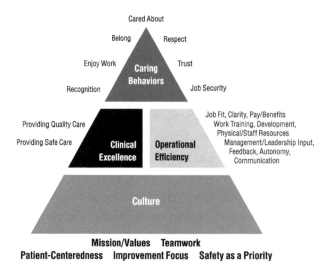

**FIGURE 11.5** Compassionate Connected Care for the Caregiver.

When affinity diagramming was completed, six themes for the caregiver were identified (Dempsey & Assi, 2018):

1. **Acknowledge the complexity and gravity of the work.** Caregivers need to receive recognition for the work they do by leaders and colleagues. Rewards may be tangible or intangible.

2. **Support caregivers with emotional, material, and human resources.** Management has a duty to provide support in the form of material, human, and emotional help. Leaders create a positive and healthy work environment.

3. **Foster teamwork as a vital component for success.** Team members support one another. Multidisciplinary teamwork is organized around patient needs.

4. **Model empathy and trust.** Trust is built on accountability, integrity, and fidelity at levels of the organization. Caregivers demonstrate empathy to each other and patients.

5. **Reduce compassion fatigue through a positive work-life balance.** Caregivers feel their work is meaningful. Their perception of a positive work-life balance reduces compassion fatigue. Leaders identify caregivers who exhibit burnout and intervene appropriately.

6. **Communication at all levels is foundational to success.** Listening is a critical component of communication. Communication and transparency are fundamental for the demonstration of empathy and trust.

Ensuring that we care for caregivers has never been more critical. As a profession, we are challenged with a healthcare workforce that has been on the front lines of the COVID-19 pandemic over an extended period of time. Caregivers have experienced incredible stress, compassion fatigue, and burnout due to the many challenges encountered during the pandemic, but they continue to come back to care for patients day after day. The Compassionate Connected Care for Caregivers model is a framework for action that leaders can leverage to focus on what is most important to those who provide care (Dempsey, 2021).

# THE BROADER CASE FOR COMPASSIONATE CONNECTED CARE

Earlier discussion in this chapter focused on some of the significant factors that have contributed to a healthcare system that focuses more on clinical processes of care than on prioritizing caring and empathy in the provision of care. Not surprisingly, a literature review demonstrates a sizeable body of research related to compassion, caring, and empathy in healthcare.

National survey data from the Schwartz Center for Compassionate Healthcare (2017) revealed that only 60% of patients, 48% of physicians, and 42% of nurses felt that the US healthcare system provided compassionate care. Further, 63% of nurses and physicians felt that communication and emotional support had declined in the past five years. This survey suggests that healthcare systems need to prioritize compassionate care as a critical component of a successful patient experience improvement strategy. To achieve this, leaders must assess current organizational culture and the health and well-being of caregivers to be sure that the appropriate structures and processes are in place to create and sustain a positive and healthy work environment and to support compassion and care in clinical practice

It has been postulated that empathy cannot be learned. People either have it or they don't. However, research does not support that hypothesis. Bas-Sarmiento et al. (2017) studied the impact of an empathy training program on a cohort of 48 nursing students. Using validated empathy scales to measure both caregiver and patient perceptions of empathy pre- and post-training, researchers found statistically significant improvement in all study variables after empathy training was completed. Riess et al. (2012) noted similar findings in a randomized controlled trial of 99 medical residents and fellows. Fifty-four residents participated in an empathy training program, and 45 were assigned to the control group. Patient ratings for empathy significantly increased for those that attended empathy training.

In a scoping review of the healthcare literature that focused on compassion (Sinclair et al., 2016), several studies demonstrated positive outcomes for both patients and caregivers associated with compassionate care. Patients conveyed that receiving compassionate care made them feel understood and heightened their sense of ownership concerning self-care. Both physicians and nurses reported that compassion in practice resulted in better patient compliance and disclosure of information.

Pereira et al. (2016) found that an empathic, patient-centered approach to care for patients in the ambulatory procedural setting improved patient satisfaction and had a significant positive impact on patient reports of post-procedural pain and anxiety. Patients also had a faster recovery time and better wound healing than patients in the control group who did not receive the same patient-centered approach.

Compassion and caring in practice also impact caregivers. In a meta-analysis of 11 studies, compassion fatigue strongly correlated with nurse burnout, while higher levels of compassion satisfaction were inversely related to burnout (Zhang et al., 2018).

As discussed earlier in this chapter, critical drivers of patient experience are those correlated with, or those that "drive" global measures of patient experience, such as rate the hospital 1-10 or recommend the hospital. Through survey and extensive comment analysis, we know that more than half of the top 10 key drivers of patient experience require caregivers to create a human connection through caring, empathy, and compassion to achieve great scores. When those elements are consistently added to care, patient experience scores improve (Dempsey, 2017).

In a Press Ganey Special Report (2017a), research scientists applied cross-domain analytics across multiple databases to better understand how quality, safety, workforce engagement, and patient experience influence one another. Performance across patient experience was found to be closely associated with security, clinical quality, and financial outcomes. In addition, organizations with top quartile workforce engagement scores scored significantly higher in all domains of HCAHPs than organizations in the bottom quartile of workforce engagement. A research study from Deloitte Center for Health Solutions (Betts et al., 2016) also reported that hospitals with high patient experience scores perform better financially. The study also found that patient experience scores related to the HCAHPs measure for nursing strongly associated with financial outcomes. The relationship between patient experience scores and economic outcomes was so significant that recommendations from the research study team to healthcare leaders include investing in resources to support a robust, evidence-based patient experience strategy.

As leaders and caregivers, our ability to empathize with patients so that we more deeply understand what is truly important to those under our care is critical to any patient experience improvement efforts we may undertake. And a successful patient experience strategy must include a patient care framework that emphasizes caring, empathy, and compassion. We must use data to guide our efforts and leverage tools and technology that best support our ability to create and sustain a highly reliable compassionate caring model. New and innovative methods for gaining these critical insights should be incorporated into practice in a timely manner. The next section will discuss in detail how an innovative approach utilizing artificial intelligence to analyze patient experience survey comments provides a deeper understanding of the patient experience.

# AI-ENABLED INSIGHTS INTO HUMAN CARING FROM THE PATIENT'S PERSPECTIVE

Patients' comments reveal the rich context of what happened, between whom, where, and when from the patient's perspective in an episode of care. Patients often write about more than one topic in a single comment or unstructured response to a question. For example, a patient's comment in response to a question about how well nurses listen might start out describing how thoroughly the day-shift nurse answered the patient's questions. The same comment might continue with remarks about the day-shift nurse not relaying the patient's request for a blanket to the night-shift nurse and end with how the night-shift nurse repeatedly turned the room lights on without warning after being asked not to do so.

Leaders need to be able to act on insights from rich narrative data, which reflect the patients' own words on what excellence means and where there are opportunities for improvement in caregiving. The challenge has been the limitations of traditional analytical methods to create an evidence base over large volumes of narrative comments. AI (artificial intelligence) analysis has overcome these limitations.

AI technology mimics human thought processes. For example, AI can identify trends from commonly mentioned topics, mimicking what a human analyst would do in a line-by-line reading of narrative data. AI needs to be trained to reach the expert level of analysis in a specific domain of discourse, such as healthcare experiences. Just like a human analyst of narrative data, AI would identify the different meanings of the word "cool" in *"The temperature in my room was too cool"* and in *"My nurse was cool."* Unlike a human analyst, though, once trained, AI can continuously identify trends from thousands of narrative comments, which makes the insights drawn from these data scalable across care settings.

There are two fundamental steps in the AI analysis of narrative data: 1) sentiment analysis, and 2) categorization. Ideally, the unit of analysis should be a phrase, which is smaller than a sentence, because even a sentence might describe distinct care experiences, as in this hypothetical sentence:

*"My nurses were so understanding with me, but the doctor always seemed rushed."*

After dividing the sentence above into two phrases (separated with *but*), AI would identify the first phrase as having positive sentiment and the second phrase as having negative sentiment. The next step is categorizing each phrase under categories, themes, and subthemes. Let's suppose AI is analyzing a sentence like:

*"Nurse Jenny showed care, compassion and really alleviated my horrible suffering, what I was going through."*

After assigning positive sentiment to different phrases based on what is before and after the words like "care," "compassion," and "suffering," AI would identify that the insight from this comment is about "nurse" at the highest level of analysis (category). Healthcare-specific AI would go deeper than a high-level categorization to identify insights about the patient experience with nurses, such as "courtesy and respect" (theme) and to identify even more specific insights about nurse behavior, such as "showing empathy and compassion" (subtheme). As AI continues with the sentiment analysis and categorization of each phrase, positive and negative trends emerge from narrative data. The larger the number of distinct insights that AI can extract per comment, the better it can identify the root causes behind positive and negative care experiences and what matters most to patients (Figure 11.6).

*"Nurse Jenny showed care, compassion and really alleviated my horrible suffering, what I was going through"*

| Sentiment | Root Cause Identification | | | Attribution |
|---|---|---|---|---|
| Rating | Category | Theme | Sub-Theme | Person or Group |
| **Positive** | **Nurse** | **Courtesy and Respect** | Kindness | Dr. Jane Doe |
| Negative | Doctor | Skill/Knowledge | Helpfulnes | Nurse Tom |
| Neutral | Quietness/Distractions | Explanation | **Empathy & Compassion** | **Nurse Jenny** |
| | Cleanliness | Reliability & Scheduling | Other | All Staff |
| | Responsiveness | Listening | | |
| | Admission | Nurse Type | | |
| | Discharge | Other | | |

**Figure 11.6**  AI-enabled classification of insights from patients' comments into categories, themes, and subthemes.

By allowing us to hear what patients say in large volumes, AI makes it possible to create a narrative evidence basis for the science and practice of human caring. Using AI, leaders can detect early signals about patients' perceptions of caregiving in moments of uncertainty, such as the outbreak of a pandemic (Guney et al., 2020). Seeing the distinct patterns of positive and negative themes from patients' comments, leaders can implement evidence-based actions to consistently provide positive care experiences and prevent negative care experiences (Guney et al., 2021). AI can also show leaders and clinicians what patients value the most in caregiving.

# LEADERSHIP'S ROLES IN LEVERAGING THE PATIENT VOICE: WHAT PATIENTS SAY ABOUT EXCEPTIONAL HUMAN CARING

AI presents a great opportunity for visionary leaders to learn from and act on the patient voice to advance nursing science and practice. Two studies in the literature illustrate this opportunity. Clavelle et al. (2019) used patented AI technology (NarrativeDx, a Press Ganey Solution) to analyze patients' comments about extraordinary nursing care across three hospitals. McCulloh Nair et al. (2021) used the same technology to identify common themes from patients' comments about excellent nursing that one health system collected over 18 months. Both studies leveraged a first-of-its-kind evidence base of narrative data—one across multiple care settings, the other collected longitudinally across a large system.

Clavelle et al.'s (2019) study presented the empirical evidence for what clinicians have known from experience: Patients value the caring aspect of nursing significantly more than the knowledge aspect. Courtesy and respect emerged as the top theme of extraordinary nursing care, being mentioned in 64% of the comments NarrativeDx analyzed. Patients described courtesy and respect as showing empathy and compassion, helpfulness, kindness, attentiveness, and emotional comfort. Skill and knowledge appeared in 10% of the comments, emerging as a distant second theme in patients' narratives of excellent nursing.

McCulloh Nair et al. (2021) identified a similar pattern in their study, where patients described caring behaviors much more than technical skill and knowledge in their narratives about excellent nurses. Patients appreciated nursing care that made them feel safe and secure, both emotionally and physically. From the patient's perspective, excellent nurses frequently checked on the patient's comfort and needs, answered questions or facilitated answers, and treated visitors and family members with respect and compassion. When patients described how excellent nurses provided comfort and compassion, they commented on the nurse's ability to maintain a sense of humor during difficult experiences.

While we might have known from clinical experience that compassion matters to patients, AI analysis of narrative data shows us how important compassion is in exceptional human caring from the patient's perspective. AI can also give leaders deeper insights into what actions and behaviors patients describe as showing compassion.

Patients positively comment on nurses frequently checking a patient's comfort level, which has been a best practice of nursing. Patients also describe behaviors like providing emotional comfort through humor, which has not been commonly recognized as a behavior of compassion. AI amplifies the patient voice and provides previously unknown insights into patients' perceptions for a patient-centered view of what is exceptional human caring.

Previous research has defined *compassionate care* as a convergence point between the science of medicine that shows how to treat patients and the art of medicine that focuses on how to take care of patients (Trzeciak & Mazzarelli, 2019). Leveraging AI-enabled insights, leaders can bring compassionate care closer to the domain of evidence-based medicine. If patients are telling us in large volumes that compassion is what they value the most in their caregiver, it is the role of visionary leadership to act on this evidence and create environments of human caring where compassion—in all the different ways patients experience it—is recognized and operationalized as the driver of excellence.

# IMPLICATIONS FOR PRACTICE

There are many theoretical models of nursing care that include constructs such as caring, empathy, and compassion as critical components of nursing practice (Percy & Richardson, 2018). Assumptions are often made that people who choose to become nurses, physicians or other types of professional caregivers are also caring and empathetic by nature. However, as discussed earlier, both patients and caregivers in the US perceive that these qualities are too often lacking among healthcare professionals.

Some of the challenges in healthcare today—such as scarcity of resources, lack of training, and failure to emphasize human connection in the provision of patient care—were discussed earlier in the chapter. In addition, healthcare professionals may not believe that compassion and empathy are as important as academic preparation and clinical competence (Trzeciak & Mazzarelli, 2019, pp. 217–218). Caregivers have other concerns as well. In talking with leaders and team members in dozens of hospitals across the country, they acknowledge that Compassionate Connected Care is important to both patient care and caregiver well-being. So, what is holding us back? When participants are asked what the biggest barrier is to providing compassionate care, they do not hesitate in answering: time. There is not enough time to be able to sit with patients to create the kind of human connection that will build trust and a sense of safety. But lack of time need not be a barrier. Research has demonstrated that it takes less than a minute to establish a human connection (Dempsey, 2017), and the intentional selection of certain words and phrases can completely change the tone and outcome of a patient encounter (Trzeciak & Mazzarelli, 2019, p. 251).

A white paper on high-performing nurse managers (Press Ganey, 2017b) provided insights from nurse leaders across the country on the elements and traits of top performers that contributed to exemplary nurse practice and work environments. An unwavering focus on patient quality and safety, creating and maintaining a culture of respect, strong nurse manager support, and transparent communication were all identified as critically important. A healthy and positive work environment is necessary to support a patient-centered model of care that includes empathy, caring, and compassion. However, it often necessitates a change in culture as well, which starts with leadership. If we expect team members to demonstrate these behaviors, leaders must create an environment in which caregivers can be successful and hold staff and each other accountable for caring behaviors.

For reasons previously stated, we cannot assume that caregivers are skilled in providing compassionate care. The work of leaders at all levels must include operationalizing a caring model by defining caring and empathetic behaviors and providing the appropriate training for staff and leaders. This can be accomplished through workshops, simulation, role-play, and other varied approaches. Once training is completed, periodic observation by leaders should be employed to validate that the caring behaviors are being used reliably in practice. Other ways of evaluating whether an organization's caring model is having the desired impact are to include relevant questions during leader rounding on patients and/or by adding questions to the patient experience survey that capture the patient's perception of whether they received compassionate care.

# SUMMARY

Compassion, empathy, and caring are considered core values in nursing practice. They are critical components in leadership practice and patient care delivery. This chapter introduced the Compassionate Connected Care model and described ways to implement the model to improve patient and caregiver outcomes. We would like to end with a quote by Dempsey, 2021:

> "The reduction of suffering is why the Compassionate Connected Care model came into being. It's the action model to reduce suffering for both patients and the people who care for them. The name Compassionate Connected Care was chosen very carefully. It's not enough to be compassionate, and it's not enough to give great clinical care. It's the connection between compassion and care and the connection we have

with one another and our patients that makes what we do meaningful. There is no light between clinical quality, patient safety, and patient experience. It's all the same thing. Suffering, both for patients and caregivers, is reduced when great care is provided by compassionate and connected caregivers." (C. Dempsey, personal communication, July 5, 2021)

# REFLECTIVE QUESTIONS

1.   What is an important distinction between empathy and compassion?

2.   Why are patient experience surveys important to patient care?

3.   *It takes less than one-minute to establish a human connection.* How can using this technique in clinical practice improve patient care?

4.   Why is AI important to analyze patients' comments?

5.   How does AI make it possible to create a narrative evidence basis for human caring?

---

# NARRATIVE

## APPLICATION OF COMPASSIONATE CONNECTED CARE TO PRACTICE

Community General Hospital is experiencing a downward trending over the past two years for both patient experience and caregiver engagement scores. Organizational annual goals have included targets for selected patient experience key performance indicators such as nurse communication scores and likelihood to recommend the hospital, and intent to leave the organization as a global measure of workforce engagement. Leaders used a number of tactical approaches to improve both engagement and patient experience scores. While efforts have sometimes resulted in temporary improvement, these gains do not last. Staff and leaders are frustrated as they are working hard to provide good patient care and to engage and support staff and caregivers. How might they change their improvement approach to achieve success?

# AUTHOR BIOGRAPHIES

**Mary Jo Assi, DNP, RN, NEA-BC, FAAN,** Associate Chief Nursing Officer, Press Ganey, is responsible for leading strategies to achieve nursing and caregiver excellence by delivering Compassionate Connected Care, strengthening caregiver resilience and engagement, and improving the healthcare practice and work environment, within a framework of high reliability and safety. During her more than 35 years of nursing experience, she has worked as a clinician, nurse educator, advanced practice registered nurse, and nurse executive. More recently, Assi held the position of Director of Professional Practice and Magnet Program Director for 10 years in both community hospital and academic medical center settings, and during that period was appointed to the Commission on Magnet Recognition—a position she held for six years. As the Vice President for Nursing Practice and Innovation at the American Nurses Association, she led several groundbreaking nursing initiatives at the national level, including the creation and launch of the Healthy Nurse, Healthy Nation Grand Challenge, a social movement aimed at improving the health of the nation's 4.3 million nurses.

**Senem Guney, PhD, Vice President of** Language Analytics, Press Ganey, was the Co-Founder and Chief Experience Officer of NarrativeDx before joining Press Ganey. Founded in 2013, NarrativeDx created the industry-leading AI platform for experience management in healthcare and grew to support 14 of the top 20 *US News and World Report* health systems before being acquired by Press Ganey in early 2020. Guney's published work on insights into patient-centered care from the AI analysis of patient narratives appeared in *NEJM Catalyst*, *HBR* and *JONA*. Her publications in *JONA* leveraged a first-of-its-kind evidence basis of nursing excellence based on AI-enabled insights. Prior to entrepreneurship, Guney served on the faculty of College of Computing and Information at SUNY, Albany and was a Fellow at the Center for Technology in Government.

# REFERENCES

Bas-Sarmiento, P., Fernández-Gutiérrez, M., Baena-Baños, M., & Romero-Sánchez, J. M. (2017). Efficacy of empathy training in nursing students: A quasi-experimental study. *Nurse Education Today*, *59*, 59–65.

Betts, D., Balan-Cohen, A., Shukla, M., & Kumar, N. (2016). *The value of patient experience: Hospitals with better patient-reported experience perform better financially*. Deloitte Center for Health Solutions. https://www2.deloitte.com/content/dam/Deloitte/us/Documents/life-sciences-health-care/us-dchs-the-value-of-patient-experience.pdf

Clavelle, J. T., Sweeney, C. D., Swartwout, E., Lefton, G., & Guney, S. (2019). Leveraging technology to sustain extraordinary care: A qualitative analysis of meaningful nurse recognition. *JONA*, *49*(6), 303–309.

Dempsey, C. (2017). *The antidote to suffering: How compassionate connected care can improve safety, quality, and experience*. McGraw-Hill Education.

Dempsey, C. (2021). The impact of compassionate connected care on safety, quality, and experience in the age of COVID-19. *Nurse Leader*, *19*(3), 269–275.

Dempsey, C., & Assi, M. J. (2018). The impact of nurse engagement on quality, safety, and the experience of care: What nurse leaders should know. *Nursing Administration Quarterly*, *42*(3), 278–283.

Dempsey, C., Wojciechowski, S., McConville, E., & Drain, M. (2014). Reducing patient suffering through compassionate connected care. *JONA: The Journal of Nursing Administration*, *44*(10), 517–524.

Guney, S., Childers, Z., & Lee, T. H. (2021, April 2). Understanding unhappy patients makes hospitals better for everyone. *Harvard Business Review*. https://hbr.org/2021/04/understanding-unhappy-patients-makes-hospitals-better-for-everyone

Guney, S., Daniels, C., & Childers, Z. (2020). AI to understand the patient voice during the Covid-19 pandemic. *NEJM Catalyst*.

The Joint Commission. (2021, July). *History of performance measures*. https://www.jointcommission.org/measurement/measures/

McCulloh Nair, J., Merring, P., Jones, B., & Guney, S. (2021). An exploration of characteristics and behavioral traits of DAISY honorees and nominees. *JONA*, *51*(1), 26–32.

Oxford Learners Dictionary. (2021). https://www.oxfordlearnersdictionaries.com/

Pereira, L., Figueiredo-Braga, M., & Carvalho, I. P. (2016). Preoperative anxiety in ambulatory surgery: The impact of an empathic patient-centered approach on psychological and clinical outcomes. *Patient Education and Counseling*, *99*(5), 733–738.

Percy, M., & Richardson, C. (2018). Introducing nursing practice to student nurses: How can we promote care compassion and empathy. *Nurse Education in Practice*, *29*, 200–205.

Press Ganey. (2017a). *Achieving excellence: The convergence of safety, quality, experience and caregiver engagement*. https://healthcare.pressganey.com/2017-Strategic-Insights?s=White_Paper-PGPost

Press Ganey. (2017b). *Nursing special report: The influence of nurse manager leadership on patient and nurse outcomes and the mediating effects of the nurse work environment*. http://healthcare.pressganey.com/2017-Nursing-Special-Report?s=White_Paper-Web

Press Ganey. (2021, May 11). *Celebrating and supporting nurses: An interview with Dr. Jean Watson*. https://healthcare.pressganey.com/2021nursesweekwebinarondemand

Riess, H., Kelley, J. M., Bailey, R. W., Dunn, E. J., & Phillips, M. (2012). Empathy training for resident physicians: A randomized controlled trial of a neuroscience-informed curriculum. *Journal of General Internal Medicine*, *27*(10), 1280–1286.

The Schwartz Center for Compassionate Healthcare. (2017, June 27). *National survey data presented at the Compassion in Action Conference show mixed reactions on state of compassion in U.S. healthcare*. https://www.theschwartzcenter.org/media/2019/05/Natl-Poll-and-Conf-Press-Release-Final.pdf

Sinclair, S., Norris, J. M., McConnell, S. J., Chochinov, H. M., Hack, T. F., Hagen, N. A., McClement, S., & Bouchal, S. R. (2016). Compassion: A scoping review of the healthcare literature. *BMC Palliative Care*, *15*(1), 1–16.

Trzeciak, S., & Mazzarelli, A. (2019). *Compassionomics: The revolutionary scientific evidence that caring makes a difference*. Studer Group.

Zhang, Y. Y., Zhang, C., Han, X. R., Li, W., & Wang, Y. L. (2018). Determinants of compassion satisfaction, compassion fatigue and burn out in nursing: A correlative meta-analysis. *Medicine*, *97*(26), e11086.

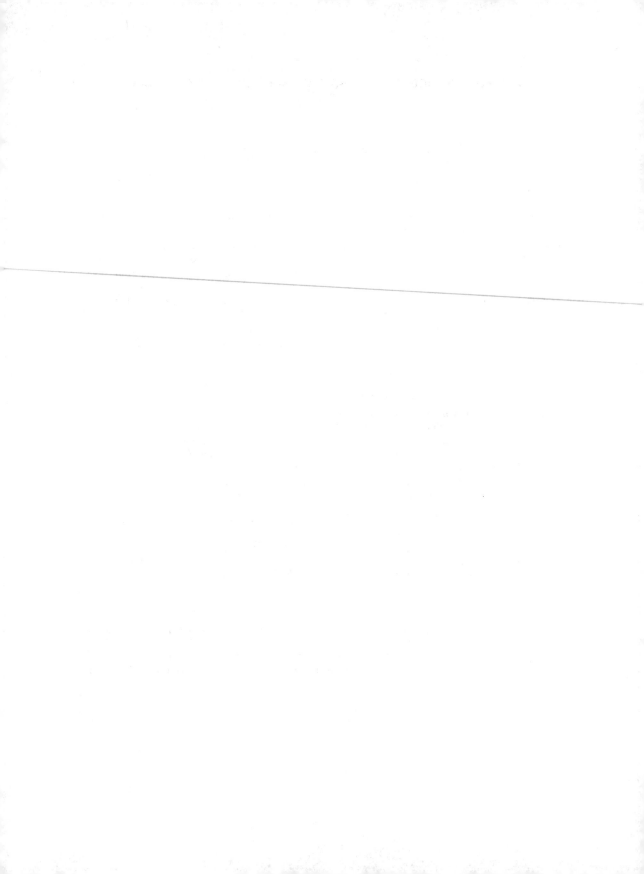

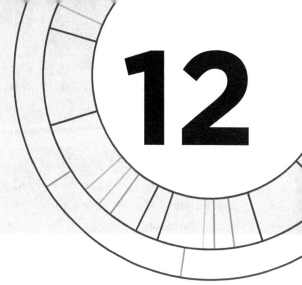

# 12

# APPLYING COMPLEXITY SCIENCE IN PROMOTING COMMUNITY AND POPULATION HEALTH

Donna Lake, PhD, RN, NEA-BC, FAAN
Dame Donna Kinnair, MA, RGN, HV, LLB, PGCE
Crystal Oldman, EdD, MSc, MA, RN, RHV, QN, FRCN, CBE
Kefang Wang, PhD, RN, FAAN
Kenichi Yamaguchi, PhD
Holly Wei, PhD, RN, NEA-BC, FAAN

## LEARNING OBJECTIVES

After completing this chapter, readers will:

- Understand the concepts of complexity science and adaptive systems

- Explain population and community health from a complexity science perspective

- Apply the principles of complexity science in population health nursing leadership

- Recognize nurse leaders' roles in global population and community health

# OVERVIEW

Current healthcare organizations need to operate and balance in legal, economic, and technical settings within the growth of globalization. The increase in globalization interactions (e.g., medications/vaccines, biomedical equipment, workforce recruitment, changing demographics within countries, etc.) has caused a growth in international trade and the exchange of ideas, beliefs, culture, partnerships, and new challenges. In addition, globalization has added to healthcare systems' complexity and limitations of linear cause-and-effect logic in establishing and assessing healthcare interventions. Health systems, including global, public, population, and community health, are complex adaptive systems.

Approaches that attempt to organize actions and coordinate among stakeholders face an enormously interwoven and complex global system. It is essential to use a complexity theory's perspective to recognize the intricacy we encounter in health organizations, create coherence in global health governance, engage in health policy, and operate in a complex system to generate transformational change. Healthcare leaders and nurses need to shift their leadership perspectives and practices to fit stakeholders' needs with deeply embedded structures and processes. This chapter will discuss complexity science, nurse leadership in complex health systems, community and population health in the face of global growing threats, and how nurses can participate in health policies and governance networks to improve the community and population health.

# POPULATION AND COMMUNITY HEALTH FROM A COMPLEX ADAPTIVE SYSTEM PERSPECTIVE

## COMPLEXITY SCIENCE AND ADAPTIVE SYSTEMS

As we look closer into the science, complexity occurs with the intricacies of inter-relationships, interactions, and interconnectivity within and between systems and their environments. *Complexity science* is the inquiry of living systems, studying the uncertainty, unpredictability, and non-linearity of living systems (Uhl-Bien & Arena, 2017). Complexity science refers to a group of concepts, heuristics, and analytical tools, emphasizing interactions and feedback loops of the constantly changing systems. Complexity science and theory propose that living systems are bound by order-generating rules while complicated, chaotic, uncertain, and unpredictable (Olsson et al., 2020; Uhl-Bien & Arena, 2017).

A *complex adaptive system* (CAS) is a complex system involving dynamic networks of interactions; the behaviors and interactions of the ensemble may be uncertain and unpredictable. A CAS is a dynamic system that can adapt and evolve with changing environments. A complex system and its environment are intertwined without separation. The system constantly adjusts to the ever-changing environment, which makes up an ecosystem in which nurses routinely work (Uhl-Bien et al., 2020). A CAS has several characteristics, including distributed control, connectivity, and co-evolution (Uhl-Bien & Marion, 2009):

- **Distributed control:** The interactions and interrelationships between system elements generate coherence. There is not one single centralized control governing system behaviors. The overall system performance is not simply the sum of individual actions.

- **Connectivity:** Complexity occurs because of system elements' interrelationship, interaction, and interconnectivity and between systems and environments. A change by any part of a system affects its related sections in various forms and degrees.

- **Co-evolution:** System elements change contingent on their interactions with one another and the environment. The behavior patterns can change over time. Thus, change can be considered as a necessity of co-evolution of the system and its environment.

- **Emergent order:** There are continuous actions and reactions among agents and between agents and environments. Nothing in the system is fixed, and there is always the possibility for emergent behaviors in the unpredictable, complex system. Each agent rests in the environment constructed by its interactions with other agents and the environment.

- **Non-linear causality:** In CAS, causality is not a case of straightforward cause-and-effect. Non-linear causality is indicated by various positive and negative feedback loops, external constraints, and sensitivity to initial conditions.

# HEALTHCARE AS A COMPLEX SYSTEM

Healthcare organizations are commonly governed by bureaucratic models under authoritarian hierarchy and control (Khan et al., 2018; Uhl-Bien & Arena, 2017). Historically, healthcare organizations operate as a manufactory and machinery, with strict hierarchical power, rules, and assembly lines. Leaders use top-down processes to manage, control, and attain top efficiency (Arena & Uhl-Bien, 2016). Therefore, an agile leader who can lead teams by understanding complexity science could find new planning and management processes that foster accelerated innovation. Thus, providing a quick response to changing needs while being disciplined and accountable could change interprofessional collaborative team design, digital communication, new access to care models (Crotty et al., 2019), or disaster responses.

The traditional rigid and hierarchical organizational structures offer little flexibility and adaptive space for innovation or creation or the potential to facilitate crucial inner- or inter-system dynamics, including self-organization and collaboration. This type of leadership focuses on controlling for order and depends on certainty and predictability, which are often lacking in the current society (Uhl-Bien & Arena, 2017). Like in pandemic situations, regular orders are broken, and systems fall into crises. When leaders are faced with complexity, they commonly go to an order response, denying that problems are happening and thinking that the troubles will settle down and things will go back to the old routine. Another order response is that leaders feel that the current systems and structures can handle the crises. The current COVID-19 pandemic is an example of the order response and the importance of understanding nurses' psychological changes as well during complex situations (World Health Organization [WHO], 2021; Zhang et al., 2020).

Leaders need to recognize the complexity of the systems, create an adaptive space for creation and innovation, and institutionalize the adaptions into new norms, which are the Complexity Leadership Theory's core values (Arena & Uhl-Bien, 2016; Uhl-Bien & Marion, 2009). When there is a complexity event, the complexity pressure loosens up some organizational structures, creating an adaptive space, an opportunity for change and transformation. During this time, we may see things change quickly. For example, during the COVID-19 pandemic, online platforms, such as telehealth and online meetings and education, were accepted and happened quickly, a classic complexity event with the adaptive space opening up.

Because the adaptive space only opens for a limited time before systems lock back up, agile leaders need to seize the opportunity to make changes and get them in the form of a new order. Leaders need to institutionalize the changes to be embedded and become part of the new system to make the changes stick. Instead of controlling and forcing order, leaders need to facilitate and enable adaptation and emergence change, which drives system change, improvement, and resilience.

## GLOBAL POPULATION AND COMMUNITY HEALTH AS A COMPLEX ADAPTIVE SYSTEM

Population and community health science is an integral part of academic curricula and is adopted in healthcare around the world (Apostolopoulos et al., 2020). There is now a need to revise interventions grounded in complex systems science, leading to innovative policies and interventions, including the redesign of community health systems (Apostolopoulos et al., 2020). There is a need for clinical linkages between community public health centers and other clinical sectors such as hospitals, clinics, or home health services to enhance community health services. However, it will take new system remodeling and nurses' contributions to health system reforms. This will take creativity, risk-taking, understanding of complex adaptive systems, and engagement in health policy as we tackle healthcare changes.

Population and community health is a CAS that possesses central principles and behaviors, such as open boundaries, multiple levels, control constraints, adaptation, emergence, and non-linear causality. Population and community health has open or less-defined instead of fixed boundaries. In global and population health, the openness or the adaptive space varies depending on the nature of the systems. Like living systems, organizations also have multiple levels, including sub- and supra-systems at various levels. Population and community health involves manifold levels, including individuals, teams, local, state, national services, and global organizations (Mager & Conelius, 2019). Each health system level has its unique control parameters, laws, regulations, and cultural boundaries. A dynamic policy process with minimum specifications can be a great facilitator, granting legitimacy in global and population health.

As in biological systems, body chemicals adjust and adapt based on their needs and environments. Organizations and team members' rules should also change and adapt according to their environment or context over time (Uhl-Bien et al., 2020). It also becomes structurally coupled, meaning that individuals and systems adapt to one another and coevolve. For health systems, population and global systems can change one another's structure, organization, and environments. Because the global population and community health are adaptive systems, nurse leaders need to recognize the characteristics of CAS and create an adaptive space for organizations and team members to perform creatively and innovatively.

# HEALTHCARE LEADERSHIP TO IMPROVE COMMUNITY AND POPULATION HEALTH

## NURSE LEADERSHIP IN COMPLEX HEALTH SYSTEMS

Nurse leaders should be involved and engaged in community and population health. They can apply their expertise and voice in new health policies to achieve more significant equity through new service delivery systems and increase their capacity to meet greater demands. Nurse leaders can build new interprofessional health teams (e.g., nurses, physicians, social workers), integrating medical treatment with clinical psychology care as we blend physical and mental health in the care of an elderly population (Apostolopoulos et al., 2020; Wei & Watson, 2019). It is essential for nurse leaders to understand complexity leadership and collaborate with multi-level stakeholders for optimal health outcomes (Wei et al., 2018; Wei et al., in press).

Complexity science provides a theoretical base for the nurse who functions in a dynamic healthcare system within other complex systems such as in hospital settings, disaster emergency management, or community health services. Nurses practice between science and the art of caring and must rely on knowledge and skills related to interpersonal abilities, communication competencies, clinical nursing skills, leadership, and critical thinking skills embedded in their nursing practice. Nurses are agile, skilled leaders—from the bedside to governance in the boardroom to the community—who have the confidence to lead teams during complex times impacted by a globalized world. Historically, nurses continually adjust in response to multidimensional situations using creativity leading to innovation and flexibility, which are valued nursing attributes. When nurses understand the principles of complex systems and apply them during these times of confusion, they may open spaces for new norms and innovation. For example, the COVID-19 global pandemic has sped up massive intensive care units specialized in respiratory care or massive public health vaccination programs. Leadership is situational based on context and organizations. Leaders who recognize the systems' complexity can create an adaptive space for creativity and innovation and institutionalize the adaptations into new norms (Arena & Uhl Bien, 2016).

Population health management that includes assessments and strategies for communities can lead to the public health delivery of care to improve health outcomes within communities (Mager & Conelius, 2019). Population health can be accomplished within public health systems. Each country may have its own public health service delivery. For example, the Nicaragua Ministry of Health directs nursing practice that conducts public health clinics and home health visits within villages (Rogers et al., 2018). The nurse does much of the community's patient education, care, and surveillance. Various nurse partnerships and exchanges can develop between nurses from various countries.

# NURSES LEADING DURING CHAOTIC TIMES

The year of 2020 was an example of how health systems and professionals, especially nurses, responded during chaotic times. We can learn from this and prepare nurses to lead during constant complex change. The spread of the SARS-CoV-2 virus was declared a pandemic and named COVID-19 by the WHO (Cucinotta & Vanelli, 2020). The role of nurses became visibly critical to the world during this pandemic. Millions of people have now been infected and have died. This global public health crisis has since provided extensive challenges for leaders around the world, threatening both the health and economy of populations. The contributions of nurses during the COVID-19 pandemic have been heroic. Worldwide, the images of nurses providing lifesaving and emotional care to those dying alone without family members are sketched in our memories. The media highlighted nurses sacrificing their own lives to save others, and the public's recognition of the critical nurse's role worldwide was evident. Less visibly, nurses engaged in their communities, contacting government and political leaders about patient needs and the lack of critical resources. During the pandemic, nurses were involved in rapid, new health policies at various levels within federal and regional governments.

The International Council of Nurses (ICN), an organization of international leaders, believes that nurses are vital to improving access to quality and cost-effective care and enhancing populations' health. To this end, it is essential that nurses can effectively influence change at local, organizational, systems, regional, national, and international levels. The ICN represents 20 million nurses focusing on nursing and health policy and seeks to align and integrate nursing with global health priorities, and is a crucial resource for nurses worldwide (ICN, 2021). An example of ICN involvement during COVID-19 was during the 74th World Assembly, 2021. The ICN called on member states to ensure vaccine equity in distribution among low-, middle-, and high-income countries to protect the most vulnerable, including nurses and healthcare workers (ICN, 2021).

Nurses globally are learning extensively how to deal rapidly with multiple, complex issues during disasters such as a global pandemic, fires in Australia, the tsunami and nuclear reactor leak in Japan, earthquake in Haiti, and increased terrorist attacks on innocent citizens, to name a few. These large-scale events present high levels of uncertainty and require collaborative actions between multiple sectors and agencies, and interdependencies between healthcare and social systems, which are part of complex adaptive systems (Munro et al., 2020).

Therefore, the dynamic and collaborative process of disaster management lends itself to complexity science and its basic principles: emergency, self-organization, non-linearity adaptiveness, and connectivity (O'Sullivan et al., 2013). O'Sullivan's Canadian team studied at the micro-level five communities' capacity and what occurred to facilitate collaborative action and promote health among high-risk populations, ultimately to promote population health and resilience. Complexity theory was utilized and found helpful among healthcare organizations, social services, community stakeholders, and partnerships in these five communities in Canada with diverse geographic and linguistic groups.

The study demonstrated that emergency management factors during the phases of a disaster are multidirectional and interact with the culture. Political priorities influence funding structures and priorities and connect to the municipal level, which influences political decision-making. Expanding knowledge, skills, social networks, understanding emergent opportunities, and partnerships can lead to a successful adaptive response. The communities demonstrated a high trust level when they connected and were aware of one another's needs based on situational awareness, public health understanding and skills, political awareness, and partnerships with the political leaders.

In disaster management and building the social infrastructure of adaptive response, intervention strategies at the micro-level can promote population health and community resilience. Nurses are known to be able to use their people skills and public health competency skills. They can adapt new technologies for interoperability of new information systems with ease and communicate in a disaster vertically and horizontally, formally and informally. In these changing times, the area of most need is for nurses to understand their role in health policy and acquire skill acquisition to maneuver within public governing systems and political systems to enhance social service decision-making (access to public health/emergency services for community members). Nurses' expertise and participation in public health policy identification and creation can lead to crucial funding decisions within health policy infrastructures to ensure care services are delivered for those in need.

## POLICY AND PRACTICE RESPONSES: NURSE LEADERS' ACTIONS IN THE FACE OF A GLOBAL THREAT

Nurses' awareness of federal health policies at the national and local levels is critical. As a profession, nurses need to be aware of government policies, learn about the many roles performed during global threats such as COVID-19, and possibly identify new roles involving significant health events. Here is an example of nurse leaders' actions in the United Kingdom (UK) during the COVID-19 pandemic.

Nurses in the UK welcomed the Prime Minister's announcement in March 2020 for a national lockdown. It was evident to all nurses delivering care in the hospital and the community that there was an urgent need for decisive action against COVID-19. Scientists predicted that the National Health Service (NHS) would be overwhelmed within weeks, and the intensive care units would struggle to cope with those requiring ventilation. Nurses have witnessed this prediction in their communities, and they also recognized and supported the necessary lockdown. During this critical time, nurse leaders of four UK countries rapidly formed a leadership group and worked alongside the Royal College of Nursing (RCN) and the Nursing and Midwifery Council (NMC) to change health policy, modify regulations, and mobilize actions. It was recognized that nursing in these extraordinary circumstances would require cohesive and strong leadership across the system to ensure immediate changes to nurse regulation (e.g., allowing student nurses to enter onto an NMC emergency register) and equality in healthcare access (Kale/Kinnair, 2020)

In addition, nurse leaders identified a critical need for cultural changes. Nurses recognized that any sign of feeling unwell would require a period of sick leave to minimize the risk of spreading the infection to colleagues and vulnerable patients. This required a change in mindset—the requirement to isolate was mandatory and essential in preventing the spread of the virus. Also, the UK COVID-19 experience emphasizes the significant roles that nurses play in community health. Nurses are a substantial part of the workforce, delivering services throughout all health and social care settings. Another UK lesson learned in decision-making included preventing hospitals from being overwhelmed. Community settings, including care homes, need to be part of the health systems response to keep down hospital admissions as seen in the COVID-19 pandemic. During these growing population health threats, as seen during this crisis, UK District Nursing teams observed a doubling of the number of people receiving care at home at the end of their lives (Collins, 2021).

People chose not to go to hospitals or hospices as they might have done before the pandemic, electing to stay at home with loved ones who would otherwise have been denied visiting rights. Thus, the astute UK nurses quickly assessed that the virus was spreading rapidly in the community, and a public health response was needed. However, the relentless focus on hospitals and capacity for ventilation, against a backdrop of years without a suitable and robust community nursing workforce plan, meant that nurses struggled to deliver care to the increased numbers of people being cared for outside of hospitals. In the UK, these out-of-hospital services are in primarily nurse-led services, dispersed across communities with the leadership skills and clinical competence to take a comprehensive approach to deliver care. Such care was initially hampered by the fact that the NHS had no planned strategy to engage systematically with many independent nursing and care homes. It took community nurses themselves to organize support to these homes locally, ensuring that those skilled in infection prevention and control delivered expertise and advice wherever needed. This is just one country's successful approach of nurse leaders making complex decisions during a horrific pandemic.

Nurses leading during constant change with global threats take various leadership skills, such as the above UK examples. The recent leadership literature also emphasizes agile leadership styles that can implement rapid changes to benefit an organization and a mission, especially during crises (Crotty et al., 2019). Being an agile, skilled leader in healthcare can lead to timely global and local policy changes during times of unpredictability. Healthcare organizations are inherently complex adaptive systems; therefore, being an agile leader who can apply the framework of complexity science is seen as a successful way to transform healthcare delivery.

# POPULATION HEALTHCARE: A GLOBAL COLLABORATIVE EFFORT

Since 2000, the United Nations General Assembly, ICN has worked with national nurses' associations to support and promote international collaboration. The growing need for medical services in Nicaragua, the expanding role of nurses, and a longstanding partnership between a US and Nicaraguan University provided an innovative opportunity involving hospital and public health delivery of care systems. This trusted partnership and exchange led to a Nicaragua and US community health education project utilizing a community engagement model (Lake et al., 2017). This Nicaragua example started as a nursing study abroad educational experience that quickly turned into an international collaboration between two countries: nurse leaders and educators learning about each other's population health delivery systems, various health policies, and the complexity of governance and professional practice. This experience helped US nurse educators learn how to develop culturally sensitive public health case studies related to low-wealth community members during home health visits from their Latin American nurse colleagues. In addition, the Nicaraguan nurses demonstrated the importance of community health home visits and public health delivery practices and policies to be woven into US academic entry-level nursing programs. During this rich international collaboration, the US nurses shared with their partners various teaching modalities within simulation learning lab scenarios and assisted with funding resources to advance their ability to conduct simulation labs.

As seen in the above narrative, governments play a significant role in citizens' daily lives protecting the public's health. Within the US Public Health Service, the government actions include services such as registration of births and deaths, public health surveillance of disease and injury, outbreak investigations, research and education, free health access for the poor and elderly, enforcement of laws and regulations, evaluation of health promotion programs, and assurance of a competent, healthy workforce. An important part of this is the public health economics and the economic role of government in public health. Therefore, nurses will find learning about public funding, legislation (laws), and public policies important to understanding public health services. Analytical tools have been applied to estimate the economic impact of diseases and injuries and address the cost, cost-effectiveness, and cost-benefit of interventions to prevent disease and promote health (US Department of Health and Human Services [DHHS], 2021). However, each country has its own public health services. Nurses should become more aware of their responsibilities, structures, workforce, and capacity to provide care, especially if they are hospital-based nurses with little understanding of community health.

For nurses to understand community health as a public health advocate or clinical practicing nurse in the community, the role is to promote public wellness overall (Mager & Conelius, 2019; World Economic Forum, 2021). In this capacity, nurses focus on helping underserved and at-risk individuals gain access to the care they need. The main goal is to help prevent disease and reduce health risks at the population level through evidence-based care and education. Public health is also an opportunity to learn how to build interprofessional collaborative teams (Rogers et al., 2018). This type of work is where nurses' involvement with governance networks, local elected officials, or government leaders can impact health policy or institutional governance, leading to the improvement of population health or disease management. Nurses' understanding of health policy, government reactions, political tensions, and changes in government structures or one's own healthcare institution can provide opportunities for nurses to be engaged in governance management and networks. Nurses need to be aware of advocating for access to quality healthcare within their countries, territories/cities/villages, or communities.

From a complexity science perspective, nurses can learn the intricacies of these interrelationships, interactions, and interconnectivity within health systems, government entities, and social support networks (churches, etc.), and the importance of partnerships. It is critical for nurses to become engaged advocates for health policy and think globally, especially when facing so many global threats (e.g., pandemics, climate changes leading to weather disasters, migration issues, and increased poverty). Nurses need to allocate time to rediscover their professional past experiences during chaotic times, build on the successes of today, and develop new roles for the future. Nurses play a significant role in promoting community health, practice, health policy, and redesigning health systems from a population health perspective.

# LEARN AND PONDER: LOOKING TO THE PAST TO VISUALIZE THE FUTURE

Sometimes we need to look back into history to appreciate and learn from our past to plan for future professional endeavors, especially when it comes to governance and nurses engaged in political activities and public policy. An example of an adaptable and flexible nurse leader who led massive change at the national level during a chaotic time comes from a legendary Japanese nurse leader, Nobu Madanbashi—the first Okinawan recipient of the Florence Nightingale Medal. Madanbashi contributed to the post-war construction of nursing education and medical institutions, impacting many islands around Okinawa, Japan. This was during 1945 when institutions were destroyed due to war. She started a nursing education program when Japanese institutional practices were terminated by the war. In 1946, she became a director of the nursing school attached to the Okinawa Central Hospital (Madanbashi, 1972). It was the time when medical facilities were installed in Quonset huts and tents, and there were only about 20 licensed nurses and 40–50 nursing assistants in Okinawa (Madanbashi, 1972).

Madanbashi's adaptability skills and social capital (networking) propelled post-war nursing education in Okinawa, where educational and human resources were scarce. Madanbashi built partnerships and extensive political networks between the US and Japanese government officials to acquire scarce resources, propel post-war nursing education during this time, develop new hospital management, and establish professional nursing skills (Madanbashi, 1972). The key to this historical story is Madanbashi demonstrated valued networking skills that lead to new policies and institutional governance at a high level within the government. She was vital to securing the beginning of professional nursing in Okinawa and Japan. This story illustrates how a nurse leader who mentored other nurses was adaptive, agile, and flexible. This is a model case on how one nurse could realize empowerment and provide institutional stability during a post-war period and had an extensive impact in Japan.

# IMPLICATIONS FOR PRACTICE

## ACTIONS NURSES CAN TAKE NOW

Nurses can seize opportunities to engage in various population health initiatives, thus improving the health of communities worldwide. With increased interest in the exciting area of population health, nurses can start volunteering or seeking governance roles in the hospital, current positions, or new projects in community health. Another approach is learning how to conduct community assessments determining public health needs, health interventions, and services to impact positive health outcomes. Preparing nurses to lead policy changes utilizing CAS may need to include new academic and clinical partnerships to facilitate innovative public healthcare models to ensure improved health equity and access for vulnerable populations. Nurses being more engaged in policymaking includes increased nurse political participation in civic activities, nurses on boards or commissions, or even nurses seeking political appointments themselves or fostering partnerships with elected officials. This involvement can ensure that health policies and laws are updated, revised, or added to ensure patient safety and better health. The following provides four suggested actions that nurses can take to increase their participation in population health management and health policy.

First action: Learn about population health management based on Healthy People 2030 (US DHHS, 2021), specifically to enhance health interventions to address health inequities through social determinants of health (Mtenga et al., 2016; Newman et al., 2015). *Social determinants of health* (SDOH) are determined by access to social and economic opportunities such as resources and supports available in our homes, neighborhoods, and communities; the quality of our schooling; the safety of our workplaces; the cleanliness of our water, food, and air; and the nature of our social interactions and relationships (US DHHS, 2021).

The second action: Pick a topical area you are comfortable and interested in and learn about the interrelationships and how population health systems approach this situation, and what connects organizations to government networks. Explore government networks in this context (federal, national, state, village, or community government officials) that could be partners to address this challenge by exchanging information, coordinating policies and collaborative efforts. Investigate informal and formal structures and relationships at each level of society that are engaged in this challenge. One can see this example during the beginning of the COVID-19 vaccination program among low- and high-wealth countries or within cities.

The third action: Assess the healthcare systems conducting health services and determine if they are aware of the community's needs, starting by picking a small program to evaluate. As in the case of population health, the health outcomes of a defined group of people need to be measured after an intervention. For example, hospitals and healthcare systems should include these five distinct goals in their population health strategies (US DHHS, 2021):

1.   Increase preventive health services through coordinated care across the healthcare continuum

2.   Provide culturally and linguistically appropriate care

3.   Promote healthy behaviors

4.   Coordinate hospital-based interventions with community stakeholders and other key partners through mature collaborative partnerships

5.   Track population health metrics against dashboard targets based on Healthy People 2030

The fourth action: Read about CAS, systems approach transformational leadership, population health, and how to influence health policy (Apostolopoulos et al., 2020). From a global perspective, there have been increased global joint planning sessions related to population health among social, medical, and political science experts. For example, an international conference assembled population health experts to conduct a plan on population health intervention research to foster interprofessional information exchanges (Moore et al., 2019). This successful meeting explored ways to facilitate further evidence-based decisions and population health interventions and promote sharing experiences between researchers, clinicians, and policymakers. The emphasis was on using theory-driven research and encouraging all disciplines to collaborate and conduct health policy together. Therefore, the time is now to position nursing influencers in policy decision-making roles to redesign collaborative population health initiatives.

# NURSING PRACTICE: LOOKING AHEAD

Nurse leaders play a crucial role in articulating complex healthcare systems to others and have a long tradition of leading healthcare services (Olsson et al., 2020; Solbakken et al., 2018; Wei & Watson, 2018). In addition, nurses are responsible for implementing organizational governance procedures, especially in hospital settings. They can use these experiences by being involved in planning opportunities, nursing role expansions, or changes to enhance public health outcomes in disaster event responses for new global threats. Many nurses are already engaged in disaster planning. Still, nurses need to be more visible in governance roles in clinical and non-clinical settings, especially in public policy discussions. There are many opportunities for nurses to be involved in mitigating global health threats, including climate change, food insecurity, displacement of people, pollution, clean water, violence targeted at certain groups, sexual assault, and global poverty (Institute for Health Metrics and Evaluation, 2021).

From the global perspective, "the COVID-19 pandemic has a disproportionate impact on the most vulnerable and marginalized communities around the world" without affordable healthcare and increased poverty (Mirchandani, 2020, para. 5). Other areas that nurses can be involved include environmental protection and humanitarian work. It is reported that the year 2020 was the warmest year on record globally, and summits in Glasgow, Scotland, and Kunming, China, discussed what the world needs to do to prevent floods, droughts, and climate and biodiversity changes. Another area is the worst humanitarian crisis predicted by the World Food Programme, that 235 million people need humanitarian assistance and protection during 2021, a near 40% increase from 2020 (Mirchandani, 2020, para. 18). Therefore, nurses need to be visionary and seize opportunities to lead to safer communities and improved health outcomes.

# RESOURCE TOOLS

Seeking resources to assist with complex health issues can provide guidance on how to conduct assessments and reimagine new public health systems. The complexity leader must create an adaptive space for innovation, and institutions must allow for creativity. Driving system improvements through learning can open boundaries between individuals, teams, local and state and national services to global organizations. This will enable new policies and provide space for new leaders to emerge. This is nursing's time to be involved in new health policy changes at the local organization, government, or community levels, utilizing the following resources:

- Centers for Disease Control and Prevention (CDC) Policy Analysis Key Questions for implementing policy. This document could be an effective worksheet in the assessment (CDC, 2015).

- *Public Health Service Activities—10 Essential Public Health Services* (CDC, 2021).

- *The US Future of Nursing 2020–2030: Charting a Path to Achieve Health Equity* (2021). A consensus study from the National Academy of Medicine. This is an example of a national strategic plan for the next decade of nursing to address racial inequity. It includes strategies nurses can employ to improve health outcomes, expand nurses' scope of practice, and enhance disaster preparedness. This document is an example of a national policy plan (National Academy of Medicine, 2021).

# SUMMARY

Nurses thinking boldly can be a catalyst for transforming healthcare delivery, improving the quality of care, and promoting population health policy changes by applying complexity theory science to complex issues. Nurses are in a position to participate within governance structures to redesign healthcare policies, leading to better health initiatives. Participating within government health policy development could mean legislative work with a nurses association, work with elected officials, or applying for a public office position or civic involvement on community boards/commissions.

Nurses can be influencers in their individual work and/or via their country's nurses associations, which can be a key vehicle for influencing policy, both nationally and globally. Nurses' extensive knowledge and involvement in essential services and their understanding of the link between the environment and social determinants of health provide opportunities to be engaged in policy development. Too often, nurses traditionally have to implement policies that nurses were not involved with creating. Therefore, to ensure a caring healthcare delivery system and health equity, nurses must develop new skills and advocate for healthy public policies as we deal with complex health and increased global threat challenges now and in the future.

# REFLECTIVE QUESTIONS

1. From your knowledge and experience, how would you describe healthcare as a complex system and the relationship to complexity theory?

2. Describe population and community health as a complex adaptive system from a nurse leader's perspective as described in this chapter.

3. Describe global threats and/or disaster examples that can benefit from complexity leadership as described in this chapter.

4. Identify at least two actions suggested in the chapter to assist with skill acquisition or increased participation in population health initiatives or health policy development.

5. What is at least one resource you can utilize from this chapter to assist you with conducting health policy assessments and foster your participation in health policy development?

# NARRATIVE

## NURSES LEADING CHANGE IN CHINA TO IMPROVE BREASTFEEDING OF PREMATURE NEWBORNS

The Chief Nursing Officer, Senior Charge Nurse, and staff nurses of the obstetric department in a China children's hospital collaborated with a US nurse scientist in a research project in Qingdao, China (Yu et al., 2021). The nursing team identified the breastfeeding rate (17.9%) in their hospital was much lower than the national rate in China (23%), which is a work in progress toward the World Health Organization goal of 50% by 2025 (WHO, 2014). Utilizing project data, the exclusive breastfeeding rate of premature infants was 1.8% and contributed to the separation between mothers and premature infants who were admitted to the Newborn Intensive Care Unit (NICU). From a population health perspective, the team understood, breastfeeding is associated with decreased risk for many early-life diseases and conditions, such as otitis media, respiratory tract infections, asthma, and sudden infant death syndrome. The project team identified gaps between best practice and current practice and the components involved in breastfeeding NICU newborns. From a complex adaptive system perspective and process review, interviews with 17 staff nurses revealed a lack of breastmilk storage equipment in the unit. Interviews with 70 mothers demonstrated they had limited visitation time which restricted their breastfeeding time in the NICU. These system components, relationships, and interconnections provided a better understanding of the issue's complexity and ultimately encouraged new ways of thinking and practices within this unit. Innovative changes achieved increased education for nurses and mothers on breastfeeding; new processes led to new governance (policies); and improved health outcomes are yielding an improvement in breastfeeding among premature newborns rates from 17.9% to 52.7% (exceeding the WHO goal of 50%), and the exclusive breastfeeding rates from 1.8% to 4.1% over a three-year period. In addition, this case demonstrated international nurses collaborating in critical research, which improved health outcomes.

# AUTHOR BIOGRAPHIES

**Donna Lake, PhD, RN, NEA-BC, FAAN,** is a Clinical Professor at East Carolina University in North Carolina. Specialty areas include Leadership, Health Policy, and Community Health. She has taught 900 Master of Science in Nursing, PhD, and medical students, and health sciences faculty. Also, she has published 19 peer-reviewed articles, five book chapters, contributed to obtaining $7 million in grant-funded research, and conducted 850 scholarly international, national, and state presentations. She served as the only nurse representative on the American Medical Association Grant ($11 million) from 2014-19, Accelerating Change in Medical Education. Prior to ECU, Lake had a 25-year career in the US Air Force, which provided international public health leadership experiences in the Middle East, Europe, Latin America, and Africa. During 2020, she was recruited to run for state senator and the unsuccessful run led to further research and advocacy for more nurses to be engaged in health policy. She is currently an ECU Innovations Lab and Curriculum Consultant to build stronger workforce capacity for nurse practitioners, midwives, and nurse specialists in primary care in rural and underserved areas.

**Dame Donna Kinnair, MA, RGN, HV, LLB, PGCE,** is the Chief Executive and General Secretary of the Royal College of Nursing. She has demonstrated operational leadership in a number of roles throughout her career, none more so than through this recent COVID-19 pandemic, where she has been a constant voice both in the media and to ministers ensuring that nursing staff and patients are protected. Kinnair is a qualified nurse, health visitor, and lecturer in medical and child law. She has held many director posts in acute trust, community care, and commissioning and is Past Editor of *Nursing Management*. She wrote a monthly editorial on nursing issues, strategic planning, commissioning articles, and advising on content

**Crystal Oldman, EdD, MSc, MA, RN, RHV, QN, FRCN, CBE,** has been the Chief Executive of the Queen's Nursing Institute (QNI), the oldest nursing charity in the world, since 2012. After qualifying as a nurse and a Health Visitor, Oldman worked in NHS community services for 18 years, supporting some of the most deprived communities in west London. She then enjoyed an academic career for a further 18 years, completing her higher education career as Dean, where her role included the development of partnerships with external agencies to promote research and assist in workforce development. Oldman's interest in leadership and management inspired her doctoral studies into the knowledge, skills, and attributes of middle managers, research that was completed in 2014. She was awarded a CBE in the Queen's Birthday Honours List in 2017 for services to community nursing and her leadership of the QNI, and in 2020 was awarded Fellowship of the Royal College of Nursing.

**Kefang Wang, PhD, RN, FAAN,** Dean and Professor, School of Nursing and Rehabilitation, Shandong University, China, has a sustained and distinguished record of research funding from multiple national funding agencies in China that mirrors her research priorities: chronic condition management and elder care. Wang demonstrated her impact in nursing education through contributions to curricular development and implementation. She has transformed the disease-focused curriculum model to a health-centered model by creating multiple courses. The impact of these courses has been recognized by three national-level course excellence awards. Her excellence and contribution in education has been recognized as Distinguished Educator in Gerontological Nursing by the National Hartford Center of Gerontological Nursing Excellence, 2019. Wang has published more than 100 articles in peer-reviewed journals and delivered more than 60 presentations at international and national scientific conferences, demonstrating her outstanding and sustained impact on nursing research and education.

**Kenichi Yamaguchi, PhD,** is an Associate Professor at the Okinawa Prefectural College of Nursing in Japan. He teaches introductory sociology and sociology of the family at this college. With his research interests in Japanese colonialism and modernization projects, he started his research on history of modern medical institutions and governance in Okinawa and Taiwan. In 2019, he received four-year research funding from the Ministry of Education, Culture, Sports, Science and Technology, Japan (Reference Number: 19K13886) to conduct this research project. His academic accomplishments include a PhD degree in Sociology from the University of Saskatchewan and a MA degree in Social Studies from the University of Regina in Canada. His PhD thesis investigated post-World War II governance in Okinawa with reference to analytical insights of Michele Foucault and Giorgio Agamben. He was awarded the 2015 Outstanding Graduating Student Award by the Canadian Sociological Association.

**Holly Wei, PhD, RN, NEA-BC, FAAN,** is a Professor and Assistant Dean for the PhD program at the University of Louisville School of Nursing. Her overarching research focuses on healthcare organizational culture, leadership development, clinician well-being, stress genomic biomarkers, and patient care quality. She is known nationally and internationally for her nursing practice models and a Convergent Care Theory. Multiple healthcare systems have used Wei's nursing models to guide practice and promote organizational culture and patient care with significant improvements in nursing practice and patient care quality.

# REFERENCES

Apostolopoulos, Y., Lemke, M. K., & Hassmiller Lich, K. (2020). *Complex systems and population health*. Oxford University Press.

Arena, M. J., & Uhl-Bien, M. (2016). Complexity leadership theory: Shifting from human capital to social capital. *People & Strategy*, 39(2), 22–27.

Centers for Disease Control and Prevention. (2015). *CDC policy process*. https://www.cdc.gov/policy/analysis/process/

Centers for Disease Control and Prevention. (2021). *10 essential public health services.* https://www.cdc.gov/publichealthgateway/publichealthservices/essentialhealthservices.html

Collins, A. (2021, April 15). The ward round: Moving from hope to commitment. *Health Service Journal.* https://www.hsj.co.uk/workforce/the-ward-round-moving-from-hope-to-commitment/7029891.article

Crotty, B. H., Somai, M., & Carlile, N. (2019, August 15). Adopting agile principles in health care. *Health Affairs.* https://www.healthaffairs.org/do/10.1377/hblog20190813.559504/full/

Cucinotta, D., & Vanelli, M. (2020). WHO declares COVID-19 a pandemic. *Acta Biomedica, 91*(1), 157–160. https://doi.org/10.23750/abm.v91i1.9397

Institute for Health Metrics and Evaluation. (2021). *Global Burden of Disease Study 2019 (GBD 2019) reference life table.* http://ghdx.healthdata.org/record/ihme-data/global-burden-disease-study-2019-gbd-2019-reference-life-table

International Council of Nurses. (2021). *Nursing policy.* https://www.icn.ch/nursing-policy

Kale, S. (2020, June 10). Prof Donna Kinnair on racism in the NHS: 'In every community, BAME patients suffer the most.' *The Guardian.* https://www.theguardian.com/world/2020/jun/10/donna-kinnair-racism-nhs-if-you-arent-white-your-illness-isnt-taken-as-seriously

Khan, S., Vandermorris, A., Shepherd, J., Begun, J. W., Lanham, H. J., Uhl-Bien, M., & Berta, W. (2018). Embracing uncertainty, managing complexity: Applying complexity thinking principles to transformation efforts in healthcare systems. *BMC Health Services Research, 18*(1), 192. https://doi.org/10.1186/s12913-018-2994-0

Lake, D., Engelke, M. K., Kosko, D. A., Roberson, D. W., Jaime, J. F., López, F. R., Rivas, F. M. P., Salazar, Y. M., & Salmeron, J. J. (2017). Nicaraguan and US nursing collaborative evaluation study: Identifying similarities and differences between US and Nicaraguan curricula and teaching modalities using the community engagement model. *Nurse Education Today, 51*, 34–40. https://doi.org/10.1016/j.nedt.2017.01.004

Madanbashi, N. (1972). Medical and nursing care in Okinawa. *The Japanese Journal of Nursing, 36*(4), 454–469.

Mager, D. R., & Conelius, J. (2019). *Population health for nurses: Improving community outcomes.* Springer Publishing Company.

Mirchandani, R. (2020, December 23). *Five global issues to watch in 2021.* United Nations Foundation. https://unfoundation.org/blog/post/five-global-issues-to-watch-in-2021/

Moore, G., Cambon, L., Michie, S., Arwidson, P., Ninot, G., Ferron, C., Potvin, L., Kellou, N., Charlesworth, J., & Alla, F. (2019). Population health intervention research: The place of theories. *Trials, 20*(1), 285. https://doi.org/10.1186/s13063-019-3383-7

Mtenga, S., Masanja, I. M., & Mamdani, M. (2016). Strengthening national capacities for researching on social determinants of health (SDH) towards informing and addressing health inequities in tanzania. *International Journal for Equity in Health, 15*(1), 23–23. https://doi.org/10.1186/s12939-016-0308-x

Munro, S., Kornelsen, J., Wilcox, E., Kaufman, S., Bansback, N., Corbett, K., & Janssen, P. (2020). Implementation of shared decision-making in healthcare policy and practice: A complex adaptive systems perspective. *Evidence & Policy, 16*(3), 393–411. https://doi.org/10.1332/174426419X15468571657773

National Academy of Medicine. (2021). *The future of nursing 2020–2030.* https://nam.edu/publications/the-future-of-nursing-2020-2030/

Newman, L., Baum, F., Javanparast, S., O'Rourke, K., & Carlon, L. (2015). Addressing social determinants of health inequities through settings: A rapid review. *Health Promotion International, 30 Suppl 2*(suppl 2), ii126–ii143. https://doi.org/10.1093/heapro/dav054

Olsson, A., Thunborg, C., Björkman, A., Blom, A., Sjöberg, F., & Salzmann-Erikson, M. (2020). A scoping review of complexity science in nursing. *Journal of Advanced Nursing, 76*(8), 1961–1976. https://doi.

org/10.1111/jan.14382

O'Sullivan, T. L., Kuziemsky, C. E., Toal-Sullivan, D., & Corneil, W. (2013). Unraveling the complexities of disaster management: A framework for critical social infrastructure to promote population health and resilience. *Social Science & Medicine*, *93*, 238–246. https://doi.org/10.1016/j.socscimed.2012.07.040

Rogers, R. R., Owen, J. A., Lake, D. M., Durham, C. F., Latham, T. G., Sherwood, G., & Golding, C. S. (2018). Developing an innovative statewide infrastructure and model for delivering continuing interprofessional education: The North Carolina AHEC Initiative. *The Journal of Continuing Education in the Health Professions*, *38*(4), 282–292. https://doi.org/10.1097/CEH.0000000000000215

Solbakken, R., Bergdahl, E., Rudolfsson, G., & Bondas, T. (2018). International nursing: Caring in nursing leadership: A meta-ethnography from the nurse leader's perspective. *Nursing Administration Quarterly*, *42*(4), E1–E19. https://doi.org/10.1097/NAQ.0000000000000314

Uhl-Bien, M., & Arena, M. (2017). Complexity leadership: Enabling people and organizations for adaptability. *Organizational Dynamics*, *46*(1), 9–20. https://doi.org/10.1016/j.orgdyn.2016.12.001

Uhl-Bien, M., & Marion, R. (2009). Complexity leadership in bureaucratic forms of organizing: A meso model. *The Leadership Quarterly*, *20*(4), 631–650. https://doi.org/10.1016/j.leaqua.2009.04.007

Uhl-Bien, M., Meyer, D., & Smith, J. (2020). Complexity leadership in the nursing context. *Nursing Administration Quarterly*, *44*(2), 109–116. https://doi.org/10.1097/NAQ.0000000000000407

US Department of Health and Human Services. (2021, July 5). *Healthy People 2030*. Office of Disease Prevention and Health Promotion. https://health.gov/healthypeople

Wei, H., Horns, P., Sears, S. F., Huang, K., Smith, C. M., & Wei, T. L. (in press). A systematic meta-review of systematic reviews about interprofessional collaboration: Facilitators, barriers, and outcomes. *Journal of Interprofessional Care*.

Wei, H., Sewell, K. A., Woody, G., & Rose, M. A. (2018). The state of the science of nurse work environments in the United States: A systematic review. *International Journal of Nursing Sciences*, *5*(3), 287–300. https://10.1016/j.ijnss.2018.04.010

Wei, H., & Watson, J. (2019). Healthcare interprofessional team members' perspectives on human caring: A directed content analysis study. *International Journal of Nursing Sciences*, *6*(1), 17–23. https://doi.org/10.1016/j.ijnss.2018.12.001

World Economic Forum. (2021). *The Global Risks Report 2021*. http://www3.weforum.org/docs/WEF_The_Global_Risks_Report_2021.pdf

World Health Organization. (2014). *Global targets 2025. To improve maternal, infant and young child nutrition*. www.who.int/nutrition/topics/nutrition_ globaltargets2025/en/accessed 2021

World Health Organization. (2021). *WHO coronavirus (COVID-19) dashboard*. https://covid19.who.int/

Yu, G., Liu, F., Zhao, Y., Kong, Y., & Wei, H. (2021). Promoting breastfeeding and lactation among mothers of premature newborns in a hospital in China. *Nursing for Women's Health*, *25*(1), 21–29. https://doi.org/10.1016/j.nwh.2020.11.005

Zhang, Y., Wei, L., Li, H., Pan, Y., Wang, J., Li, Q., Wu, Q., & Wei, H. (2020). The psychological change process of frontline nurses caring for patients with COVID-19 during its outbreak. *Issues in Mental Health Nursing*, *41*(6), 525–530. https://doi.org/10.1080/01612840.2020.1752865

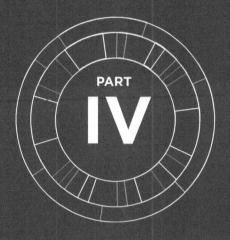

PART

# IV

# LEADERSHIP IN COLLABORATION, LEADING CHANGE, AND INNOVATION

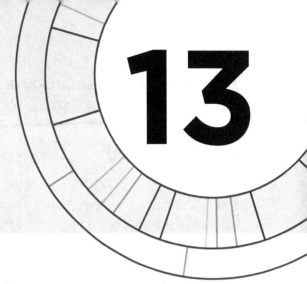

# 13

# ASSEMBLING A UNIFYING FORCE: INTERPROFESSIONAL COLLABORATION TO IMPROVE HEALTHCARE

Teddie M. Potter, PhD, RN, FAAN, FNAP
Stephanie D. Gingerich, DNP, RN, CPN
Diana Drake, DNP, APRN, WHNP, FAAN, FNAP

---

## LEARNING OBJECTIVES

After completing this chapter, you should be able to:

- Define interprofessional collaborative practice

- List key concepts of interprofessional education

- Discuss embedding interprofessional collaborative practice experiences in clinical education of health professionals

- Discuss a population health model that applies interprofessional practice at the local/neighborhood level

- Expand interprofessional education and practice to include transdisciplinary education and practice

---

# OVERVIEW

The SARS-CoV-2 (COVID-19) pandemic made it painfully obvious that the greatest threats to human health are extremely complex and constantly evolving. In addition, we saw on full display the impact of a fragmented healthcare system compounded by failed communication and flawed strategies. We are coming to realize that disciplinary excellence, once the hallmark of healthcare in America, is insufficient to ensure populations' health. More and more, we understand that the path forward will require highly effective interprofessional collaboration. This chapter briefly describes the history and guiding principles of Interprofessional Education and Collaborative Practice (IPECP). Then, it provides examples of local and global interprofessional education and collaborative best practices. It concludes with a call for the evolution of interprofessional collaborative practice to transdisciplinary collaborative practice and for visionary nurses to lead the way in addressing current and emerging global health crises.

# BRIEF REVIEW OF INTERPROFESSIONAL EDUCATION AND COLLABORATIVE PRACTICE

Since the arrival of modern healthcare, there have been examples of physicians, nurses, pharmacists, and others collaborating for the good of patients, but these interprofessional partnerships were the exception. To normalize interprofessional collaboration, the Institute of Medicine (IOM, 1972) issued a report, *Educating for the Health Team*. This was the first report to propose that high-quality care for patients living with chronic illness requires a team approach. The World Health Organization (WHO, 1988) drew a similar conclusion in *Learning Together to Work Together for Health*. Both papers acknowledge that single-discipline solutions are no longer adequate for complex healthcare needs. However, Interprofessional Education and Collaborative Practice (IPECP) did not gain significant traction until the IOM (2001) report, *Crossing the Quality Chasm: A New Health System for the 21st Century*, provided a wake-up call for healthcare organizations.

It is important to note that the move toward interprofessional collaboration was not happening only in the United States. In 2008, a survey of 193 WHO member states found that over 41 nations utilized interprofessional education to some degree in their countries (Rodger & Hoffman, 2010). In 2010, the WHO took another step toward normalizing interprofessional education and collaborative practice through the *Framework for Action on Interprofessional Education and Collaborative Practice.* This report formally defines *interprofessional education* (IPE) as an experience "when students from two or more professions learn about, from and with each other to enable effective collaboration and improve health outcomes" (p. 10).

The purpose or goal of IPE is stated most clearly in the *Lancet* report, "Health Professionals for a New Century: Transforming Education to Strengthen Health Systems in an Interdependent World" (Frenk et al., 2010):

> All health professionals in all countries should be educated to mobilize knowledge and to engage in critical reasoning and ethical conduct so that they are competent to participate in patient and population-centered health systems as members of locally responsive and globally connected teams. The ultimate purpose is to assure universal coverage of the high-quality comprehensive services that are essential to advance the opportunity for health equity within and between countries. (p. 1924)

The Interprofessional Education Collaborative (IEC) defined four core competencies for interprofessional collaborative practice. These competencies were updated in 2016 and included (IEC, 2016, p. 10):

- Competency 1: Work with individuals of other professions to maintain a climate of mutual respect and shared values.

- Competency 2: Use the knowledge of one's role and those of other professions to appropriately assess and address patients' healthcare needs and promote and advance the health of populations.

- Competency 3: Communicate with patients, families, communities, and professionals in health and other fields responsively and responsibly, supporting a team approach to promoting and maintaining health and preventing and treating diseases.

- Competency 4: Apply relationship-building values and the principles of team dynamics to perform effectively in different team roles to plan, deliver, and evaluate patient/population-centered care and population health programs and policies that are safe, timely, efficient, effective, and equitable.

These essential competencies prepare health professionals with the necessary knowledge of values, roles and responsibilities, and principles of communication to practice collaboratively.

Of the four competencies, nurses may find the second competency most challenging, not because nurses are unaware of the roles and responsibilities of other health professions, but because nurses sometimes struggle to convey to others their unique contribution to interprofessional practice. Too frequently, nurses can be heard saying, "I'm just a nurse…"

These words are not a sign of humility; they indicate inadequate knowledge about nurses' unique role on the interprofessional team.

What is the contribution of nursing to interprofessional practice? Nurses frequently spend more time with patients and families than other health professionals. Therefore, they are most likely to hear the patients' stories about the cause of their condition, the meaning of illness, and their perceived response to treatments and treatment plans. Nurses bring these stories to interprofessional team meetings and use these narratives to advocate for the patient when they cannot advocate for themselves. Thus, the unique contribution of nurses is that they ensure that the patient, family, and/or community is a full partner in making healthcare decisions (Eisler & Potter, 2014).

Eisler and Potter (2014) added an additional interprofessional education and collaborative practice competency to address the fact that health professions have traditionally been implicitly, and often explicitly, ranked in hierarchies with unequal power and influence. This pattern of power imbalance prevents the development of the type of relationships that promote interprofessional collaboration. The authors propose that effective IPECP can only occur when hierarchies of domination are transformed into partnership-based practice.

Domination-based relationships are rigidly ranked; communication flows one way: top-down; and leaders in domination systems maintain the status quo by using shame, blame, and fear. On the other hand, partnership-based relationships are identified by mutual respect for all members, communication that flows both ways, and leaders who use their power and influence to raise everyone in the system to their highest potential. Partnership-based relationships encourage innovation, engagement, and collaboration toward a shared goal.

Eisler and Potter (2014) describe critical practices that can promote partnership-based interprofessional education and collaborative practice. These practices must occur at every level of relationship, including attitudes and behaviors toward ourselves, other members of our discipline (intra-professional), other professions (interprofessional), the patients and communities we serve, and even the environment on which health depends. Key practices include (Eisler & Potter, 2014):

- Understand the roles and responsibilities of each profession.

- Develop an awareness that the system depends on the contributions of each profession.

- Learn that the disciplines cannot be ranked as each makes a unique contribution to the health of the people and communities that we serve.

- Partnership-based healthcare organizations must address old patterns of domination that may still exist in hiring, human relations, and policies.

- Leaders in partnership-based systems are appointed based on expertise rather than discipline.

Visionary nursing leaders have a significant role to play in shaping highly effective healthcare systems. One of the first steps is identifying and addressing patterns and structures of domination that inhibit healthcare employees' full potential. When dominance persists, the organizational culture is based on fear, shame, and blame. People feel safer maintaining the status quo and therefore do not work toward transformative change. In systems of domination, professional hierarchies persist, and the unique contribution of each profession is overshadowed by the professions with the most power and authority. In systems of domination, patients are ranked the lowest and therefore must settle for being a passive recipient of care.

Visionary nurse leaders promote and support partnership-based interprofessional collaborative practice. Each profession brings its unique knowledge and contributions to the team. Dialogue is mutually respectful, and patients, families, and communities participate as full partners. In this milieu, complex individual and population health issues can be addressed, and effective solutions proposed. In summary, effective interprofessional collaborative practice "optimizes health-services, strengthens health systems, and improves health outcomes...In both acute and primary care settings, patients report higher levels of satisfaction, better acceptance of care, and improved health outcomes following treatment by a collaborative team" (WHO, 2010, p. 18).

The following case studies demonstrate excellence in partnership-based interprofessional education and practice. They illuminate the many ways that IPECP contributes to improved population health outcomes, decreased cost of care, and improved care experiences for patients and health professionals.

# EDUCATION NARRATIVE

## PREPARING HEALTH STUDENTS FOR INTERPROFESSIONAL COLLABORATION TO IMPROVE WOMEN'S HEALTH

Educating healthcare students with a combined interprofessional education curriculum and clinical practice rotation offers students comprehensive, immersive experiences in learning and practicing interprofessional care. Interprofessional education provides a critical pedagogical approach to preparing healthcare students for collaborative team environments (Buring et al., 2009). The exposure of students to a collaborative culture also shifts systems toward a partnership paradigm. In the partnership paradigm, patients are integral participants, team members are valued equally, and healthcare providers are supported to practice to the full extent of their education, certification, and experience and accept accountability for their practice (Kendig, 2016).

Ideally, interprofessional education is integrated vertically and horizontally throughout the entire curriculum and learning includes not only training to understand people anatomically but also functionally across the life span. When both classroom and student immersion experiences in interprofessional practice settings exemplify partnership-based healthcare, students are better prepared for their future careers as effective interprofessional team members and leaders (Buring et al., 2009)

## INTERPROFESSIONAL WOMEN'S HEALTHCARE

An example of the necessity of interprofessional collaboration can be found in women's healthcare. It has been reported that as a nation of highly trained specialists, the lack of interconnectedness of healthcare providers leads to a fragmented system, particularly for women (McClellan, 2019). Team-based efforts that recognize the importance of access to gender-focused care within the contextual realities and demands of women's lives can best address these increasing complexities. The US primary healthcare system does not effectively meet women's needs as they age and transition through stages of life. Barriers preventing the healthcare system from meeting women's needs include gaps in medical training, biases, time constraints, lack of focus on social factors, access barriers related to language, culture, and lack of a regular source of primary care. Women's under-representation in healthcare leadership and policymaking and in the politicization of women's health issues continue to be barriers and challenges (Zephyrin et al., 2020).

High-risk pregnancies are a unique healthcare challenge involving multiple healthcare specialists; team and partnership-based care are essential to address the complexity of healthcare needs (American College of Obstetricians and Gynecologists' Task Force on Collaborative Practice, 2016). In the most recent US maternal mortality rate data, the ratio is 17.4 deaths per 100,000 pregnancies in 2018 (Declercq & Zephyrin, 2020). African American women have 2.5 times the ratio of maternal mortality than White women. A team-based approach that supports active patient engagement, personalized care, and shared decision-making in interprofessional collaboration is one key strategy to improving women's health outcomes and addressing the disparities in maternal health (Kendig, 2016).

It is not uncommon to see physicians and APRNs representing multiple specialties, pharmacists, psychologists, sonographers, genetic counselors, and integrative therapists in women's outpatient settings. Nevertheless, simply sharing clinic space does not result in interprofessional collaboration. If interprofessional collaboration aims to reach the highest level of quality and safety to attain this goal, there needs to be a collaboration between providers before it can be called "interprofessional" (Rayburn & Jenkins, 2021).

An *interprofessional education* offering can be defined as an activity undertaken when members of two or more health or social care professionals learn with, from, and about each other, focusing on improving collaboration and quality of care. Linked to this definition, the following core educational concepts are described (Reeves et al., 2007):

1. Promote collaboration, not only between learners but among developers, facilitators, and patients

2. Egalitarian (or equal) learning

3. Learner-led and team-oriented

4. Use real-life clinical problems to motivate learners

5. Shared reflection to provide opportunities for learners to discuss and debrief the successes and challenges in their clinical work

A systematic review of 64 articles with a focus on physicians and nurses in interprofessional collaboration found that professionals contribute informally to collaboration with each other through three essential actions: bridging professional and social gaps between each other, negotiating overlapping roles and tasks, and creating spaces to be able to do so (Schot et al., 2019).

An example of these three key elements is a nurse-led interprofessional collaboration based in a large academic women's health clinic. Born out of a need to provide more comprehensive healthcare services to mid-life women, an interprofessional team at the clinic collaborated on a healthcare education model. Team members included an advanced practice nurse leader, physicians, a health coach, integrative therapists, nutritionists, and healthcare students rotating throughout the clinical setting. The goal was to improve adherence to age-appropriate preventive screenings, promote sustainable lifestyle transitions, and empower health decision-making through a six-week interactive educational and experiential program. In addition, the model provided a framework for providers and students to foster interprofessional relationships in their practice and learning through collaborative course planning, participation, evaluation, and, ultimately, improved patient outcomes.

Each team member provided education and counseling to the patient participants based on their expertise. Provider team members overlapped roles in the class sessions to bridge gaps in care delivery for the participants. Patients also had an active role in co-creating learning experiences with the providers through intention setting of priorities and class agendas. The group sessions occurred in a quiet clinic conference room after traditional work hours, and this was felt to contribute to the informal and smooth collaboration between professionals and patients (Pechacek et al., 2015).

The skills learned from interprofessional education and practice experiences during clinical education help foster competencies in the learner for teamwork, leadership, consensus building, and addressing patient care goals.

## PRACTICE NARRATIVE: THE CUBAN HEALTHCARE MODEL— INTERPROFESSIONAL COLLABORATION IN EVERY NEIGHBORHOOD

Over the past several years, medical and health professionals from the University of Minnesota have collaborated with MEDICC, a nonprofit organization with a mission to "promote US-Cuba health collaboration and highlight Cuba's public health approaches to inform the quest for health equity and universal health world-wide" (MEDICC, 2020). This partnership provided opportunities to visit Cuba to learn about their public health, prevention-focused approach to healthcare and population health management. One major point of focus on these trips has been to see Cuba's highly effective primary care model known as the *consultorio*, which is described below by one of the authors and a participant on the trip.

Tucked away within a small neighborhood in Cuba, the breeze flows through the three-room community clinic known as a consultorio. Tall trees, thick grass, and flowers surround the building, while the sweet smell of flowers enters the small five-chair waiting room where you can hear the birds chirping and smell the recent rain in the air. The nurse and physician along with their families live above the clinic on the second and third floors.

The neighborhood consultorio is the foundation of Cuba's highly effective population health system. Each neighborhood has a consultorio staffed with a nurse and physician dyad who live within the community, get to know their patients and their families closely as community members, and work in partnership with the community they serve. The nurse/physician interprofessional partnership is evident in their philosophy that working together will best serve their community.

The nurse-physician dyad in each neighborhood consultorio cares for up to 40 patients per day and is responsible for between 700 and 1,500 residents. During the morning, the physician and nurse see patients by appointment or walk-in, and in the afternoon, they make house visits, either to care for those who are unable to travel to the clinic or to assess the family unit. Every year, the physician and nurse reevaluate the health of individuals as well as the health of the entire household so that emerging issues can be detected and addressed in a timely manner. This holistic approach contributes to exceptional population health outcomes.

Across Cuba, the level of care provided within the consultorios includes basic primary care, health education, annual physical assessments, and chronic care with an established plan. In addition, health data are collected and reported nationally. The physician and nurse address patient concerns and reinforce the value and importance of health and well-being. Patients seek healthcare as needed and when recommended. When asked how the providers encourage community members to access the services provided and recommended, one physician laughed and said, "People come because they know it is important for them to stay healthy. We don't need to make them come; they just do."

Consultorios offer primary care within the community, and this is the first tier within the Cuban healthcare system. The second tier includes the *polyclinicas*, where patients receive more advanced levels of care that the community clinics are not equipped to deliver. Providers in this tier serve a larger region and provide services such as laboratory, radiology, cancer treatment, dental care, reproductive services, and holistic and alternative medicine. Often, the community physician or nurse will accompany patients to the polyclinica and maintain communication with the various providers to ensure seamless care across the healthcare continuum.

The third tier in the Cuban healthcare system includes more specialized care, such as hospitals and specialty institutes. The institutes include nationwide specialty care such as cardiology and diabetes. Once patients have returned to an optimal level of health, they return to their community nurse and physician dyad in their neighborhood consultorio.

Communication is paramount within this tiered system. One way to maintain good communication is through daily reporting from the nurse/physician dyad to national health officials. The nurses and physicians assess the health of the community daily. Local health concerns are identified and reported to the National Administrator of Public Health, and concerns are also communicated across the country to ensure early detection and awareness of public health trends. As issues emerge, data are shared across the various tiers and around the nation so that quick and adaptive changes can be made to ensure positive results and early impact. This approach is similar to syndromic surveillance techniques used for public health in other countries worldwide (May et al., 2009).

Public health approaches are integral to maintaining healthy individuals, communities, and the nation. With limited resources, the Cuban healthcare system prioritizes health maintenance, education, and prevention to maintain health and prevent illness instead of focusing primarily on treating illness after it has occurred. This system of prevention is woven through other aspects of society as well. The Cuban government provides health literacy through television advertisements and posters placed in the consultorios, polyclinicas, hospitals, and specialty institutes. In addition, nutrition and basic health principles are taught in schools, communities, and various public health programs. With such a strong emphasis on disease prevention and population health and the strong support of these messages by healthcare providers, Cubans have a basic understanding of maintaining health.

In a country with limited economic resources, maintaining health and preventing costly illness takes on added importance. This national prevention- and health-oriented national healthcare system has enabled the country to realize such healthcare outcomes as infant mortality rates of 3.8/1,000 live births (The World Bank, 2021c) compared to the worldwide median rate of 14.7/1000 live births (The World Bank, 2021b). Furthermore, in 2019, life expectancy rates in Cuba averaged 79 years compared to the worldwide average of 72.7 years (The World Bank, 2021a).

It is important to note that Cuba has achieved these outcomes through its established public health system. While other countries could learn and adapt their systems based on this model, they need to consider their unique economy, healthcare infrastructure, available resources, and political and legal systems when attempting to apply strategies from other countries to their own. Simply transplanting the Cuban model directly to another country may not be effective.

In summary, the Cuban healthcare system is a government-run population health system accessible to everyone. Communities benefit from the nurse/physician dyad model and the holistic approach inclusive of human, community, and environmental health. In part, Cuba's impressive health outcomes are due to interprofessional education and collaborative practice and patients, families, and communities participating as full partners in health maintenance and disease prevention.

# PLANETARY HEALTH: MOVING TOWARD TRANSDISCIPLINARY COLLABORATION

Interprofessional education and practice can improve the current healthcare system. However, visionary nursing leaders understand that we need to not only improve but transform the system to advance the health of populations. Significant developments such as social determinants of health (SDOH) help us see that health and well-being are much more complex than simply the absence of disease. Furthermore, global initiatives like the United Nations Sustainable Development Goals (SDGs) advance the call for equity based on the understanding that our choices today impact the options of future generations. With these frames in mind, we believe it is time for nurses to implement transdisciplinary collaboration to improve planetary health.

# TRANSDISCIPLINARITY

Transdisciplinary collaboration represents the most recent advancement in cross-sector collaboration. While interprofessional collaboration encourages people from different healthcare disciplines to work together, transdisciplinary collaboration invites all fields to come together to advance the health of populations.

Transdisciplinarity seeks new knowledge and insights, which would not be available if healthcare professionals only look through a disciplinary or a traditional interprofessional practice lens. Broad systems thinking and inclusive collaboration are necessary to redefine health and innovate transformational change. From drafting a new policy to designing a new care delivery model, transdisciplinary thinking offers complete knowledge to address complex issues.

# PLANETARY HEALTH

Few challenges are more complex than planetary health. Planetary health is both ancient and rapidly emerging. It represents a way of knowing, valuing, and living common to Indigenous people through history. It also represents an emerging field of science, an ecosystem-oriented value system, and a lifestyle and practice movement for today. Planetary health recognizes that humans cannot flourish if the health of Earth's natural systems is in peril because, essentially, the health of humans and the health of the planet are deeply interconnected.

The modern planetary health movement gained momentum following the publication of "Safeguarding Human Health in the Anthropocene Epoch: Report of The Rockefeller Foundation–Lancet Commission on Planetary Health" (Whitmee et al., 2015). This paper documents the consequences of the human-caused disruption of Earth's natural systems and the impact on human health now and for generations to come. Increased loss of biodiversity, climate change, disrupted biogeochemical flows, and other ways humans exceed the planet's boundaries or life support systems put all our public health gains over the last century at risk.

Planetary health offers a way of thinking that not only includes public health, one health, eco-health, and global health, but also emphasizes the critical need for transdisciplinary research to create effective solutions. Planetary health recognizes that there must be a great transition of all aspects of human society to address the rapidly accelerating destruction of Earth's natural systems. We need to redesign how we produce and consume food, products, and energy. We need to reimagine cities and create sustainably built environments to live and work. We also need to transform our relationships with nature and with one another from hierarchies of domination, extraction, and oppression to partnerships to ensure that future generations have a habitable planet.

Nursing is particularly well-equipped to lead and promote planetary health. Since the earliest days of the profession, nursing has recognized that the environment and nature are part of the healing paradigm. Nursing is also a profession that excels in systems thinking. From acid-base balance and gas exchange to safe housing and air quality, nurses understand that every part of the system is interconnected. We cannot have healthy humans when the environment is damaged.

Today, nursing leaders are using the cross-cutting principles for planetary health education (Stone et al., 2018) to redesign curricula to give future nurses the necessary knowledge to practice effectively and responsibly in a rapidly changing eco-system (Potter, 2019). In addition, the *Planetary Health Education Framework* (Faerron Guzman & Potter, 2021) proposes a transdisciplinary curriculum to facilitate collaboration to restore planetary health.

*Nurses Drawdown* (NDD), a partnership between Project Drawdown and the Alliance of Nurses for Healthy Environments, is another planetary health initiative. Nurses Drawdown teaches nurses about evidence-based solutions to drawdown greenhouse gases contributing to climate change. The NDD solutions have the co-benefit of improving the health of humans and the planet. Visionary nursing leaders understand that an orientation toward planetary health combined with transdisciplinary collaboration equips us to address our most urgent global health challenges quickly. ˙

# PLANETARY HEALTH RESOURCES FOR VISIONARY NURSING LEADERS

Every emerging field has foundational resources to support its growth. The following are key links for nursing leaders who want to address the urgent planetary health crisis:

- **Alliance of Nurses for Healthy Environments:** A nursing professional organization promoting education and advocacy of nurses related to care of the environment. https://envirn.org

- **Nurses Drawdown:** A global nursing movement to promote evidence-based solutions to drawdown greenhouse gasses contributing to climate change. https://www.nursesdrawdown.org

- **Planetary Health Alliance:** A collaboration of over 240 organizations working to promote planetary health research, education, and practice. https://www.planetaryhealthalliance.org/planetary-health

- **The Promise of Planetary Health** (10-minute video): https://www.youtube.com/watch?v=9cZ0zBSJz_g

- **Planetary Health Education Framework:** A global framework to support planetary health education and curriculum design in higher education disciplines. https://www.planetaryhealthalliance.org/education-framework

# IMPLICATIONS FOR PRACTICE

We have several decades of data supporting interprofessional team-based care to strengthen health systems and improve health outcomes for patients. There are also implications for nursing practice, including evidence that the nursing profession can influence team-based culture and assume interprofessional leadership roles at all levels.

Nursing represents the largest health profession sector in direct contact with patients (IOM, 2011). Despite challenges in diverse healthcare settings, distinct professional domains, and unequal power and hierarchical governance issues, nursing has a history of being integral to delivering team-based, patient- and family-centered care. In 2015, the National League for Nursing created a document outlining the importance of interprofessional education and practice in nursing (NLN, 2015). This document utilized the Interprofessional Education Collaborative's (IPEC Expert Panel, 2011) core competencies to create a toolkit for nursing educators and leaders. In addition, the American Association of Colleges of Nursing (AACN), a founding member of the IPEC, regularly provides nursing faculty with IPECP education and support. The nursing profession recognizes the importance of promoting excellence in interprofessional education and the implications for nursing practice that align with societal needs in a changing healthcare landscape.

Historically, most studies about the impact of interprofessional practice on nursing have focused on hospital settings and healthcare teams working together to care for an acutely ill patient. However, these studies demonstrate that acute care delivery requires ongoing negotiations among multiple professionals (e.g., social workers and nurses), and coordination is necessary between them. However, other forms of collaborative relations are gaining prominence, and the work settings can play a vital role in collaboration (Dow, 2017).

Interprofessional nursing practice is multifaceted and occurs across diverse settings. Examples include an electronic collaboration among diverse professionals doing telehealth visits, an interprofessional group collaborating in a community clinic effort for a patient with multiple psychosocial needs, or nurses on cancer care teams building key patient support contacts with outside agencies. These examples suggest that interprofessional and transdisciplinary partnerships are critical in promoting health outcomes. The nursing profession can become a role model in a partnership-based culture that supports equal power, respect, accountability, and trust, setting an example for the entire interprofessional team. Nurses and nurse leaders play an integral role in expanding meaningful interprofessional education and practice.

# SUMMARY

The data are clear that interprofessional collaboration is having a significant impact on global health outcomes. However, collaborative practice does not happen spontaneously; it requires all health profession students (WHO, 2010). Collaborative practice also requires healthcare organizations to be willing to empower interprofessional teams to function and do their unique work to advance health. These organizations must orient toward partnership, with full recognition of the value and contributions of each profession. They must also support structures and processes that allocate time and resources to support team development and practice. Interprofessional collaboration is advanced through disseminating examples of highly effective, partnership-based interprofessional collaborative practice. The examples of interprofessional teams promoting population health indicate that the interprofessional collaborative approach can move nations from illness care to healthcare.

Complex global health issues such as emerging infectious diseases, the increased number and severity of natural disasters, and the global refugee crisis call us to realize that the health of humans is deeply interconnected with the health of the planet. We must move beyond interprofessional collaborative practice to a transdisciplinary collaborative approach where all disciplines work together to address these urgent issues. It is time for visionary nursing leaders to step forward and assemble a unifying force for the health of all people and the planet.

# REFLECTIVE QUESTIONS

1.  Eisler and Potter (2014) applied cultural transformation theory to healthcare systems and described those systems fall along a continuum from domination- to partnership-based systems.

    *Question*: List characteristics specific to a domination-based system.

    *Question*: List characteristics specific to a partnership-based system.

2.  Consider how a domination system impacts the patient experience within healthcare environments. Read the following example and then answer the following question.

    Emely was 5. She and her mother, Lydia, were scared. Emely was admitted to the hospital for chronic leg pain and they both had a lot of questions. As a non-native English speaker, Lydia did the best she could to understand the nurses and physicians when they told her that Emely would have labs done, various tests, and possible treatments. The healthcare team made little attempt to ensure that Lydia understood what they were saying, and rarely included her in any decisions. She continued to ask questions and seek partnership from the team during the journey but didn't even know what questions to ask. Behind closed doors, the physicians discussed the cancer diagnosis and asked that the nurses not discuss it with the family. They withheld the information for four days. On a Friday afternoon, the healthcare team took 10 minutes to tell Lydia that Emely was diagnosed with cancer. Lydia was alone in the room with Emely, no support person present. She was left with more questions than she initially had and felt too rushed to ask anything. Whom could she turn to about her fears when so far no one had made the effort to listen, to work in partnership, to truly care for them? Lydia and Emely felt alone.

    *Question*: List some ways in which the healthcare team exhibited domination characteristics during the care of Lydia and Emely.

3.  Given this example, consider if the care provided was within a partner-ship-based system. Read the following example from a partnership-based perspective and then answer the following questions.

Emely was 5. She and her mother, Lydia, were scared. Emely was admitted to the hospital for chronic leg pain and they both had a lot of questions. The healthcare team immediately recognized the need for an interpreter and arranged one to be present as they discussed with Lydia all the labs that could be done, various tests, and possible treatments. They asked her if she needed other resources or support during this time. Lydia and Emely discussed their fears with the healthcare team. Each day the healthcare team would discuss any new information or change in plans, including them in all the decisions. Once they identified that it was in fact cancer, the healthcare team held a meeting to discuss the information with Lydia as her family surrounded her. They supported Lydia as she asked her questions and provided her with resources in case more questions came up afterwards. Lydia and Emely knew they could turn to their healthcare team at any time with their fears and questions as the team had made every effort to listen, to work in partnership, and to truly care for them. Lydia and Emely felt safe.

*Question*: List some ways in which the healthcare team exhibited partner-ship-based characteristics during the care of Lydia and Emely.

*Question*: How can partnership-based systems be used to transform healthcare at the bedside, in communities, across nations, and even the health of the planet?

# NARRATIVE

You are the Director of Public Health for a county in Northern California. Climate change is causing frequent and severe heat waves with high temperatures throughout the day and very little relief in the evenings. You are aware of numerous families living in older apartment buildings without air-conditioning and their indoor temperatures are continuing to rise.

In addition, heavy winter snows led to massive growth of brush which has now dried and is fueling predictions that this will be a very severe fire year. You are aware that your county has an aging population with many chronic health issues. In addition to wildfires and severe heat, fires bring days with unhealthy air quality, which can be especially dangerous for people with asthma and other chronic lung diseases.

Climate change impacts the health of populations, but it also impacts the health of individuals. Recently one of the county's visiting nurses raised a concern about an insulin dependent diabetic. The packaging for the insulin says "keep it at room temperature of 20–25°C (68–77°F) after opening. DO NOT store in the refrigerator." Without air-conditioning, indoor temperatures are no longer less than 77 degrees. Is this patient safe?

# AUTHOR BIOGRAPHIES

Teddie M. Potter, PhD, RN, FAAN, FNAP, Clinical Professor, University of Minnesota School of Nursing, is a Fellow in the National Academies of Practice and the American Academy of Nursing, where she chairs the Environment and Public Health Expert Panel. She is a member of the Coordinating Committee of Columbia University's Global Consortium on Climate and Health Education and a Fellow in the Institute on the Environment at the University of Minnesota. She chairs Clinicians for Planetary Health (C4PH) and is a member of the Steering Committee of the Planetary Health Alliance at Harvard. Working in partnership with Project Drawdown, Potter co-created *Nurses Drawdown*, which inspires nurses around the world to decrease greenhouse gas emissions and create a healthier future for humans and the rest of the planet. In 2019, she was appointed the first Director of Planetary Health for the University of Minnesota School of Nursing and is also the specialty coordinator for the Doctor of Nursing Practice in Health Innovation and Leadership. Her scholarship includes co-authoring *Transforming Interprofessional Partnerships: A New Framework for Nursing and Partnership-Based Health Care*, which received a 2014 AJN Book of the Year Award and the 2015 Capstone International Nursing Book Award.

**Stephanie D. Gingerich, DNP, RN, CPN,** is a Clinical Assistant Professor at the University of Minnesota School of Nursing and also leads the Health Care Design and Innovation post-baccalaureate certificate program within the university. Her scholarly focus is on global healthcare studies, partnership approaches to academic and professional nursing, and leadership. As part of her global healthcare interest, Gingerich has had the opportunity to study the healthcare systems within several countries including Cuba. She holds a Doctor of Nursing Practice in Health Innovation and Leadership from the University of Minnesota and a Bachelor of Science in Nursing from the University of Iowa. She holds certificates in Health Care Design and Innovation from the University of Minnesota and Pediatric Nursing from the Pediatric Nursing Certification Board. Gingerich is a registered nurse, dedicated professor to her students and colleagues, and active community member.

**Diana Drake, DNP, APRN, WHNP, FAAN, FNAP,** Clinical Professor, Director of Women's Health Gender-Related Nurse Practitioner specialty, University of Minnesota School of Nursing, holds faculty appointments at the University of Minnesota School of Nursing and the Earl Bakken Center for Spirituality and Healing. She is the current Chair of the National Association of Women's Health Nurse Practitioners (NPWH) and has served as a member of NPWH Board of Directors since 2016. Her ongoing work represents the intersectionality of women's health practice, teaching, and leadership with a focus on midlife care and the impact of gender, race, and ethnicity on health equity. With over three decades in the nursing profession, she has provided patient care and leadership in private, academic, and community clinics and led an annual Afro-Brazilian women's health study program in Salvador, Brazil. Drake's scholarly work continues to be grounded in developing and sustaining interprofessional practice models, integrative healthcare options, and advocacy for women's health issues across the life span.

# REFERENCES

American College of Obstetricians and Gynecologists' Task Force on Collaborative Practice. (2016). Collaboration in practice: Implementing team-based care. *Obstetrics & Gynecology, 127*(3), 612–617. https://www.acog.org/-/media/project/acog/acogorg/clinical/files/task-force-report/articles/2016/executive-summary-collaboration-in-practice.pdf?la=en&hash=5AEC403EB3C068FB7D1BA5336798177C

Buring, S., Bhushan, A., Broeseker, A., Conway, S., Duncan-Hewitt, W., Hansen, L., & Westberg, S. (2009). Interprofessional education: Definitions, student competencies and guidelines for implementation. *American Journal of Pharmaceutical Education, 73*(4), 59. doi: 10.5688/aj730459

Declercq, E., & Zephryrin, L. (2020). *Maternal mortality in the United States: A primer.* The Commonwealth Fund. https://www.commonwealthfund.org/publications/issue-brief-report/2020/dec/maternal-mortality-united-states-primer

Dow, A. W., Zhu, X., Sewell, D., Banas, C. A., Mishra, V., & Tu, S.-P. (2017). Teamwork on the rocks: Rethinking interprofessional practice as networking. *Journal of Interprofessional Care, 31*(6), 677–678. doi:1080/13561820.2017.1344048

Eisler, R., & Potter, T. (2014). *Transforming interprofessional partnerships: A new framework for nursing and partnership-based health care.* Sigma Theta Tau International.

Faerron Guzman, C. A., & Potter, T. (2021). *The planetary health education framework*. Planetary Health Alliance. https://planetaryhealthalliance.org/education-framework

Frenk, J., Chen, L., Bhutta, Z. A., Cohen, J., Crisp, N., Evans, T., Fineberg, H., Garcia, P., Ke, Y., Kelley, P., Kistnasamy, B., Meleis, A., Naylor, D., Pablos-Mendez, A., Reddy, S., Scrimshaw, S., Sepulveda, J., Serwadda, D., & Zurayk, H. (2010). Health professionals for a new century: Transforming education to strengthen health systems in an interdependent world. *The Lancet, 376*(9756), 1923–1958.

Institute of Medicine. (1972). *Educating for the health team* [Conference report]. Washington, DC: National Academies.

Institute of Medicine. (2001). *Crossing the quality chasm: A new health system for the 21st century*. Washington, DC: National Academies.

Institute of Medicine. (2011). *The future of nursing: Leading change, advancing health*. Washington, DC: National Academies.

Interprofessional Education Collaborative. (2016). *Core competencies for interprofessional collaborative practice: 2016 update*. Washington, DC: Author.

Interprofessional Education Collaborative Expert Panel. (2011). *Core competencies for interprofessional collaborative practice: Report of an expert panel*. Author. https://ipec.memberclicks.net/assets/2011-Original.pdf

Kendig, S. (2016, June 2). Collaboration in practice: A framework for team-based care. *Women's Healthcare: A Clinical Journal for NPs*. https://www.npwomenshealthcare.com/collaboration-practice-framework-team-based-care/

May, L., Chretien, J. P., & Pavlin, J. A. (2009). Beyond traditional surveillance: Applying syndromic surveillance to developing settings—opportunities and challenges. *BMC Public Health, 9*(242). doi: 10.1186/1471-2458-9-242

McClellan, S. (2019). *Women's health is more than gynecology*. https://qz.com/1763135/how-us-healthcare-is-failing-women/

MEDICC. (2020). *Our mission*. https://medicc.org/ns/wp-content/cache/all/ns/about/index.html

National League for Nursing. (2015). *Interprofessional collaboration in education and practice*. http://www.nln.org/docs/default-source/default-document-library/ipe-ipp-vision.pdf?sfvrsn=14

Pechacek, J., Drake, D., Terrell, C. & Torkelson, C. (2015). Interprofessional intervention to support mature women: A case study. *Creative Nursing, 21*(3), 34–43. doi: 10.1891/1078-4535.21.3.134

Potter, T. (2019). Planetary health: The next frontier in nursing education. *Creative Nursing, 25*(3), 201–207.

Rayburn, W., & Jenkins, D. (2021). Interprofessional collaboration in women's health care: Collective competencies, interactive learning, and measurable improvement. *Obstetrics and Gynecology Clinics of North America, 48*(1), 1–10. https://doi.org/10.1016/j.ogc.2020.11.010

Reeves, S., Goldman, J., & Oandasan, I. (2007). Key factors in planning and implementing interprofessional education in health care settings. *Journal of Allied Health, 36*(4), 231–235.

Rodger, S., & Hoffman, S. J. (2010). Where in the world is interprofessional education? A global environment scan. *Journal of Interprofessional Care, 24*(5), 479–491.

Schot, E., Tummers, L., & Noordegraaf, M. (2019). Working on working together. A systematic review on how healthcare professionals contribute to interprofessional collaboration. *Journal of Interprofessional Care, 34*(3), 332–342. https://www.tandfonline.com/doi/full/10.1080/13561820.2019.1636007

Stone, S. B., Myers, S. S., & Golden, C. D. (2018). Cross-cutting principles for planetary health education. *The Lancet – Planetary Health, 2*, e192–e193.

Whitmee, S., Haines, A., Beyrer, C., Boltz, F., Capon, A. G., de Souza Dias, B. F., Ezeh, A., Frumkin, H., Gong, P., Head, P., Horton, R., Mace, G. M., Marten, R., Myers, S. S., Nishtar, S., Osofsky, S. A., Pattanayak, S. K., Pongsiri, M. J., Romanelli, C., Soucat, A., . . . Yach, D. (2015). Safeguarding human health in the Anthropocene epoch: Report of the Rockefeller Foundation – *Lancet* Commission on Planetary Health. *The Lancet*, *386*(10007), 1973–2028. https://doi.org/10.1016/S0140-6736(15)60901-1

The World Bank. (2021a). *Life expectancy at birth, total (years)*. https://data.worldbank.org/indicator/SP.DYN.LE00.IN

The World Bank. (2021b). *Mortality rate, infant (per 1,000 live births)*. https://data.worldbank.org/indicator/SP.DYN.IMRT.IN

The World Bank. (2021c). *Mortality rate, infant (per 1,000 live births) – Cuba*. https://data.worldbank.org/indicator/SP.DYN.IMRT.IN?locations=CU

World Health Organization. (1988). Learning together to work together for health: Report of a WHO study group on multi-professional education of health personnel – the team approach. *World Health Organization Technical Report Series*, *769*, 1–72.

World Health Organization. (2010). *Framework for action on interprofessional education and collaborative practice*. WHO Press.

Zephyrin, L., Suennen, L., Viswanathan, P., Augenstein, J., & Bacjrach, D. (2020). *Transforming primary health care for women – Part 1: A framework for addressing gaps and barriers*. The Commonwealth Fund. https://www.commonwealthfund.org/publications/fund-reports/2020/jul/transforming-primary-health-care-women-part-1-framework

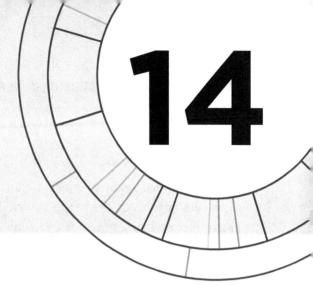

# 14

# LEADERSHIP IN DISASTER PREPAREDNESS AND RESPONSE

Carol Ann King, DNP, MSN, BSN, FNP-BC, RN, NHDP-BC
Gabrielle Dawn Childs, MA, MPH, RN
Michelle Taylor Skipper, DNP, FNP-BC, NHDP-BC, FAANP

---

## LEARNING OBJECTIVES

After completing this chapter, you should be able to understand:

- Contemporary global disasters and health implications

- Essential concepts and common language of disaster management

- Roles and responsibilities of nurses as leaders related to disaster planning and management

- Nurses' roles in promoting and advocating disaster management policies

- Training and education programs to promote disaster management

- Implications to nursing practice related to interprofessional disaster planning and management

---

# OVERVIEW

Disasters happen, many of which are unavoidable or uncontrollable and have significant impacts on the health and well-being of individuals and communities. Hurricanes/cyclones, tornadoes, earthquakes, droughts, wildfires, landslides, volcanoes, and tsunamis are all potentially life-threatening natural disasters that happen with minimal or no advanced notice. Man-made disasters, whether intentional or accidental, also threaten the public's health and safety, including nefarious acts of terrorism or human and mechanical errors resulting in catastrophes, such as the malfunctioning of a nuclear powerplant. With minimal advanced notice of impending disasters, communities and organizations must focus on disaster assessments, preparation, and proactive planning. Nursing leaders are vitally important to successful disaster planning and risk mitigation and need to be integral members of community emergency and disaster management teams. Nursing leaders also play a pivotal role in the development of competent nurses ready to respond when disasters strike (McNeill et al., 2020).

# DISASTERS AND THEIR IMPACTS

As defined by the International Federation of Red Cross and Red Crescent Societies (IFRC, 2021), a *disaster* is "a sudden, calamitous event that seriously disrupts the functioning of a community or society and causes human, material, and economic or environmental losses that exceed the community's or society's ability to cope using its own resources" (p. 1). A disaster is not determined by the size of the event but rather the magnitude of the impact on the community that exceeds its current response capacity. A minor flood could produce significant negative consequences for a community, threatening health and safety and disrupting essential functioning. Globally, disasters contribute to injury, death, destruction, and financial costs that impact the ability of communities to maintain essential functions for safety and access to life-sustaining necessities such as clean drinking water, safe food, safe sanitation, and essential healthcare. Death rates from both natural and man-made disasters vary by year, ranging from around 8,000 reported in 2020 (excluding COVID-19 pandemic deaths) to nearly 400,000 in 1970 (Swiss Re Institute, 2020). The COVID-19 pandemic is considered the most catastrophic disaster in recorded history that affected much of our global population, with over 170 million confirmed cases and over 3.5 million deaths as of June 2021 (World Health Organization [WHO], 2021).

Disaster management prepares in advance and assumes there will be future catastrophic events. It is proactive in planning and reactive when necessary. Emergency and disaster planning are specialized areas of education and training with an all-threats/hazards approach to promote collaboration between organizations, communities, states, and countries through mutual aid agreements. The primary driving goals of disaster management must prioritize efforts to reduce loss of life, minimize property and environmental damage, and protect communities from all hazards. A well-developed disaster management plan includes the key missions of prevention, protection, mitigation, response, and recovery (Federal Emergency Management Agency, [FEMA], 2020a).

Disaster management is a complex process that requires communication and coordination among many different agencies, organizations, and municipalities and the development of a comprehensive plan that includes policies and procedures that require training and a list of available and needed resources. Once the disaster plan is developed, training and simulation exercises, based on the crawl/walk/run process, must begin, starting with classroom education and progressing to table-top exercises followed by larger-scale exercises within the health system or community, depending on the focus of the disaster plan. Disaster plans need continual review and updating, including an updated list of available resources, equipment, personnel, and facilities (Songwathana & Timalsina, 2021).

The all-threats/hazards approach to community emergency management and disaster planning attempts to identify and address all potential threats to the health and well-being of the population and jurisdictions of interest. In the United States (US), FEMA developed the National Threat and Hazard Identification and Risk

Assessment (THIRA) to guide communities through an all-threats/hazard assessment; it serves as an important resource for nursing leaders in organizational risk assessments (FEMA, 2019). Nursing leaders must have a firm understanding of the methodology to identify disaster threats and hazards, assess the potential severity of the threat or hazard, and be able to accurately assess vulnerabilities to community health to be effective in disaster planning efforts.

# CONTEMPORARY GLOBAL DISASTERS AND HEALTH IMPLICATIONS

The current global COVID-19 pandemic has highlighted the global disparity in health and healthcare. Vulnerable populations—including those with low socio-economic resources, minorities, and the elderly—have been disproportionally affected by the devastating health effects of the COVID-19 virus due to its inequitable spread in areas of dense population and limited mitigation capacity due to the high prevalence of chronic conditions or poor access to high-quality public health and medical care. Additionally, the pandemic has not only affected global physical and mental health but has also impacted global economies and the social aspects of society, compounding the effects of the pandemic disproportionately against poor and vulnerable populations. The interventions to mitigate the pandemic restricted movements and forced different levels of quarantine that impacted social and mental connections and everyday routines. Businesses closed, employees lost wages, schools and daycares closed, and life as the world knew it was changed. With the introduction of mass vaccinations and herd immunity, a new normal began to develop, but life will never return to pre-pandemic norms (Shadmi et al., 2020).

While the COVID-19 pandemic was a global catastrophe, most disasters affect a specific region of the world, such as the east coast of the United States from Hurricane Florence or the 2010 Haitian region earthquake. The Haiti-region earthquake killed over 316,000 people and affected millions of others through injuries, loss of homes, and limited access to essential resources, stressing the region's response and recovery capabilities far beyond the resources available (Fisher & Kramer, 2012). Regional disasters stress the survival capabilities of the affected regions but provide prime opportunities for unaffected regions to collaborate and offer assistance for response and recovery. Nurse leaders are vital advocates for regional disaster mutual aid planning, response, and recovery and must assert themselves to be included as part of disaster planning.

# CONTEMPORARY ISSUES IN DISASTER MANAGEMENT

When considering disasters, nursing leaders need to understand the subsequent short-term and long-term impacts on people's health and well-being due to the compounding effects of the disaster. Beyond the devasting effects of the initial disaster impact, communities experiencing disasters face secondary risks to health and well-being that emerge soon after the initial impact, such as the cholera outbreak following the earthquake in Haiti, which infected over 500,000 people resulting in 7,000 deaths (Fisher & Kramer, 2012). The short-term aftereffects of disasters include unsafe drinking water, limited access to safe food, limited access to essential healthcare, limited money to buy essential goods, loss of homes and safe living and sleeping areas, and increase in opportunistic criminal activity, including profiteering due to supply and demand imbalance (Raker et al., 2020).

Businesses that provide essential services, such as grocery stores, gas stations, pharmacies, and medical supply companies, may be closed due to disruption in utility services and unsafe community conditions. These businesses are unable not only to provide their products and services but also may be unable to pay employees. Unemployment, both short-term and long-term, along with loss of homes, can produce significant psychological stress for community members, which becomes evident in the short-term recovery period, with depression, anxiety, insomnia, increased substance use, and post-traumatic stress (Wilson-Genderson et al., 2018).

Long-term effects from disasters can include a loss of income and economic insta-bility, physical health declines, and long-term psychological health declines includ-ing, most commonly, post-traumatic stress disorders, depression, and anxiety (Es-terwood & Saeed, 2020). Businesses may be temporarily or permanently closed, whole communities may be permanently uninhabitable, and loved ones may not have survived the disaster. People's lives are changed with minimal to no advanced notice, and these changes stress individuals' and communities' ability to adapt and cope with the impacts of the event. Those individuals with pre-existing behavior-al health and substance abuse conditions are at higher risk than others without pre-existing conditions for adverse psychological outcomes and increased morbid-ity and mortality. Nurse leaders need to clearly advocate for pre-disaster planning that includes identifying at-risk populations and linking those at increased risk with needed services, information, and support (Morganstein & Ursano, 2020).

Nurse leaders must examine the past to help plan for future disasters. Contempo-rary issues in disaster management include considerations of the potential of the *perfect storm*—an emergency management concept that presents the compounded effect of multiple disaster events occurring simultaneously or cascading to increase the complexity of response and recovery. For example, cascading events that were considered the perfect storm involved the Fukushima Japan events in 2011, in which an earthquake created a tsunami and subsequent compromise of the Fukushima Daiichi nuclear power plant. Deaths and destruction occurred from the impact of the earthquake initially, and then additional deaths and injuries that overwhelmed the healthcare system, with extensive property damage from the subsequent tsunami. Then the nuclear power plant was damaged, which required evacuations that created further disruption in the social capital and economy. Due to the evacuation, people migrated away from the affected areas, and communi-ties suffered a significant economic and social decline, dying with all the people lost. Five of eight hospitals in the surrounding areas had to close due to staffing shortages. The perfect storm presents challenges that stress even the most resilient people and communities. Planning for all hazards and threats that may occur in a cascading manner is vital to successful response and recovery (Morita et al., 2017).

When considering psychological stress related to disasters, nurses must recognize the impact of the role of communication through cellular and internet service, including social media. Additionally, all electronic devices require a power source for recharging, including electricity that is often disrupted in many disasters. Society has become very dependent on mobile communication through advanced cellular and internet services and relies on those services to connect with family members and reunification efforts, receive essential disaster communications, locate available services and goods, and remain connected with the greater social media community (Stieger & Lewetz, 2018). When people are unable to access social media, they may experience withdrawal effects of anxiety, loss of control, insecurity, and cravings for social media.

Additionally, when internet and social media access is available, community members are affected by the false information that is posted, including inaccurate hazards, threats, and effects of the disaster event. For example, people who might be missing have been inaccurately reported as being deceased, causing significant distress for family and friends. Resources have been reported as being available when, in fact, they were not. Events were reported, such as a chemical bioterrorism event, that did not happen, but the public panics based on the false information. Nurse leaders must be aware of the importance of connectivity through the internet and social media, prepare for the impact of disruption on the community, and act to promote the circulation of accurate and helpful information through social media and mass communication efforts.

This disruption tests the resiliency of those affected and strains the resources available for response and recovery. Community members lose a sense of control and experience insecurities for which they may not have existing coping skills. For example, families may rely on electronic debit cards for state or federal funds for unemployment benefits or supplemental food programs, and cash on hand may be limited. When banks are closed and stores that sell essential goods, such as gas and food, will only take cash due to lack of electricity and internet services, families may not be able to obtain needed supplies. This loss of security is compounded by the potential of displacement, loss of routine, and uncertainty in the immediate future return to pre-disaster life. Nurse leaders who understand the psychological impacts of disasters can help prepare their communities through resiliency training, proper disaster planning and preparation, and centralized coordination of goods and services. Nurses can ensure people know where to turn for help and be part of the recovery that can promote post-disaster community growth.

Community disaster shelters are an important part of response and recovery efforts. Emergency shelters are intended to help support basic human needs, including food, water, bedding, hygiene, and information. In the US, the American Red Cross and local health departments typically lead the sheltering process as requested and directed by the disaster incident commander. When the need for shelters is identified, the incident command will request shelter coordination from the health director or appointed shelter leader in collaboration with the American Red Cross lead, who typically have representation on the incident command team. The local educational system lead and a faith-based community representative may also be involved, as schools, churches, and other large gathering places are typically designated as shelters due to the size and structure of schools and available resources. The number, size, and type of shelters needed are based on the impact of the disaster. There are three general types of shelters:

- **Cooling/warming stations** are available for independent community members and require minimal supervision, basically providing food, water, rest, information, and a respite from the climate.

- **General population shelters** provide enhanced services for those people with minimal medical needs who are able to independently attend to their own activities of daily living.

- **Medical assistance/special needs shelters** provide shelter for persons who require medical assistance or other special needs. These shelters have additional healthcare resources and supervision, typically provided by nurses who help coordinate the healthcare needs of the shelter occupants.

When considering the types and numbers of shelters needed for a given disaster, nurses need to consider the diversity of the population affected, including language barriers, cultural and religious practices (including as they relate to dietary practices), women who may be breastfeeding, and the elderly. Nurses need to know their community to be able to anticipate community needs to enable adequate planning. The county public health department is an excellent resource for the latest community assessment, which typically includes basic population demographics and populations served by the health department. While one can never anticipate every potential situation, nurses need to be armed with as much community information as possible to reasonably plan sheltering requirements.

Some shelters accept certain types of pets, but not all shelters will accept every type of pet. Service animals are typically allowed, but other animals may be excluded. Since many shelters will not allow pets, many community members have a serious dilemma, as many will not leave their pets behind and will stay in an unsafe situation to remain with their pets. Nurses can be instrumental in disaster preparation and include the importance of planning for the needs of family pets with at least a week's supply of food and water per pet. Also, nurses can help advocate for shelters that will accept pets to help keep all community members as safe as possible. For additional information and specific details on shelter organization, please refer to the American Red Cross Sheltering Handbook (https://crcog.org/wp-content/uploads/2017/12/American-Red-Cross-Sheltering-Handbook.pdf).

# DISASTER NURSING AS AN EVOLVING CONCEPT

Nurses have specialized education and training in healthcare assessment and care planning in partnership with patients and families across the lifespan and are skilled in responding in times of crisis. Typically, nurses are experts in crisis management in acute care settings with individuals and families. However, with additional education and training, nurses can be vital resources to communities during stressful, life-changing disasters. Nurse leaders are well-posed to facilitate the translation of these specialized nursing skills and clinical reasoning to disaster planning, mitigation, response, and recovery and promote nurses as key members of the interprofessional disaster team.

Globally, the nursing profession's disaster preparation and readiness to respond varies greatly between countries. While developed countries may have opportunities for education and training, nurses' perception of disaster preparation and readiness remains low overall. Disaster training includes much more than the basic health system emergency response plans and drills and includes key areas of community assessments; recognition of risks, hazards, and threats; community triage skills; and specific actions during the response and recovery phases (Songwathana & Timalsina, 2021).

Expanding the education and training of nurses to include disaster planning, response, and recovery is essential to prepare them to function as key members of the emergency management team. The International Council of Nurses (ICN, 2019) developed core disaster nursing competencies and differentiated the different levels of nursing practice with associated expected competencies. Level 1 nurses are those who have completed a basic nursing education program with authority to practice based on the country's requirements. Level II nurses meet the Level 1 requirements and receive additional training to qualify them as a responder within the healthcare system in the event of a disaster. Level III nurses meet the requirements for both Level 1 and II and have advanced education, training, and experience to prepare them to be part of the disaster management interprofessional team with the capability of responding to disasters in the community.

The ICN identified eight domains for nursing competency:

1.  Preparation and planning

2.  Communication

3.  Incident management systems

4.  Safety and security

5.  Assessment

6.  Intervention

7.  Recovery

8.  Law and ethics

Explaining the domains and expected competencies is only the start, and more work must be done. Measuring and evaluating competencies is still under development and expanding slowly in nursing curricula. The American Medical Association has developed core disaster competencies for public health and disaster medicine that nurse leaders may consider as they develop community disaster training (Walsh et al., 2012). Nurses need specific training and practice opportunities to allow for evaluating competency through exercises, building to real-life disaster experience. Nurses need to participate in disaster after-action reviews for evaluation of practice and improvement. While measurement and evaluation of specific nursing disaster competencies may be vague, nurse leaders need to continue these discussions and promote ongoing nursing education.

Disaster nursing is an evolving specialty, and integrating an international program for disaster nursing poses many challenges. The first challenge is the lack of universal standard nursing scope of care and standards of practice. Each country has its own regulatory body for nursing that defines the nursing scope of practice, and one must be cognizant of the varying standards and legal limitations to practice. Additionally, to work in another country may require a nurse to seek local licensure and validation of their current licensure before practicing in that country. Therefore, the expectation of what skills and abilities nurses can bring to disaster nursing has to be based on a common basic understanding among international boards of nursing. The ICN is the organization to help define those boundaries and ensure a shared understanding. Morrison (2010) developed the Scope of

Nursing Practice and Decision-Making Framework Toolkit, which concluded the following:

> International Council of Nurses (ICN) has held a clear position about the importance of regulation in assuring safe and competent nursing practice in order to protect the public. The way in which the scope of nursing practice is defined, outlines the very parameters and boundaries within which nurses practice. It is vital that the profession can clearly articulate its practice parameters in order to ensure that nursing practice can accommodate and respond to the current needs of society. Otherwise, there is a risk that practice may become restricted and constrained, thereby leaving needs unmet or care delivery fragmented (p. 5).

When planning for disasters and the role of nurses in the disaster management process, a clear understanding of healthcare resources, the distribution of resources, and the integration of the various government organizations is critical. The international standard for disaster planning and healthcare is based upon the United Nations (UN) doctrine, which requires all disaster personnel to have a clear understanding of health and disaster concepts and processes, including paid responders and volunteers alike. The UN echelons of care for peacekeeping missions are based on codified levels of care that clearly outline the provision of healthcare from the point of injury to definitive care.

In an international disaster, the medical response may be a mixture of government agencies, non-governmental organizations (NGOs), civilian disaster response agencies, and military medical response. The UN has provided guidance for international disaster management and clearly defines the healthcare personnel who make up the care continuum and their designated roles. Nurse leaders must have a clear understanding of the levels of care, the accepted scope of practice for nurses, and the required competency and training needed to integrate into the disaster management process globally (United Nations Medical Directors, 2020).

An example of a UN model of care for COVID-19 pandemic response is included in Table 14.2 (Disaster Training and Resources for Nurses).

# STATE OF HEALTHCARE LEADERSHIP IN THE DISASTER CONTINUUM

Most nursing programs prepare nurses to work in the acute care hospital setting primarily. While public health may be part of the nursing curriculum, it is only a brief exposure and experience, falling far short of the needed community health education and training needed to be effective in disaster management. Nursing integration into the greater community is lacking, remaining in their own silo. Nurses need to be present in community assessments and planning for more than a triage, response, and recovery. Nurses engage when disasters strike and tend to staff shelters and maintain inpatient and outpatient healthcare. Nursing leaders need to promote the expansion of the nursing role and be active in local, state, national, and global risk assessments, preparation, budgeting, policy-making, and ethical and legal considerations. Nurses also need specific education, training, and experience related to integration into an interprofessional team.

Disaster response teams are very diverse, including many non-healthcare-related professionals. Communication, negotiation, and collaboration are essential professional skills nurses need to be respected members of the interprofessional team (Hoying et al., 2017). Also, nurses need to recognize that they may be called upon to assist in areas of which they have little experience, such as managing volunteers, filling sandbags to prevent flooding of essential buildings, or helping rescue farm animals.

Nurse leaders may have education and training on disaster management processes and plans, especially related to healthcare systems, hospitals, and outpatient healthcare organizations, such as dialysis centers. However, leaders may not have experience in community disaster planning and actual disaster response and recovery referred to as *crisis leadership*, which encompasses all the essential disaster management functions of planning, preparation, training, risk mitigation, response, recovery, including the coordination of resources and assignments of required roles and responsibilities. Additionally, nurses need specific training and practice in the after-incident evaluations that begin the cycle of disaster preparation again. Nurses never know when they may be thrust into a leadership role on the incident command team. Even with adequate planning, formally appointed leaders of an organization or community may not be able to respond, leaving a gap that could result in negative outcomes if not addressed (Millet & Porche, 2017). For example, the lead public health nurse at the local health department is unable to assume their appointed role on the incident command team due to flooding, and the only available nurse is a junior faculty at the nearby community college. Nurses need to be prepared to assume leadership responsibilities and integrate as essential members of the interprofessional team.

The US continues to experience a nursing shortage overall, and nurses are working in a very stressful healthcare system. Nurses work long hours and face their own fatigue and burnout, leading to an increased number of nurses leaving the profession. Asking nurses to do more, work harder, and study longer is not sustainable. Nurse leaders need to be advocates for balance within the nurses' lives, helping nurses remain dedicated to improving the lives of people in their communities.

# LEADERS' ROLES IN DISASTER PREPAREDNESS

Nurse leaders must start the disaster management process by first having their own personal preparations for themselves and their families and have a plan to ensure personal sustainability in the response and recovery phases. Disaster response and recovery can vary from a few days to months or even years, depending on the type and magnitude of the disaster, and can happen without advanced notice. Everyone needs a personal and family disaster plan that includes adequate supplies (including food, water, medications, gasoline, and paper goods) and a reunification plan should family members become separated. Moral conflicts may arise when nurses are called upon to help their neighbors and community while having to entrust the care of their own families to other people. Self-care is vital to remaining mentally and physically ready to respond when disasters happen and sustain health during disaster recovery. Good hydration and nutrition, personal hygiene, times of rest, personal medications, and emotional support are important in initial response phases as well as ongoing recovery management. Nurse leaders need to first take care of themselves and their families, then ensure the nurses working with them do the same (Heagele et al., 2020).

Part of the nurse leader's role in disaster management involves learning the language and processes involved. Leaders must seek the knowledge and education needed to effectively contribute to disaster preparation, mitigation, response, and recovery. Nurses cannot be satisfied with participating in the response and recovery efforts as traditionally assigned, such as manning a disaster shelter. Learning the language and processes involved in disaster management requires time and energy (see Table 14.1 for common disaster terminology and Table 14.2 for training resources).

The US has developed a stellar emergency management system with specific training and plans that are easily adapted by local communities, states, and regions. FEMA's National Preparedness Plan and Incident Management System provide guidance for communities and the nation, with specific tools, training, and guidance to promote a unified, coordinated disaster management plan (FEMA, 2020b). Disaster training can easily be integrated into nursing education curricula utilizing the many online educational resources available. Nurse leaders must prepare nurses to be able to communicate effectively using the language of emergency management and to promote policies and plans that include nurses in all levels of disaster planning, mitigation, response, and recovery.

**TABLE 14.1** Sample Disaster Management Definitions

| | |
|---|---|
| All-Hazards Approach | Consider a wide range of disasters of various types, duration, size, and cause for well-designed disaster plans. Must also consider the possibility of the "perfect storm" of cascading/co-existing disasters |
| Perfect Storm | A term used to describe cascading or co-occurring disaster incidents, such as an earthquake causing a tidal wave, which then causes massive flooding that destroys crops and contaminated the water supply |
| Emergency Operations Planning (EOP) | The formal process and structure organizations and communities can use for disaster planning and responding that can be tailored to the specific needs of the organization or community |
| Command, Control, & Communication | "C3" includes the designated authority/lead of the disaster management team, verifying or correcting activities to ensure the goals of the command are accomplished, and liaison communication between the tactical and strategic commands. All three areas are essential for effective disaster management |
| NIMS | National Incident Management System—a framework that provides guidance and structure over a variety of hazards/threats that includes common terms/definitions and standards for overall incident management. See NIMS website: https://www.fema.gov/emergency-managers/nims |
| Incident Command | One of the 3 Cs in command, control, & communication—key people with expertise in dealing with the specific type of disaster are assigned to the Incident Command team, led by an Incident Commander. The designated incident commander is the lead authority in disaster management and is determined by the type of incident and personal expertise. |
| Continuity of Operation Plan (COOP) | Plans to ensure continuity of essential functions of communities, hospitals, healthcare systems, or businesses—include key "if/then" contingency plans and needed resources |
| Disaster Epidemiology | Health surveillance systems planned to be fully operational 2-6 hours after a disaster, focusing on tracking communicable diseases, environmental health risks, injuries, and subsequent chronic diseases |
| Mass Casualty Incident | Casualties exceed the available resources and are determined not by the number of casualties, but the resources needed to respond |

| | |
|---|---|
| Mutual Aid Agreement | Formalized agreements between towns/cities/states/countries and organizations/agencies to be available to provide or exchange resources based on needs |
| Geographic Information System (GIS) | Computer system that collects and displays specific earth surface data that can be used for modeling, including plume and vector forecasts. It can help the IC determine the potential impact of an event, such as a chemical release. |
| Bioterrorism Attack | Nefarious intentional release of viruses, bacteria, or other germs intended to cause illness and injury |
| Chemical Emergency | A chemical has been released that is potentially toxic, such as a major chlorine spill |
| Health System Resilience | The system's capacity to effectively and efficiently prepare for and respond to a disaster while maintaining core functions |

*For additional definitions, see the FEMA glossary at https://training.fema.gov/programs/emischool/el361toolkit/glossary.htm*

The true key to nursing leadership in a local community setting during a healthcare emergency or disaster crisis is advanced preparation, including critical evaluation of resources. This includes much more than basic medical supplies; it should also include a formal or informal evaluation of a community's infrastructure, including physical and human resources. Using FEMA standardized language and an all-hazards approach is ideal, but particularly in the initial phases of disaster response, local leaders are more likely to provide a first-line critical response. Nurse leaders need to have trusted relationships already established with more than their immediate healthcare community (Wyte-Lake et al., 2016). Nurse leaders must also know elected officials, education system leaders, and community administrators. Nurses need a basic understanding of the businesses and industries in their town and know the risks and resources those industries may provide.

**TABLE 14.2** Disaster Training and Resources for Nurses

| TRAINING | WEB LINK |
| --- | --- |
| FEMA Emergency Management Modules are available free online through the Independent Study tab. Recommend first: IS-100-c, IS-200-c, IS-700-b, & IS-800-d | https://training.fema.gov/is |
| World Health Organization Environmental Health in Emergencies. Recommend: Vulnerable groups, displaced people, medical aspects, and healthcare facilities | https://www.who.int/environmental_health_emergencies/preparedness/en |
| American Red Cross Disaster Training | https://www.redcross.org/take-a-class/disaster-training |
| National Center for Disaster Preparedness | https://ncdp.columbia.edu/practice/training-education/online-face-to-face-training |
| TRAIN website with many free training courses. Recommend: Caring for Older Adults in Disasters | https://www.train.org/main/course/1059666/ |
| Medical Service Corps Development Tools. Recommend: MRC Volunteer Core Competencies and MRC Volunteer Training Plan | https://www.naccho.org/uploads/downloadable-resources/2019-MRC-Core-Competencies-and-Training-Plan.pdf |
| Community Emergency Response Team training website | https://www.ready.gov/cert |
| The United Nations Medical Directors' UN Model of Care Checklist for UN Duty Stations in Response to COVID-19+ Pandemic | https://www.un.org/sites/un2.un.org/files/un_model_of_care_checklist_and_matrix.pdf |
| American Red Cross Sheltering Handbook 2017: step-by-step guide for planning and implementing shelters | https://crcog.org/wp-content/uploads/2017/12/American-Red-Cross-Sheltering-Handbook.pdf |
| National Voluntary Organizations Active in Disaster (VOAD)—a coalition of non-government organizations that provide disaster response and recovery services | https://www.nvoad.org/ |

Nurse leaders must actively assert themselves within the community emergency preparedness process. While not exhaustive, the list below includes key questions nurse leaders need to consider:

1. Who are my local elected officials? (required to authorize disaster response)

2. Who are my local school officials? (can be used for shelter and food resources)

3. Who are my local public health nurses, and what services have they been authorized to initiate?

4. Who are other medical personnel available, including local pharmacists, for emergency dispensation of medications?

5. What vulnerable populations live in the community? Who will need oxygen, dialysis, or glucose monitoring? Are there group homes or other long-term care facilities that might need evacuation or specialized shelter?

6. What local buildings have gas, electricity, or backup generators? Is the infrastructure safe to provide temporary healthcare or housing needs?

7. Are highways passable? Are emergency personnel available to assist with critical transportation needs?

8. Are local non-governmental organizations or faith communities prepared to assist in response?

9. Where are my community's flood zones? How are my community's water sources protected?

10. What community faith-based organizations are willing to respond, and what can they provide?

A nurse leader must also know what may not be needed in a local emergency. Often during an emergency, community members feel the need to donate food or clothing items that may be substandard. Professional discernment is quickly needed to pair resources with critical needs. By far, monetary donations and safe drinking water are key donations needed. Clothing, furniture, and perishable food items are not needed in the initial response, and recovery phases can become a hazard or threat for others and can drain vital resources to manage these donations. Nurse leaders need to know the local emergency management personnel, the leads of local agencies and organizations who will respond to disasters, and available resources. These needed relationships and discernment cannot be effectively established after a disaster strikes and must be developed in the disaster planning process (Ramsbottom et al., 2018).

Nurses should also be aware of vulnerable populations, such as the elderly, children, persons who require complex medications or medical treatments in the home, and community members with various limitations to mobility. For example, the elderly represented 75% of the deaths from Hurricane Katrina in 2005 while representing only 15% of the affected population at the time (Morita et al., 2017). Not all community members are able to evacuate or have the resources to transition to emergency shelters due to their medical needs. Often, they forego necessary medical treatments due to the healthcare system being overwhelmed by the effects of the disaster. After Hurricane Florence in 2018, a small coastal town was without electricity and safe drinking water, healthcare offices and pharmacies were closed, roads were blocked due to flooding, but people still needed their medications and supplemental oxygen to survive. Elderly persons were alone in their homes without electricity, food and water, and transportation in a hot, humid climate. Nurses were pivotal disaster team members, knew the community health needs, and quickly coordinated services to address the needs of these vulnerable people. Specific actions included community distribution of water and food, welfare checks on the elderly, securing necessary medications like insulin and respiratory inhalers from a variety of sources, and helping to maintain the health of all community response workers. As a result of a strong nursing presence and leadership, the community rebounded well without any loss of life (A. King, personal communication, March 2019).

Nurse leaders must consider the complexity of the community to include cultural diversity, special healthcare needs, limitations to mobility, and needed medical supplies, and strive to coordinate available resources to sustain life following a disaster. Evacuation costs money, and hotels/motels are most likely full if they are even open. Roads may be congested with evacuation traffic. Many people must remain in their homes for various reasons, and nurses need to assist those who remain in a nonjudgmental manner, linking them with vital goods and services. Nurses must understand the cultural diversity of their population, plan for language interpretation services, and institute measures to ensure disaster response team members are respectful of the diversity within the population (Harada et al., 2021).

Nurses have many resources available when the community pulls together and prepares for disasters, knowing that disasters happen locally, and the local area is responsible for the first response efforts. When a disaster's impact exceeds local capabilities, additional resources are enlisted through mutual aid agreements. Nurse leaders can be essential in negotiating these mutual aid agreements with surrounding cities and municipalities, states, and countries. Once the disaster's impact exceeds the capabilities of mutual aid, then other national and international organizations can aid. The list of potential contributors is extensive and includes the following: FEMA, American Red Cross/IFRC, community emergency response teams (CERTs), US Department of Homeland Security, US Small Business Administration, Samaritan's Purse, United Way, World Vision International, Save the Children Foundation, Medical Service Corps, Office of Foreign Disaster Assistance/USAID, Catholic Charities, Baptist Men on Missions, Methodist Disaster Response Teams, Feed the Children, Volunteers of America, US Army Corps of Engineers, Hope Worldwide, and Operation Blessing International.

# IMPLICATIONS FOR PRACTICE

Currently, many nurses have minimal training regarding disaster or emergency management and would not be considered competent in emergency and disaster preparedness, response, and recovery processes. Barriers include the expense and complexity of simulation experience and the lack of qualified disaster management faculty (Loke et al., 2021). This lack of training and competency development poses a risk to our communities, especially with response and recovery efforts. For example, nurse leaders should be well-versed in the use of social media for disaster communication, knowing how to inform the public effectively and efficiently on key disaster response efforts, including the current state of the situation, location of resources, and health education that could prove to be lifesaving. If the drinking water source is contaminated, people can easily get sick without the proper information to protect themselves. Through social media and various web-based applications (apps), such as local news and weather apps, people have been able to access essential pre-disaster warnings and information for preparation, response, and recovery in real-time. Additionally, nurse leaders are recognizing the deficit in disaster nursing resources and are developing specific disaster resources, such as the TriService Nursing Research Program *Battlefield and Disaster Nursing Pocket Guide*, which offers a comprehensive resource for nurses through all phases of disaster management (Bridges & McNeill, 2020).

One key policy and legal issue surrounding nursing is the ability for nurses to practice at the full scope of their capability and licensure in different states or countries. In the US, states grant nursing licenses, and the issuing state has the legal authority over the nursing practice in the state. In disasters, nurses may be needed in neighboring states but may face challenges with crossing state lines to perform nursing acts even with state-to-state license agreements. Nurses must be versed on the Nurse Practice Act in their state of licensure and any other state in which they may practice. Nurses who volunteer for disaster response and recovery must maintain the same nursing practice standards and ethical responsibilities, focusing on doing no harm and the greater good for all those affected by the disaster.

Nurse leaders need to advocate for all nurses to be able to practice to the full scope of their capabilities and understand any implications of volunteer work on registered nurses or advanced practice nurses' roles. Advanced practice nurses, such as nurse practitioners, midwives, nurse anesthetists, and clinical nurse specialists, have significant barriers to providing care within their expertise, training, and competency due to state requirements for physician collaboration/supervision in some states within the US, and they face challenges practicing legally within other countries. One resource to help address these barriers is the Medical Service Corps, an organization that provides a process of credential verification and applications to practice in different states and countries while maintaining a list of qualified volunteers ready to respond when disasters occur. In disasters, nurses need to respond quickly and need the legal protection and capability to do so without being delayed by administrative applications. Nurses can save lives when they are skilled in disaster planning, mitigation, response, and recovery and can deploy as part of the interprofessional disaster management team.

# SUMMARY

Disasters, large and small, will continue to occur, and nurses can assume a pivotal role in planning, preparatory actions, quick response, and resilient recovery to reduce morbidity and mortality. As seen with the COVID-19 pandemic most recently, nurses are essential personnel who give selflessly to their patients and communities. Nurse leaders need to support and empower nurses through self-care, help nurses develop competency in disaster management, promote the standardized scope of nursing practice, and assist nurses in being active members of interprofessional disaster management teams.

Nurse leaders must be present in the local, state, regional, national, and global disaster planning process and not merely volunteer to assist after disasters. Nurses need the necessary education and training to be competent in disaster nursing, learning the emergency management language, threat/risk assessment process, assisting with community emergency response planning, advocating for vulnerable populations, and being ready to respond quickly in a disaster. Resources are readily available and should be included in nurses' continuing education. Nurse educators should promote disaster education within nursing curricula and encourage nursing students to pursue expertise in disaster planning, response, and recovery. Nurses can do so much more than work in disaster shelters and need to be advocates for policies that allow nurses to practice to their full scope and capabilities wherever disasters strike.

---

**SMALL GROUP ROLE-PLAY AND DISCUSSION ACTIVITY**

Assign students to small groups of four to five students considering the diversity and different learning styles of students. Ask students to review the scenario below and then identify the resources needed to respond to the disaster effectively. Each student will assume a different incident command leadership role based on the community needs they identify and present their request for resources based on what they believe is necessary to safely assist their community.

---

# REFLECTIVE QUESTIONS

1. Consider the personal and moral conflicts for disaster nurses that may occur in disaster response and recovery and ways to minimize these conflicts.

2. During disaster response and recovery, nurses may be asked by the Incident Commander to be a part of a non-healthcare-related disaster team or asked to complete tasks that are not nursing-related, such as debris removal or food distribution. Think about how nurse leaders should respond to these requests and the potential implications of both accepting and declining the assignment.

3. Discuss vulnerable populations and special considerations nurse leaders must include in disaster preparation, mitigation, response, and recovery.

4. Community members have many spiritual, cultural, and ethnic differences. Consider your community population and their ethnic and cultural differences and how you would plan for these differences in the disaster preparation process.

5. What are your community's strengths and resources for disaster preparation? What are key challenges and mitigation measures to address those challenges?

# NARRATIVE

Emerald Place is a small, quaint coastal community with a population of 3,000 people. It enjoys tourists from all over the world in the summer months. During the summer months, the population increases to over 10,000, including visitors. The town has a popular waterfront area, which sits at sea level, with many locally owned retail shops that sell local crafts, clothing, coffee, and baked goods, along with several excellent seafood restaurants. Tourists enjoy staying at the many beds and breakfasts and historic homes rented through online rental websites. The town has a mayor, five town commissioners, a town manager, and support staff. They have a combined police, fire, and rescue department with eight police officers, 10 paid firefighters with two fire trucks, and two rescue squads manned with emergency medical technicians. The electricity is operated by a large corporation located four hours away. The town has a district public water plant that supplies 90% of the population. The remaining 10% have personal wells. There is one main internet provider who services the area. There are three schools—one elementary, one middle, and one high school. The nearest hospital is 30 miles away in a larger city. There are two primary healthcare offices, two pharmacies, and one dentist in the town. There are two grocery stores, one locally owned hardware store, and a lumber store. Most residents travel to other towns to work, with a 30-mile commute at a minimum. The local population is predominately English-speaking, with 50% of the residents under the age of 65.

On August 20th, a hurricane has formed in the Atlantic Ocean. As the storm nears, it strengthens. The projected path is within 50 miles of Emerald Place, with anticipated landfall in 96 hours. Based on the information provided, you are responsible for forming a disaster response team and making initial preparations. Here are some questions to consider:

1.  What are the hazards, threats, and risks?

2.  Who would you need on your team?

3.  What resources do you need?

4.  What are the concerns you identify that would need to be addressed?

5.  What are the priorities for the disaster management team?

Think about what needs to happen and who needs to be involved. Assign specific roles to each group member. Each group member will present their role, their key responsibilities, and the resources they need to protect their community and prepare for the approaching storm.

# AUTHOR BIOGRAPHIES

**Carol Ann King, DNP, MSN, BSN, FNP-BC, RN, NHDP-BC,** Clinical Professor, East Carolina University, has decades of experience in emergency and disaster management as a public health nurse in underserved, rural communities. As a Major in the US Army Reserves, King is training in emergency response, including bioterrorism. She was on the front lines in Italy at the onset of the COVID-19 global pandemic, responsible for clinical operations and a key nurse leader of the incident command team. She holds the American Nurse Credentialing Center's board certification as a National Healthcare Disaster Professional. King currently teaches in the East Carolina University Doctor of Nursing Practice–Family and Adult-Gerontology Nurse Practitioner programs and serves as the Assistant Program Director. Her current clinical practice is at the local public health department, with past primary care experience in military and veterans' healthcare on deployments, home health and hospice care, and primary care in a rural free clinic. She volunteers as a COVID-19 vaccinator and serves on mission trips with various organizations. She completed her MSN at East Carolina University and her DNP at Duke University.

**Gabrielle Dawn Childs, MA, MPH, RN,** PhD Candidate, Program Manager, Advancing Health Professionals, Peace Corps, is retired from the US Air Force after 23 years of service as a Registered Nurse, Public Health Officer, and International Health Specialist. After retirement, she worked for the Centers for Disease Control and Prevention (CDC) as a Public Health Advisor. While with the CDC, she deployed to Sierra Leone to support the Ebola vaccine trials. In 2015, she accepted a position as a medical planner for US Army Africa. She has 10 years' experience developing medical training and engagements throughout Africa. She was accepted by the American Graduate School in Paris as a PhD candidate, International Relations and Diplomacy, with a concentration in Africa Studies. She finished the coursework in 2020. She currently works as Program Manager for the Peace Corps Response, Advancing Health Professionals program. She is also co-founder of the American Center for Strategic and International Affairs (ACSIA) and leads the Global Action program.

**Michelle Taylor Skipper, DNP, FNP-BC, NHDP-BC, FAANP,** serves as the Director of the Adult-Gerontology and Family Nurse Practitioner specialties in the DNP Program at East Carolina University. A long-time advocate for rural and international healthcare, she has combined her passion for nurse practitioner education along with service to her community, from her local area to long-term service in Nicaragua. In 2017, Skipper received the Governor's Award for Public Service, the highest award given to all state employees, for her work during Hurricane Matthew. She coordinated healthcare and community feeding efforts during Hurricanes Florence and Michael in her hometown. She was interviewed on National Public Radio as a role model of public service and was inducted in June of 2019 as a Fellow in the American Association of Nurse Practitioners.

# REFERENCES

Bridges, E., & McNeill, M. (2020). Bringing evidence to the point of care: TriService nursing research program battlefield and disaster nursing pocket guide. *Military Medicine, 185*(Suppl. 2), 50–53. https://doi.org/10.1093/milmed/usz290

Esterwood, E., & Saeed, S. A. (2020). Past epidemics, natural disasters, COVID19, and mental health: Learning from history as we deal with the present and prepare for the future. *Psychiatric Quarterly, 91*(4), 1121–1133. https://doi.org/10.1007/s11126-020-09808-4

Federal Emergency Management Agency. (2019). *National threat identification and risk assessment: Overview and methodology.* https://www.fema.gov/sites/default/files/2020-06/fema_national-thira-overview-methodology_2019_0.pdf

Federal Emergency Management Agency. (2020a). *National planning frameworks.* https://www.fema.gov/emergency-managers/national-preparedness/frameworks

Federal Emergency Management Agency. (2020b). *National preparedness system.* https://www.fema.gov/emergency-managers/national-preparedness/system

Fisher, M., & Kramer, A. (2012). *An epidemic after an earthquake: The cholera outbreak in Haiti, part 1.* Center for Strategic & International Studies. https://www.csis.org/blogs/smart-global-health/epidemic-after-earthquake-cholera-outbreak-haiti-part-1

Harada, N., Zhuravsky, L., Marutani, M., & Hickmott, B. (2021). Cultural safety in disaster nursing: Perspectives from the 2011 earthquake and tsunami in Japan and the earthquake in Christchurch featured at a forum on the importance of cultural safety in disaster nursing. *Nursing New Zealand, 27*(2), 19.

Heagele, T., McNeill, C., Adams, L., & Alfred, D. (2020). Household emergencies preparedness instrument development: A Delphi study. *Disaster Medicine and Public Health Preparedness, November,* 1–13. doi: 10.1017/dmp.2020.292

Hoying, C., Farra, S., Mainous, R., Baute, R., & Gneuhs, M. (2017). Collaboration between academia and practice: Interprofessional crises leadership and disaster management. *The Journal of Nursing Administration, 47*(2), 123–128. https://doi.org/10.1097/NNA.0000000000000451

International Council of Nurses. (2019). *Core competencies in disaster nursing version 2.0.* https://www.icn.ch/sites/default/files/inline-files/ICN_Disaster-Comp-Report_WEB.pdf

International Federation of Red Cross and Red Crescent Societies. (2021). *What is a disaster?* https://www.ifrc.org/en/what-we-do/disaster-management/about-disasters/what-is-a-disaster/

Loke, A. Y., Guo, C., & Molassiotis, A. (2021). Development of disaster nursing education and training programs in the past 20 years (2000–2019): A systematic review. *Nurse Education Today, 99,* 104809–104809. https://doi.org/10.1016/j.nedt.2021.104809

McNeill, C., Adams, L., Heagele, T., Swanson, M., & Alfred, D. (2020). Emergency preparedness competencies among nurses: Implications for nurse administrators. *Journal of Nursing Administration, 50*(7/8), 407–413.

Millet, C. P., & Porche, D. J. (2017). Overburdened systems and dealing with disaster: Nursing administrators' experiences and nursing leadership recommendations from a state-level perspective. *Nursing Administration Quarterly, 41*(2), 134–143. https://doi.org/10.1097/NAQ.0000000000000218

Morganstein, J. C., & Ursano, R. J. (2020). Ecological disasters and mental health: Causes, consequences, and interventions. *Frontiers in Psychiatry, 11.* https://doi.org/10.3389/fpsyt.2020.00001

Morita, T., Nomura, S., Tsubokura, M., Leppold, C., Gilmour, S., Ochi, S., Ozaki, A., Shimada, Y., Yamamoto, K., Inoue, M., Kato, S., Shibuya, K., & Kami, M. (2017). Excess mortality due to indirect health effects of the 2011 triple disaster in Fukushima, Japan: A retrospective observational study. *Journal of Epidemiology and Community Health, 71*(10), 974–980. https://doi.org/10.1136/jech-2016-208652

Morrison, A. (2010). *Scope of nursing practice and decision-making framework toolkit*. International Council of Nurses. https://www.icn.ch/sites/default/files/inline-files/2010_ICN%20Scope%20of%20 Nursing%20and%20Decision%20making%20Toolkit_eng.pdf

Raker, E., Arcaya, M., Lowe, S., Zacher, M., Rhodes, J., & Water, M. (2020). Mitigating health disparities after natural disasters: Lessons from the RISK project. *Health Affairs, 39*(12). https://doi.org/10.1377/ hlthaff.2020.01161

Ramsbottom, A., O'Brien, E., Ciotti, L., & Takacs, J. (2018). Enablers and barriers to community engagement in public health emergency preparedness: A literature review. *Journal of Community Health, 43*(2), 412–420. https://doi.org/10.1007/s10900-017-0415-7

Shadmi, E., Chen, Y., Dourado, I., Faran-Perach, I., Furler, J., Hangoma, P., Hanvoravongchai, P., Obando, C., Petrosyan, V., Rao, K. D., Ruano, A. L., Shi, I., de Souza, L. E., Spitzer-Shohat, S., Sturgiss, E., Suphanchaimat, R., Uribe, M. V., & Willems, S. (2020). Health equity and COVID-19: Global perspectives. *International Journal for Equity in Health, 19*(1), 104–104. https://doi.org/10.1186/s12939-020-01218-z

Songwathana, P., & Timalsina, R. (2021). Disaster preparedness among nurses of developing countries: An integrative review. *International Emergency Nursing, 55*, 100955. https://doi.org/10.1016/j. ienj.2020.100955

Stieger, S., & Lewetz, D. (2018). A week without using social media: Results from an ecological momentary intervention study using smartphones. *Cyberpsychology, Behavior and Social Networking, 21*(10), 618–624. https://doi.org/10.1089/cyber.2018.0070

Swiss Re Institute. (2020). *Victims*. https://www.sigma-explorer.com/index.html

United Nations Medical Directors. (2020). *UN model of care (MOC) checklist for UN duty stations in response to COVID19+ pandemic*. https://www.un.org/sites/un2.un.org/files/un_model_of_care_checklist_ and_matrix.pdf

Walsh, L., Subbarao, I., Gebbie, K., Schor, K. W., Lyznicki, J., Strauss-Riggs, K., Cooper, A., Hsu, E. B., King, R. V., Mitas, J. A., Hick, J., Zukowski, R. A. Altman, B., Steinbrecher, R. A., & James, J. J. (2012). Core competencies for disaster medicine and public health. *Disaster Medicine and Public Health Preparedness, 6*(1), 44–52. https://doi.org/10.1001/dmp.2012.4

Wilson-Genderson, M., Heid, A. R., & Pruchno, R. (2018). Long-term effects of disaster on depressive symptoms: Type of exposure matters. *Social Science & Medicine, 217*, 84–91. https://doi.org/10.1016/j. socscimed.2018.09.062

World Health Organization. (2021). *WHO coronavirus (COVID-19) dashboard*. https://covid19.who.int/

Wyte-Lake, T., Claver, M., & Dobalian, A. (2016). Assessing patients' disaster preparedness in home-based primary care. *Gerontology (Basel), 62*(3), 263–274. https://doi.org/10.1159/000439168

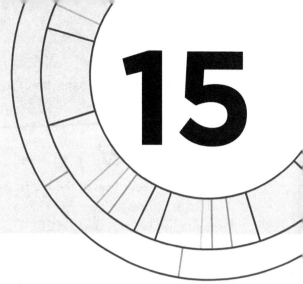

**15**

# NURSING LEADERSHIP IN THE GLOBAL HEALTH CONTEXT

Melissa T. Ojemeni, PhD, RN
Allison Squires, PhD, RN, FAAN
Judy Ngele Khanyola, MSc, BSN, RN
William E. Rosa, PhD, MBE, NP-BC, FAANP, FAAN

---

## LEARNING OBJECTIVES

After completing this chapter, you should be able to:

- Define global health, global health governance, and describe nursing's associated roles

- Describe macro-level factors that impact the nursing profession and recipients of care

- Describe the importance of nursing and midwifery leadership in Africa

- Analyze the role of leadership in the advancement of nursing and midwifery within Africa and globally

- Identify opportunities to increase leadership development

---

# OVERVIEW

Nursing is the heartbeat of the health workforce. Estimated at almost 28 million worldwide, nurses account for 59% of all healthcare workers (World Health Organization [WHO] et al., 2020). This global profession requires the cultivation of globally minded nurse leaders to guide the future of health and social care, particularly in the context of the COVID-19 pandemic, social injustice, and the evolving, dire consequences of the climate crisis. Nursing has been impacted by the rapid transformation and interdependence of globalization. Aging populations, nursing shortages, increased prevalence of and dependence on telehealth, and global health ambitions such as universal healthcare (UHC) fuel demand for more healthcare workers while creating both challenges and opportunities for nurse leaders. The rationale for the particular focus on Africa is because the authors collectively have lived and worked in numerous countries throughout the continent, and for one co-author, nursing in Africa is her area of expertise.

# CURRENT STATE OF NURSING AND NURSING LEADERSHIP

In most countries, nurses are typically the first and sometimes the only point of contact most people have with the healthcare system. They make invaluable contributions to national and international health targets and are the gatekeepers who keep health systems running due to their intimate involvement with every facet of care delivery. The heartwrenching images of nurses risking their lives to battle COVID-19 were a staple on television screens in 2020. However, beyond those powerful images, nurses remained largely excluded and overlooked amid policy decision-making related to systems delivery and patient care. Historically, nursing has been viewed as an accompanying profession, but the renewed profile and visibility of nursing in the wake of COVID-19 is an opportunity to leverage nurse leadership. Nursing voices are desperately needed and must be included as part of the interprofessional team in clinical, policy, research, and education settings.

While there is growing recognition that nurses need to be in leadership and decision-making positions, there is a lack of literature that examines initiatives geared toward preparing nurse leaders for these roles. This chapter will discuss and expand the conversation on nursing leadership in the global health context and how nursing's influence and impact can be expanded. It will briefly provide background information on the concepts of global health and global health governance (GHG) as a lens to view the current state of nursing and nursing leadership. The chapter will assess nursing within the realm of GHG while envisioning a future for nursing leadership in a globalized world.

# WHAT IS GLOBAL HEALTH AND GLOBAL HEALTH GOVERNANCE?

Although "global health" and "GHG" are widely discussed in the literature, practice, and policy, they both lack a universally accepted definition. In addition, these concepts mirror each other, as they were terms that emerged in response to the historical frustrations with international health cooperation and the evolving impacts of health and globalization (Lee & Kamradt-Scott, 2014). Until the 1990s, global health's predecessor—"international aid" or "health aid"—was rooted in the principles of colonialization and focused primarily on infectious diseases and tropical medicine in developing countries (Brown et al., 2006; Kickbusch & Buse, 2001).

International aid was centered on bilateral transactions of funds from wealthier countries to poorer countries in charity (Gostin, 2008; Oulton, 2014). During this time, the WHO coordinated most of the reporting and eradication efforts related to disease outbreaks, as the spread of emerging and infectious diseases was not as pressing as it is today (Ng & Ruger, 2011). Most industrialized countries believed they had the domestic capabilities to deal with emerging disease threats, and thus, cross-country coordination was at a much lower scale (Ng & Ruger, 2011). But this characterization of international health was flawed and too simplistic, creating a great divide between donor and recipient countries. Critics also touted that this system favored the priorities of more powerful and wealthier Western countries (e.g., the Global North) over the concerns of the countries they were attempting to assist (e.g., the Global South). Thus, the term "global health" was coined.

Building upon the shortfalls of international aid, global health sought a more inclusive, multisectoral, and cooperative approach to tackling the world's biggest health problems. An adapted definition of "global health" describes it as the health of populations that transcends the problems of national boundaries and individual countries (Gostin, 2008; Oulton, 2014). Importantly, it is a collaborative process among countries that strives to address health challenges and concerns through partnership and shared responsibility despite domestic wealth or lack thereof (O'Brien & Gostin, 2011; Oulton, 2014; Upvall & Leffers, 2018).

GHG originates from the broader concept of global governance, which is embedded in the field of international relations (Lee & Kamradt-Scott, 2014). Generally, governance is needed when collaborative action is taken to reach an agreed-upon goal. Although governance through governments (state-based institutions with recognized authority and power) is more frequently discussed in the literature, governance may also occur between both state and non-state actors (Lee & Kamradt-Scott, 2014). Non-state actors, like non-governmental organizations, are groups or individuals who hold influences but are not affiliated with or funded by a country. The non-state actors can be very prominent within GHG, and some even argue that they are more significant than traditional state actors.

GHG is defined here as the efforts to bring a more orderly and reliable response to political, social, and economic issues that go beyond the ability of a country to address individually. Although global governance implies the absence of a central authority, it seeks collaboration and cooperation among governments and non-state actors to address global issues (Gordenker & Weiss, 1995).

# GLOBAL HEALTH AND GLOBAL HEALTH GOVERNANCE LINKAGES

No global health agenda is attainable without maximizing the nursing workforce as a member of the interprofessional health team (Rosa et al., 2020). The large-scale targets, such as the "triple billion," aim to achieve one billion more people benefitting from UHC, another billion more people better protected from health emergencies, and one billion people enjoying better health and well-being by 2023 (WHO et al., 2020). From a rural health post to a district hospital to the community, nurses lead the majority of care delivery in every country. From care accessibility to combating noncommunicable and infectious diseases, to advocating for mental health, emergency preparedness, and patient safety, nurses ensure the systematic and safe delivery of patient-centered care. With over 90% of the global nursing workforce being female, further investment in their development will also provide economic opportunity for women while contributing to gender equity and improving health outcomes (All-Party Parliamentary Group on Global Health, 2016).

Unfortunately, nursing voices are largely absent within GHG structures due to a lack of nursing leadership presence at major policy and decision-making tables. Additional investments are needed. First, national and international level efforts must be made to attract, recruit, and prepare nurses across health and social care settings. There is currently a global nursing workforce shortage estimated at 6 million, the vast majority of which are in low- and middle-income countries. Second, there must be concerted multisectoral efforts to support, include, and engage nurse leadership perspectives and priorities at decision-making tables. For more than 200 years, nurses have shown their impact and significance at the bedside, in communities, and in population health. Their expertise needs to be leveraged and harnessed to influence policies, service delivery, and, ultimately, the public's welfare.

# ADVANCING THE VOICES OF NURSES IN GLOBAL HEALTH GOVERNANCE

Women constitute 70% of the global health workforce and 90% of the nursing workforce but occupy only 25% of the leadership roles (WHO, 2020). This gender imbalance suggests that even though women deliver most of the care, they do not make decisions regarding its design or delivery (WHO et al., 2019). The gender discrepancies in leadership are primarily due to power imbalances, cultural and gender norm roles, discrimination, and structural barriers that elevate one gender over another (WHO et al., 2019). These issues are further compounded by the intersection of racial, social, and ethnic injustice, which can further disadvantage women (WHO et al., 2019).

Nursing's professional socialization processes can also present challenges to inclusion in GHG structures. For example, the 19th-century gender norms that informed an attitude of subservience to physicians (historically perceived in many cultures as a man's profession) continue to pervade many nursing and non-nursing programs today. This initial socialization has only started to become dismantled through the work of emerging feminist nurse scholars and the global efforts to advance gender equity. However, the lingering effects mean that many nurses are not encouraged to assume leadership roles and may not seek out leadership training or opportunities despite possessing the necessary qualifications. These trends do not typically apply to men in nursing since they are almost uniformly promoted faster than their female counterparts and placed in leadership positions (Black et al., 2010; McMurry, 2011; Walani, 2013).

Transformative change to overcome barriers that have historically excluded nurses from GHG leadership positions requires both formal and informal strategies that can be applied at individual and institutional levels. Rao and Kelleher (2005) offer a gender-specific framework of women's empowerment to effect transformative change across societies. They note that two core processes are needed to create transformative change that increases the equity of opportunity for men and women. Shifts in consciousness, the first process, involves "overturning limiting normative beliefs and expectations that keep women locked into situations of sub-ordination and dependency, challenging restrictive cultural and social norms and contesting the institutions of everyday life that sustain inequity" (Cornwall, 2016, p. 345). The second process requires:

> Engagement with culturally embedded normative beliefs, understand-ings, and ideas about gender, power, and change. This takes the process of change beyond the level of the individual to address commonly held and taken for granted assumptions that undergird gendered inequalities in any particular cultural context... Ultimately, it is about enabling peo-ple to stand back and inspect critically the beliefs about themselves and others they take for granted, and then using this expanded understand-ing to inform an analysis of what needs to change and how they can be part of that process of change (Cornwall, 2016, pp. 345–346).

How these transformative changes can occur remains flexible in terms of format, thus enabling them to happen in ways specific to culture and context. It can, however, take years to accomplish, so changemakers must invest for the long term. In addition, these authors acknowledge that this model of change is based on a gender binary framework and does not consider the unique discriminatory lead-ership barriers confronted by gender non-binary and transgender nurses. In order to achieve gender equity in the truest sense of the phrase, we will need to invite a consciousness shift rooted in cultural humility, foster professional environments of inclusivity, and ensure that leadership opportunities are made available to all individuals, regardless of gender identity.

Mexican nursing's integration into federal levels of governance during the ear-ly part of the 21st century offers a salient example and highlights how various aspects of the Gender and Work conceptual framework can apply in the context of GHG. The North American Free Trade Agreement (NAFTA) prompted a critical comparative examination of the nursing professions of Mexico, Canada, and the United States (Gabriel, 2013). The findings in the report prompted major educa-tional changes in Mexico, moving all education to the post-secondary level. By

2001, it became clear that centralized involvement of the profession was required, resulting in the creation of the Interinstitutional Commission for Nursing. The leadership of the Institute, in effect, reinstated the Chief Nurse role in the country, something that had been eliminated in the late 1970s during the global oil crisis as part of cost-cutting measures (Squires, 2007). By 2006, the Commission was made permanent by a Presidential decree under the Calderon administration.

The emergence of nursing leadership roles at the federal level then translated into state-level leadership positions for nurses (consistently women), thus creating a nursing governance network capable of effecting transformative change based on local needs. The Mexican nursing profession advanced more in the first 20 years of the 21st century than it had in the final 40 years of the 20th because nurses were integrated into leadership and governance structures (Aristizabal et al., 2020).

# LINKAGES BETWEEN NURSING LEADERSHIP, HEALTH SERVICE DELIVERY, AND GLOBAL HEALTH GOVERNANCE

In many ways, the state, profile, and quality of nursing set the barometer for quality health services: When nurses are inadequately prepared and under-resourced, poor health access and patient outcomes are sure to follow (WHO et al., 2020). Thus, nursing leadership becomes even more crucial because, through various experiences, such as frontline providers, educators, researchers, policymakers, and community members, the profession can bring a unique perspective to improve service delivery and promote population health and outcomes. While that devotion to patients is central to the profession, a deeper understanding of how macro-level factors influence nursing's ability to deliver care and the social determinants of health needs to be heightened (Rosa et al., 2021).

Although activism and social justice are ingrained in nursing history, many nurses may disregard the politics and governance structures that directly impact the profession (Florell, 2020; Regis College, n.d.). Ironically, policy and politics are the overarching factors that shape nursing practice irrespective of country. In many settings, nurses have been mistakenly led to believe that their only obligation is at the bedside. This myopic focus prevents them from effectively addressing and dismantling the structures that restrain the profession and deter nurses from delivering optimal, quality care. The inability to recognize the systematic influences that inform bedside nursing conditions, coupled with the profession's historic fragmentation, has limited the powers of national and international nursing organizations to make a measurable change on the global stage. The competing demands faced by women in the profession further contribute to this lack of involvement.

Nurses need to be more actively engaged in viewing their profession through a socio-political lens, identifying key stakeholder interests within and outside of healthcare while speaking a stakeholder-oriented language and taking a more active role in shaping, creating, and leading policy (Salvage & White, 2020). This approach would translate to nurses having a better understanding of health issues at the intersection of socio-political, cultural, and economic considerations.

# LEADERSHIP CHALLENGES FROM THE AFRICAN LENS

Seventy percent of the population of Sub-Saharan Africa (SSA) lives on less than $2.00 per day (United Nations Economic and Social Council, 2017). In addition to this economic limitation, large portions of the population reside in rural, hard-to-reach areas. This socioeconomic context creates fragile health systems, poor health services, inequalities, and poor access to healthcare. Nurses and midwives, who form the bulk of the health workforce in SSA, provide health services amid daunting challenges every day and are often the only health professional an African will see.

In the global health context, nursing leadership is vital if Africa is to meet any of the global health targets associated with the SDGs, reduce maternal mortality, or mitigate the burden of noncommunicable diseases. In Africa, nurse leaders need to be equipped and encouraged to move away from a past characterized by subservience, inertia, and inability to speak up and readily assume leadership, responsibility, and authority.

Population health needs are rapidly changing due to economic development, technological advances, and consumer demand. The nursing leader needs to be sensitive to this contextual diversity and must pay attention to both patients' and the profession's needs (e.g., what do nurses need to build a sense of leadership identity and ownership?). Without leadership, the issues facing nursing, both within and outside Africa—severe workforce shortages caused by migration, poor retention rates, high workloads, insufficient compensation—cannot be addressed and solved.

Recognizing the gap in executive leadership preparation and accompaniment, Partners In Health (PIH) developed the Global Nurse Executive Fellowship (Ojemeni et al., 2019). It is a 12-month program geared to leadership development by creating a pipeline of nurse executives imbued with the theoretical and practical skills to succeed in leadership roles. The fellowship program includes three phases:

- **Leading self:** Allows fellows to garner a better understanding of their leadership capacity and style.

- **Leading others:** Takes a deeper dive into understanding the principles of leading and managing others.

- **Leading systems:** Focuses on garnering a macro-level understanding beyond one's organization and across health systems domestically and internationally to improve population health.

The fellowship's culmination is a capstone project to actualize the theoretical, practical, and acquired skills learned in the fellowship to improve hospital-based operations, service delivery, and/or patient outcomes at their respective sites. The program is currently open to nursing leaders and executives at six PIH sites (Liberia, Rwanda, Sierra Leone, Malawi, Lesotho, and Haiti).

# GLOBAL GOVERNANCE

Global governance in health relies on discrete, recognized bodies that contribute to the global health agenda. Nursing leadership internationally is organized around two bodies, the International Council of Nurses (ICN) and the International Confederation of Midwives (ICM), who in turn work closely with other global entities, including United Nations agencies, professional bodies, non-governmental organizations, and civil society groups. ICN and ICM together represent the nursing and midwifery voice (ICM, n.d.) and have global nursing and midwifery programs, demonstrating their recognition of the need for strong nursing leadership on the continent.

Programs such as ICN's Global Nursing Leadership Institute (GNLI) are committed to developing nurse leaders internationally by strengthening nurses' understanding of policy and politics while encouraging advocacy involvement and expanding nursing and non-nursing professional networks of influence (ICN, 2021). The GNLI program assists both emerging and established nurse leaders in understanding their influence on achieving the SDGs and advancing health equity in their local contexts (Holguin et al., 2017; Rosa et al., 2021). The GNLI curriculum emphasizes strategic communication skills, policy negotiation competencies, stakeholder engagement and coalition building, policy influence, and the abilities needed to frame the evidence base of care at local and global levels. ICN is preparing a generation of nurse leaders to actively participate in global governance through local, regional, national, and international action.

An additional example of the intersection between nursing leadership, health services, and global governance is Harvard's Global Nursing Leadership Program, launching in summer 2022. This will be a collaborative effort between the African Union, Africa Centers for Disease Control and Prevention, and Harvard's T.H. Chan School of Public Health. This certificate program will begin in Africa and subsequently expand to other continents, geared to ministry-level nurses and midwives to provide them with field experiences in global health and health management (Harvard Global Nursing Leadership Program, 2021). Graduates will receive knowledge and skills to help them excel in a) health systems strengthening, b) emergency preparedness and population health management, c) human-centered design for health and wellness, d) health financing, e) strategic communication, and f) public health law, policy, and regulations (Harvard Global Nursing Leadership Program, 2021).

# IMPLICATIONS FOR EDUCATION, PRACTICE, AND GLOBAL AGENDA

Globalization has interconnected the world through technology, migration, trade, and increased disease burden and environmental health challenges. The possibilities for nursing in this new age must be reimagined to deal with the challenges and opportunities for current and future nurse leaders in a global society. Considering what nursing went through in 2020 with COVID-19 and what is sure to come with future humanitarian crises, one must be even more cognizant that we are interlinked as a global community no matter how distant another country may appear to be. What happens in a remote village in Mongolia or a large metropolitan city like Nairobi, Kenya, has ramifications for one's own health, family, and community and vice versa (Salvage & White, 2020). Taking that broader perspective allows for knowledge attainment, curiosity, and enriching perspectives to create more dynamic nurses who lead, manage, practice, and create policy. It also positions nurses to better understand how their work influences sectors outside of health, including policy and education (Salvage & White, 2020).

The potential power of the largest group of healthcare professionals is limitless. The key is working collectively to advocate for issues with a unified voice that focuses on promoting better patient outcomes while collaborating fully with multidisciplinary stakeholders to effect change. Nurses are present on the global health scene through various networks, organizations, and WHO Collaborating Centers at universities but have yet to become major players. The absence of nursing from leadership tables has negative consequences for global health. The perspectives from the largest cadre of health professionals are missing from policy decisions that influence care delivery. This absence, however, is supported by other societal inequalities, including nursing's low position in various countries, gender disparities, race, wealth, and the lack of strong global voices from low-resource countries.

Becoming immersed in nursing leadership and policy may seem daunting when assessing GHG and global health implications, but everyone has expertise they can contribute. The key is to start where you are; think about the skill set you possess and the best way to leverage it to get to where you want to go. Table 15.1 provides tangible ways to get involved with leadership and policy within your community and professionally.

Consider reaching out to a local city councilperson, a member of parliament, or a legislator and offer your expertise on legislation relating to healthcare service delivery or any other specialty area you may have. If you do not want to call your legislator, consider writing to them consistently to discuss issues of importance to you or your community. They are often looking for constituent feedback and perspectives before making policy decisions.

**TABLE 15.1** Domestic and International Leadership and Policy Opportunities

| DOMESTIC/COMMUNITY-FOCUSED INITIATIVES | PROFESSIONAL AND GLOBAL INITIATIVES |
|---|---|
| Reach out to local legislators: offer your expertise to them, write and/or call their office on policy issues of importance | Network within and outside of nursing |
| Volunteer in local organizations that help diverse communities | Join and be active in a professional organization |
| Take more leadership positions where you live: homeowners' association in your neighborhood, town watch, school board and elected office | Blog and utilize social media to discuss issues of importance to you |
| | Follow and join international campaigns such as Nursing Now |
| | Join unit-based and organizational-based committees at your place of work |
| | Shadow nurse leaders:<br>• Deans at your college or university<br>• The nurse manager in your facility or administrator within your facility<br>• A leader in a field outside of nursing |
| | Respond to calls for comments to policy initiatives from professional and international organizations and regulatory councils |
| | Take continuing education classes and courses geared toward leadership development and policy development |
| | Seek opportunities from local community organizations, colleges, and universities centered on leadership and policy |
| | Participate in lobbying days at government entities |

*(Salvage & White, 2020)*

Join a professional nursing organization and see what opportunities they may have for you to join a committee or take on a leadership position. Network with people within and outside of nursing who have both shared and dissimilar interests to expand your network and be subjected to diverse viewpoints. From this network, seek opportunities for mentorship and further guidance to build skills that you may be currently lacking. Acquiring leadership and policy acumen requires risk-taking and initiative, but it will better position the nursing profession by raising its visibility within local, professional, and global spheres.

Regarding nursing education and practice, changes must be integrated into existing infrastructures. First, implementing mechanisms for students and nurses to be exposed to professional development opportunities outside of their direct training and exposing them to macro-level health factors. One class during undergraduate study or one lecture during a nurse residency program is insufficient. Rather, implanting those concepts of leadership and global thinking within curricula and having professional development opportunities throughout one's career is a more strategic and holistic approach to begin changing the way nurses view and think about health while equipping them with the knowledge to think globally.

Secondly, reimagining professional competencies that nurses should accrue in conjunction with clinical competencies is warranted to propel nursing into the future. Leadership and policy insight should be included in both practice and education. Immersing nurses and students into both concepts from the first day of school to the first day on the job will help begin shifting the mindset of what is expected and what is possible for the profession's future. Those transferable skills will also serve to reinforce other principles, from advocating for patients to strategizing how to best contribute to shaping, influencing, and implementing policy (ICN, 2017). A concrete example of this would be schools/colleges of nursing and workplace institutions bringing representatives from different nursing organizations quarterly to discuss the work they do on behalf of the profession locally, nationally, and internationally, coupled with the services they provide for members to continuously reinforce ways to get involved and resources to engage and be better prepared.

# SUMMARY

The influence of nursing on the global stage is rapidly evolving as demand grows for new perspectives on challenging global health issues, such as aging populations, increasing impact of climate change on health, a global workforce shortage, greater public interest in nursing, and the development of nursing specialties and advanced practice nursing (Rosa et al., 2020). Nurses are becoming policy entrepreneurs by positioning themselves to influence policy or by advocating strategically through a cohesive understanding of the relevant problems, policies, and politics (Salvage & White, 2020). The recognition of nursing is increasing through the dissemination of landmark reports, such as the *Triple Impact Report* (All-Party Parliamentary Group on Global Health, 2016) and the *State of the World's Nursing Report* (WHO, ICN, & Nursing Now, 2020) addressing nursing's impact on economic welfare, population health, and the gender equity gap. In 2017, the WHO appointed a chief nursing officer for the first time in the organization's history.

Every nurse has leadership potential, whether it is speaking up to advocate for their patient during interprofessional rounds or leading organizations or driving policy changes. Even as policy and political circumstances can constrain nurses' opportunities to grow and excel as leaders, leadership development programs allow nurses to envision their full capacity of what they could be and find their place as leaders in an increasingly globalized world. The continued investment of mentorship, practical skill development, and the willingness to speak up by advocating for the profession and patients will ensure nurses are prepared once they assume leadership positions.

# REFLECTIVE QUESTIONS

1. Please discuss why it is important for nurse leaders to understand the macro-level implications of policies.

2. How does Rao and Kelleher's (2005) gender-specific framework offer insight into empowering women and transforming change across societies?

3. What are three characteristics that would be needed of a globally minded nursing and midwifery leader?

4.   Explain the importance or lack thereof of the nursing profession within global health governance.

5.   What are three ways nurses can contribute to increasing their skill set in becoming more globally minded and politically conscious?

# NARRATIVE

Break up students into groups of four and have them go through the following exercise. Within each group, have the students assume the role of a first-time attendee at an international global health conference.

Janet is a 28-year-old staff nurse who has been a nurse for six years. She has primarily worked in an acute care setting for most of her career with older geriatric patients dealing with chronic diseases. Recently she has become more interested in working internationally and relocating abroad to use her skill set in a different country. She has seen job postings for leadership and managerial positions with global health organizations, but she is not sure how to go about gaining experience to be a viable candidate for those jobs. She does not have any experience working in global health but recently saw an advertisement for an international conference in her city and decided it might be a great way to network and meet people connected to and working in global health. This is Janet's first conference that is not specifically focused on her clinical area of expertise and not exclusively for nurses.

At the conference's networking social, she feels isolated, anxious, and inadequate since she does not have any global health experience and she does not know anyone at this event. But she also realizes this is a great opportunity as numerous international organizations with employment opportunities and major players in global health are in attendance.

# AUTHOR BIOGRAPHIES

**Melissa T. Ojemeni, PhD, RN,** is currently the Director of Nursing Education, Research and Professional Development at Partners In Health. She co-leads the Global Nurse Executive Fellowship program for the organization and serves as a board member for Rory Meyers College of Nursing Alumni board and the Global Nursing Caucus. She has over 15 years of clinical bedside nursing experience in the United States and internationally. Ojemeni has worked in Rwanda, Tanzania, and Haiti on health workforce and educational capacity building programs. Her research interests lie in health services and health systems strengthening human resources for health, capacity building, and post-conflict health reconstruction. Ojemeni holds a

PhD in Nursing from New York University Rory Meyers College of Nursing, a Master of Arts in International Peace and Conflict Resolution with a global health concentration from Arcadia University, and a Bachelor of Science in Nursing degree from Gwynedd Mercy University.

**Allison Squires, PhD, RN, FAAN,** Associate Professor & Director, PhD Program, Rory Meyers College of Nursing, New York University, is an internationally recognized expert in global health services research and immigrant health. She has led or participated in research studies and capacity building projects in over 40 countries to date. Squires also has methodological expertise in cross-language research. She has consulted for the National Council of State Boards of Nursing, Kings College London, the World Bank, and the Migration Policy Institute to name a few. She received her BSN from the University of Pennsylvania, her MSN in Nursing Education from Duquesne University in Pittsburgh, a PhD in Nursing from Yale University, and completed a post-doctoral fellowship at the Center for Health Outcomes and Policy Research at the University of Pennsylvania. Prior to moving into academia, she worked for 11 years as a staff nurse and unit-based educator in urban and rural hospitals in the US.

**Judy Ngele Khanyola, MSc, BSN, RN,** is currently the Chair for the Center for Nursing and Midwifery at the University of Global Health Equity in Rwanda, where she is working to transform nursing and midwifery education for the continent and ensure the role played by nurses and midwives is included in health decision-making. Khanyola is the Secretary of AFREhealth, the convening body for health professions education and research in Africa, and a board member of AfriPEN, the interprofessional collaborative in Africa. She was the Nursing Now Africa Representative, the global campaign to raise the status and profile of nurses. She is also an Academic Editor on the *PLOS Global Health* Editorial Board. Her clinical nursing specialties are renal, critical care, HIV, and palliative care. She is the 2019 recipient of the Association of Nurses in AIDS Care (ANAC) Global HIV Award.

**William E. Rosa, PhD, MBE, NP-BC, FAANP, FAAN,** is Chief Research Fellow in the Department of Psychiatry and Behavioral Sciences at Memorial Sloan Kettering Cancer Center. He completed his PhD and Master of Bioethics as an RWJF Future of Nursing Scholar at the University of Pennsylvania. He is the editor of four books and has contributed to more than 150 academic publications in journals and texts. He was lead researcher for the 2021 Nurses for Health Equity: Guidelines for Tackling the Social Determinants of Health policy report endorsed by the World Health Organization, among others. Rosa has been recognized with numerous distinctions, including Sigma's International Research Dissertation Award, the national Public Health Service Award for Distinguished Practice in Nursing from the American Nurses Association, and the national Excellence in Oncology Nursing Health Policy and Advocacy Award from the Oncology Nursing Society. He was most recently named to the Crain's New York Business Notable in Health Care 2021 list and is a Scientific Advisory Group Member for the Lancet Commission on Cancer and Health Systems. He serves as Associate Editor for *Palliative & Supportive Care,* the editorial boards for the *Journal of Hospice and Palliative Nursing, Journal of Pain and Symptom Management,* and *American Journal of Nursing,* and as a board/committee member for multiple global health and palliative care organizations. Rosa is a Cambia Sojourns Scholar, International Council of Nurses Global Nursing Leadership Institute Scholar, and an American Psychosocial Oncology Society Health Equity Scholar. He is a Fellow of the American Academy of Nursing, the American Association of Nurse Practitioners, and the New York Academy of Medicine.

# REFERENCES

All-Party Parliamentary Group on Global Health. (2016). *Triple impact: How developing nursing will improve health, promote gender equality and support economic growth.* https://www.who.int/hrh/com-heeg/digital-APPG_triple-impact.pdf

Aristizabal, P., Nigenda, G., Squires, A., & Rosales, Y. (2020). Regulation of nursing in Mexico: Actors, processes, and outcomes. *Ciencia e Saude Coletiva, 25*(1). https://doi.org/10.1590/1413-81232020251.28462019

Black, L., Spetz, J., & Harrington, C. (2010). Nurses who do not nurse: Factors that predict non-nursing work in the US. registered nursing labor market. *Nursing Economic$, 28*(4), 245–254.

Brown, T., Cueto, M., & Fee, E. (2006). The World Health Organization and the transition from "international" to "global" public health. *American Journal of Public Health, 96,* 62–72.

Cornwall, A. (2016). Women's empowerment: What works? *Journal of International Development, 28*(3), 342–359. https://doi.org/10.1002/jid.3210

Florell, M. C. (2020). Concept analysis of nursing activism. *Nursing Forum, 56*(1), 134–140. https://doi.org/https://doi.org/10.1111/nuf.12502

Gabriel, C. (2013). NAFTA, skilled migration and continental nursing markets. *Population, Space & Place, 19,* 389–403.

Gordenker, L., & Weiss, T. (1995). Pluralising global governance: Analytical approaches and dimensions. *Third World Quarterly, 16*(3), 357–387.

Gostin, L. O. (2008). The international migration and recruitment of nurses: Human rights and global justice. *JAMA: The Journal of the American Medical Association, 299*(15), 1827–1829. https://doi.org/10.1001/jama.299.15.1827

Harvard Global Nursing Leadership Program. (2021). *Nurses are a force for global health. You can lead the way.* https://www.hsph.harvard.edu/global-nursing/

Holguin, E., Hughers, F., & Shamian, J. (2017). Transnational nursing organizations paving the way for global health: The International Council of Nurses as exemplar. In W. Rosa (Ed.), *A new era in global health: Nursing and the United Nations 2030 agenda for sustainable development* (pp. 205–226). Springer Publishing.

International Confederation of Midwives. (n.d.). *Vision and mission.* https://www.internationalmidwives.org/

International Council of Nurses. (2017). *Nurses' role in achieving the Sustainable Development Goals.* https://onlinelibrary.wiley.com/doi/10.1111/inr.12353

International Council of Nurses. (2021). *ICN programmes: Global nursing leadership institute.* https://www.icn.ch/what-we-do/projects/global-nursing-leadership-institutetm-gnli

Kickbusch, I., & Buse, K. (2001). Global influences and global responses: International health at the turn of the twenty-first century. In M. Merson, R. Black, A. Mills, & M. Gaithersburg (Eds.), *International public health: Diseases, programs, systems and policies* (pp. 701–737). Aspen Publishers Inc.

Lee, K., & Kamradt-Scott, A. (2014). The multiple meanings of global health governance: A call for conceptual clarity. *Globalization and Health, 10*(1), 1–10. https://doi.org/10.1186/1744-8603-10-28

McMurry, T. B. (2011). The image of male nurses and nursing leadership mobility. *Nursing Forum, 46*(1), 22–28. https://doi.org/. https://doi.org/10.1111/j.1744-6198.2010.00206.x

Ng, N. Y., & Ruger, J. P. (2011). Global health governance at a crossroads. *Global Health Governance: The Scholarly Journal for the New Health Security Paradigm, 3*(2), 1–37. www.pubmedcentral.nih.gov/articlerender.fcgi?artid=PMC3983705

O'Brien, P., & Gostin, O. L. (2011). *Health worker shortages and global justice.* Millbank Memorial Fund, https://www.milbank.org/wp-content/uploads/2016/04/healthworkershortages-1.pdf

Ojemeni, M. T., Karanja, V., Cadet, G., Charles, A., Dushimimana, E., McMahon, C., Abbasi, S., & Davis, S. (2019). Fostering nursing leadership: An important key to achieving sustainable development goals and universal health care. *International Journal of Nursing Studies, 100*(103421). doi:10.1016/j.ijnurstu.2019.103421

Oulton, J. A. (2014). Special contribution: Highlights from the 2nd International Seminar of the Disaster Nursing Global Leader Degree Program. *Health Emergency and Disaster Nursing, 2014*(1), 29–33.

Rao, A., & Kelleher, D. (2005). Is there life after gender mainstreaming? *Gender and Development, 13*(2), 57–69. https://doi.org/10.1080/13552070512331332287

Regis College. (n.d.). *How to develop and maintain social justice in nursing.* https://online.regiscollege.edu/blog/social-justice-in-nursing/

Rosa, W. E., Fitzgerald, M., Davis, S., Farley, J. E., Khanyola, J., Kwong, J., Moreland, P. J., Rogers, M., Sibanda, B., & Turale, S. (2020). Leveraging nurse practicioner capacities to achieve global health for all: COVID-19 and beyond. *International Nursing Review, 67*(4), 554–559. https://doi.org/10.1111/inr.12632

Rosa, W. E., Hannaway, C. J., McAardle, C., Mcmanus, F., Alharahsheh, S. T., & Marmot, M. (2021). *Nurses for health equity: Guidelines for tackling the Social Determinants of Health.* World Innovation Summit for Health. https://www.wish.org.qa/reports/nurses-for-health-equity/

Salvage, J., & White, J. (2020). Our future is global: Nursing leadership and global health. *Revista Latino Americana de Enfermagem [Latin American Journal of Nursing], 28,* e3339.

Squires, A. (2007). *A case stufy of the professionalization of Mexican nursing: 1980–2005.* Yale University.

United Nations Economic and Social Council. (2017). *Progress towards the Sustainable Development Goals: Report of the secretary-general.* https://unstats.un.org/sdgs/files/report/2017/secretary-general-sdg-report-2017--EN.pdf

Upvall, M. J., & Leffers, J. M. (2018). Revising a conceptual model of partnership and sustainability in global health. *Public Health Nursing, 35*(3), 228–237. https://doi.org/10.111/phn.12396

Walani, S. R. (2013). Earnings of the internationally educated nurses in the U.S. labor market. *Nursing Research, 62*(3), 169–177. https://doi.org/10.1097/NNR.0b013e318286b7ac

World Health Organization. (2020). *The triple billion targets.* https://www.who.int/news-room/q-a-detail/the-triple-billion-targets

World Health Organization, Global Health Workforce Network, & Women in Global Health. (2019). *Delivered by women, led by men.* https://www.who.int/docs/default-source/nursing/delivered-by-women-led-by-men.pdf

World Health Organization, International Council of Nurses, & Nursing Now. (2020). *State of the world's nursing 2020: Investing in education, jobs and leadership.* https://apps.who.int/iris/rest/bitstreams/1274201/retrieve

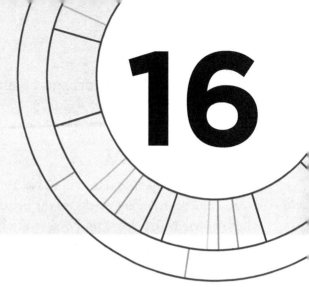

# 16

# HEALTHCARE LEADERSHIP IN PROMOTING THE USE OF EVIDENCE

Lynn Gallagher-Ford, PhD, RN, NE-BC, DPFNAP, FAAN
Laura Caramanica, PhD, RN, CNE, CNEP, FACHE, FAAN

## LEARNING OBJECTIVES

After completing this chapter, the learner will be able to:

- Describe the differences between the four domains of evidence

- Explain the critical role the nurse leader assumes in the application of evidence in the clinical setting

- Apply leadership competencies for evidence-based practice

- Justify why evidence is needed to support decision-making and clinical practice in the healthcare setting

# OVERVIEW

Healthcare organizations in the 21st century need to be capable of bringing the best and most current knowledge to the bedside, chairside, or tableside—wherever care is delivered. To achieve this, organizations must incorporate science/evidence as the underpinning for solving clinical problems. Doing so requires a thorough understanding of four domains that support best practice/care/outcomes. Each of the domains represents the use of evidence in one way or another. The domains include:

1. **Research** (the generation of new evidence)

2. **Evidence-based practice** (determination of the current, best evidence to support care)

3. **Innovation** (the ability to imagine new approaches to care based on the platform of evidence)

4. **Process improvement** (determination of the best processes to deliver the best evidence-based care)

Figure 16.1 depicts the four domains of the use of evidence.

For the contributions of these domains to be fully actualized, function effectively, and ultimately support the best care and drive best outcomes, it is imperative that leaders understand the differences between these domains and leverage their synergies as well.

Two of these domains, research and process improvement, have long histories in healthcare and are well-understood, and generally are deeply embedded in the operations of organizations. *Research* is "a systematic process used to generate new knowledge or evidence" (Melnyk & Morrison-Beedy, 2018, p. 4) that is needed to change practice, influence policy, and positively impact outcomes (Melnyk & Morrison-Beedy, 2018). Most leaders in healthcare organizations have a clear understanding of what research is, who should be conducting it, and where/how research exists in their particular organization.

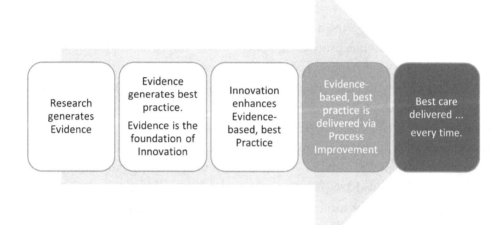

**FIGURE 16.1**   The four domains of the use of evidence.

*Process improvement* (PI) is a rigorous approach that may be used for various aims, including streamlining operations and production activities, reducing costs and billing cycles, or improving the quality of processes. In healthcare, the assumption is that all the aims of PI ultimately are associated with improving outcomes. Three of the most widely utilized process improvement methodologies employed in healthcare are Plan Do Study Act (PDSA), Six Sigma, and LEAN. Plan Do Study Act methodology features a cyclical structure for creating and assessing change. The PDSA cycle starts with determining the nature and scope of the problem, what changes can and should be made, a plan for a specific change, who should be involved, what should be measured to understand the impact of change, and where the strategy will be targeted. Change is then implemented, and data and information are collected. Results from the implementation study are assessed and interpreted by reviewing several key measurements that indicate success or failure. Lastly, action is taken on the results by implementing the change or beginning the process again.

Six Sigma methodology involves improving, designing, and monitoring processes to minimize or eliminate waste while optimizing satisfaction and increasing financial stability. The performance of a process is used to measure improvement by comparing the baseline process capability (before improvement) with the process capability after piloting potential solutions for quality improvement. The LEAN methodology often overlaps with the Six Sigma methodology but differs in that LEAN is driven by the identification of customer needs and aims to improve processes by removing activities that are non-value-added (a.k.a. waste). This methodology depends on root-cause analysis to investigate errors and then to improve quality and prevent similar errors. Steps in the LEAN methodology involve maximizing value-added activities in the best possible sequence to enable continuous operations. The steps often include: (a) systematically define the problem using root-cause analysis; (b) set goals, remove ambiguity and workarounds; (c) clarify responsibilities; and (d) develop action plans. In many organizations, PI is referred to as the "quality department." As we will see in this chapter, the quality department must house far more than PI capacity alone for quality to be delivered.

The other two domains—evidence-based practice and innovation—are relatively "new kids on the block" and are often misunderstood and rarely, if ever, embedded in organizational operations. These domains tend to be employed sporadically for special events such as for school assignments or to meet credentialing or recognition requirements. *Evidence-based practice* is a problem-solving approach that integrates the best evidence from research with a clinician's expertise and a patient's personal preferences and values (Melnyk & Fineout-Overholt, 2019, p. 8) to make clinical decisions. EBP is a rigorous methodological approach to practice improvement. Implementation of EBP results in high-quality, safe care; improved patient outcomes; and decreased healthcare costs (Melnyk et al., 2017; Woo et al., 2017; Wu et al., 2018). EBP is essential as healthcare leaders today are striving to meet multiple aims, including enhancing patients' experience of care (outcomes and satisfaction), decreasing costs, and enhancing clinician well-being. Despite the multitude of studies over the past 20 years that have clearly identified EBP as an approach to care that positively affects each of these aims, the adoption of EBP remains slow and arduous. In many healthcare organizations, leaders have failed to establish EBP as the standard of practice and evidence-based care (EBC) as the standard expectation (Harding et al., 2014; Melnyk & Fineout-Overholt, 2019; Melnyk et al., 2018). Instead, widespread variation persists, fueled by an untethered allowance of provider preference, practice based on tradition, and cultures that support and encourage "the way we've always done it here."

Innovation is often misunderstood and used to refer to activities that once were referred to as "trial and error" or "flavor of the month." This misunderstanding, misinterpretation, and possible misuse of the innovation process is a disservice to those who are true innovators and to the important contributions that innovation brings to advancing clinical practice and improving patient outcomes. *Innovation* is well described by Morrar as a "rigorous and generative process that leads to something new" (Morrar, 2014; Porter- O'Grady & Malloch, 2017, p. 4). In its true form, innovation is "creating a solution to something when a solution or evidence does not exist (emergent) or modifying an existing solution to make an improvement (incremental or process)" (Ackerman et al., 2018, p. 159; Melnyk et al., 2018; Porter-O'Grady & Malloch, 2017). Innovation-based practice comes into play when there is little or no existing practice in a particular area, resulting in a situation that warrants an innovative solution. The innovative practice leader is always grounded in the evidence and uses that evidence as to the footing from which creative energies are generated to advance and change the care experience (Porter-O'Grady & Malloch, 2017, p. 13). Creative energies for innovation include enhancement, enrichment, and intervention.

Three of these constructs—research, evidence-based practice, and innovation—create the "best practice component" of the best care. However, best care cannot be actualized unless the best practice is delivered efficiently and effectively...every time. For this to occur, the "best process component" (process improvement, PI) is required. Knowing what each of these four domains has to offer and incorporating them appropriately, depending upon the presenting question, problem, or need, is how leaders leverage the synergies of these four domains.

Each of these domains is discrete from the others, and each has unique methodological rigor, yet they co-exist; they are codependent and synergistic (Porter-O'Grady & Malloch, 2017), and together they are the elements required to be able to reap the benefits of the comprehensive "use of evidence." The EBP, Research, Innovation, and QI Alignment Model (Figure 16.2) depicts the four discrete domains of use of evidence aligning (Gallagher-Ford et al., 2021).

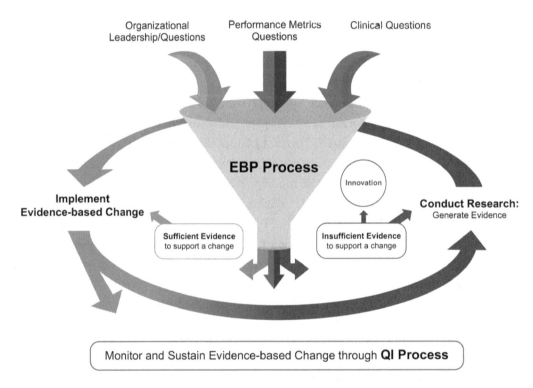

**FIGURE 16.2**   EBP, Research, Innovation, and QI Alignment Model.

For these domains to render meaningful contributions to the organization, leaders must have a solid understanding of each, recognize their dynamic and "cybernetic" (Porter-O'Grady & Malloch, 2017, p. 14) nature along a continuum, and align them synergistically. For example, the Continuous Practice and Process Improvement Model (Figure 16.3) depicts the four domains of use of evidence (research, EBP, innovation, and process improvement) conceptualized individually and synergistically (Gallagher-Ford et al., 2021).

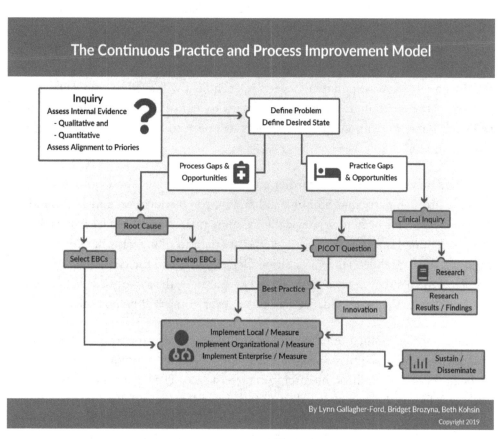

**FIGURE 16.3**  Continuous Practice and Process Improvement Model.

Leaders must value and support this continuum by creating appropriate organizational room and support for the best, evidence-based care and true innovation to exist and thrive together to deliver the best care for patients, families, and clinicians. This cannot be achieved by creating or maintaining siloes for each of these domains in an organization. Instead, leaders will need to deconstruct and reconfigure traditional "process improvement departments" and "research departments," thereby pulling together experts from each of the four domains into the same "new department." Because most clinical questions can be solved with the EBP approach, more EBP experts are needed than researcher experts. Because all practice changes must be delivered efficiently and effectively, adequate process improvement experts are needed as well. Because every best practice may have room for enhancement, true innovation experts are needed too. For all of this to be fiscally possible and sustainable, experts in each field will need to gain new expertise across the continuum. PI experts will need to learn EBP, EBP mentors will need to learn PI and innovation, and researchers will need to learn EBP and innovation, and on and on.

The good news is that gaining further competence in each of these domains is possible through participation in formal and informal education and skill-building programs. Leaders need to strategically examine their current capacity in each of the continuum domains and forge a deliberate path to filling gaps in expertise and capacity. With qualified leaders, multi-skilled experts, and the coalescing of previous departments that housed these services separately, the synergistic, cybernetic work to deliver the best, evidence-based care every time will be possible.

Building and sustaining the full use of evidence to deliver superior care takes time, and the process can be frustrating. Leaders must become emboldened and push through traditions, politics, hierarchy, and resistance, as evidenced by statements such as, "This is the way we've always done it, and it works." By doing so, these types of leaders can build capacity and synergy across the full continuum of using evidence and delivering excellence. Not doing so has resulted in the current state of affairs whereby evidence-based practice is not fully integrated into operations and is not the foundation on which many care practices and services are administered.

Evidence-based practice (EBP) was named as a required core competency for healthcare professionals by the Institute of Medicine (IOM) almost two decades ago, in 2003 (Greiner & Knebel, 2003). Since that time, there has been a tremendous amount of attention paid to the term *evidence-based practice*, but actualizing EBP in all healthcare settings has been elusive. Findings from a survey of over 1,000 nurses randomly sampled from the American Nurses Association (ANA) indicated that only one-third of the nurses reported that their colleagues consistently implemented EBP, and only one-third said they had EBP mentors. Further, the more years in practice, the fewer nurses were interested in and felt it was important to gain knowledge and skills in EBP (Melnyk et al., 2012, p. 414). Top barriers to EBP included lack of time, unsupported organizational culture hampered by politics, lack of EBP knowledge and education, lack of access to needed data, and leader or manager resistance. The identification that leaders were a major barrier to EBP prompted yet another survey of over 270 chief nurse executives (CNEs) across the US. The study revealed that although CNEs reported that their top priorities were healthcare quality and safety, EBP was a low priority. These findings revealed a major disconnect in that many CNEs did not understand that EBP is the methodological approach required to improve practice and the direct pathway to quality and safety. Other recent studies have reinforced these findings. For example, Välimäki et al. (2018) identified that the most common barriers to EBP were nursing leadership and organizational characteristics, and Pittman et al. (2019) found that nursing leadership was a key influence on organizational context and enhancing a culture of EBP within organizations. All this resistance to EBP has endured for decades, and outcomes remain less than adequate even though creating and sustaining an evidence-based enterprise is completely achievable if leaders decide it is a strategic priority.

Leaders are critical to the integration and sustainability of EBP, and therefore for the use of evidence. No organization can achieve this state without engaged leaders who have the attributes of competence, commitment, courage, and persistence to build a culture of inquiry throughout the organization and cultivate an environment where the use of evidence is an expectation (i.e., the standard of care) not the exception. Frameworks, models, assessment tools, templates, and systematic road maps are readily available, and specific research-derived competencies for EBP have been developed for frontline clinicians (Melnyk et al., 2014; Melnyk et al.,

2016) and for managers (Caramanica et al., 2022), all of which can easily be integrated into healthcare today. Many leaders, however, have not taken advantage of any of these advancements because they have not engaged in a serious journey to build and sustain EBP in their organizations. This stagnant and sometimes paralyzed situation is reflected in a study from 2016 where leaders reported that they strongly believed in the value of EBP; however, their own implementation of it was very low, and it was rated as a low priority (Melnyk et al., 2016). It is critical that nurse leaders, who oversee the largest portion of the healthcare delivery team, step up and move forward with the perseverance necessary to advance the full use of evidence in healthcare settings. Without leaders doing their part, nothing happens. In this case, the "nothing" we are talking about is quality care and desired outcomes for patients, their families, and clinicians.

# ORGANIZATIONAL CULTURE AND READINESS FOR THE USE OF EVIDENCE

For an organization to succeed in integrating the continuum of best practices and processes to deliver outcomes, organizational culture and readiness need to be assessed and addressed on an ongoing basis. Culture and readiness are not the same thing, and leaders must understand both. Organizational culture sets the context for everything an enterprise does. If leaders believe that the use of evidence is required for best practices to be delivered every time, they must share those beliefs by communicating them in a variety of ways on a continuous basis; in other words, they must create a culture that supports the use of evidence. Leaders must openly, publicly, and transparently express full support of the use of evidence through their words and actions. Supporting and resourcing only one or two of the components will not lead to success, as demonstrated in most healthcare organizations for several decades.

Readiness must be assessed and addressed as well. The Merriam-Webster dictionary defines *readiness* as "prepared mentally and/or physically for some experience or action" (Merriam-Webster, 2021). Readiness for the consistent use of evidence to guide decision-making and practice requires the development of adequate numbers of experts in all four domains that enable evidence-based practice. Readiness is complicated, takes time to achieve, and requires ongoing intentional reassessment. Several tools are available that can be used to conduct an organizational assessment including, but not limited to, the Organizational Culture and Readiness for System-wide Integration of Evidence-based Practice Survey (Fineout-Overholt & Melnyk, 2006), the Evidence-Based Practice Changes Survey (Gale & Schaffer, 2009), and the Organizational Readiness to Change Assessment instrument (Helfrich et al., 2009). Leaders must be prepared to not only build the use of evidence house; they must also be prepared to maintain or repair it when needed!

Some leaders make the mistake of thinking that if they send people to informal and formal educational programs such as LEAN training or an EBP immersion, this will be enough to make the full use of evidence happen. Nothing could be further from the truth. Instead, leaders must work together with clinicians and other key stakeholders to hardwire the use of evidence into the day-to-day operational functions of the organization. In this way, leaders and staff contribute to the organization's mission by achieving quality care and services for patients, families, and clinicians.

# MODELS AND FRAMEWORKS FOR EVIDENCE-BASED PRACTICE THAT SUPPORT THE USE OF EVIDENCE

It is not easy to build an organization that supports the use of the evidence continuum needed to deliver the best, evidence-based care every time, and it is probably even more difficult to convert an existing, tradition-based organization. Fortunately, there are many tools and resources available that can be tremendously helpful to an engaged, informed leader who *believes* that best, evidence-based care is the right thing to deliver for patients, families, and clinicians. Often, models, frameworks, and theories are perceived as esoteric and "fluff" with no true value in the "real world." In the case of evidence building, these tools and resources are exactly the opposite: they are essential. Many tools and resources such as organizational change models and practice change models have been developed to support a successful journey towards the consistent use of best evidence. These are deeply grounded in addressing what will work in the real world.

Organizational models focus on system-wide models for implementation of EBP—for example, the ARCC Model and the Integrated Promoting Action on Research Implementation in Health Services (i-PARIHS; Harvey & Kitson, 2016). The ARCC Model is one of the often-used frameworks for guiding the implementation of EBP (Speroni et al., 2020). Many studies have demonstrated that use of the ARCC Model leads to improvements in clinicians' knowledge and beliefs about the value of EBP and their ability to implement it, which is associated with greater implementation of evidence-based care and improved outcomes, both for patients and clinicians (Gorsuch et al., 2020; Levin et al., 2011; Melnyk et al., 2017; Wallen et al., 2010). Practice change models focus on guiding clinicians through the specific steps of a practice change initiative, such as the Seven Steps of EBP (Melnyk & Fineout-Overholt, 2019); Iowa Model (Buckwalter et al., 2017); or Johns Hopkins Model (Dang & Dearholt, 2017). Although there are several practice-change models from which to choose, they are all similar in many ways, and they all serve this purpose well. They all take the user through the basic steps included in EBP:

1. Identify the problem or issue to be improved

2. Formulate a searchable question

3. Search for the current, best evidence

4. Critically appraise the evidence

5. Synthesize the body of evidence

6.   Develop recommendations based on the body of evidence

7.   Implement the evidence-based change(s)

8.   Measure outcomes

9.   Disseminate the findings

Leaders who are serious about building an organization that uses evidence to support the best care all the time will need to select one of each of these types of models: one to provide the organization with an overarching road map and one to be utilized by the clinicians, experts, and mentors leading the use of evidence work to improve practice every day.

# LANGUAGE AND NOMENCLATURE

The utilization of common, shared, appropriate language and nomenclature related to the use of evidence domains is critical. The language and nomenclature of each evidence domain are specific, unique, and not interchangeable. For instance, in research, *pilot* studies are often conducted to identify problem areas related to an intervention that need to be addressed prior to launching a larger study. In EBP, there are no pilots because the research has already been conducted, and the intervention has been established as safe and appropriate. In EBP, practice changes are simply rolled out. So, it is incorrect to say that you are going to pilot an evidence-based practice change. Leaders are responsible for being well-versed in the language and nomenclature of each of the evidence domains; they must model the correct use of each domain's unique language and nomenclature, and they must coach and mentor others in the proper use of domain-specific language and nomenclature.

The field of implementation science (IS) has made significant contributions in generating evidence on effective approaches for EBP implementation in practice settings to address facilitators and barriers. The emergence of implementation science (IS) began in response to the tremendous lag between research and routine implementation of findings into clinical settings. Implementation science work has generated over 100 theories, models, and frameworks to guide the implementation process (Wensing & Grol, 2019; Westerlund et al., 2019). In this body of work, numerous trials have been conducted to examine the effectiveness of specific implementation strategies for promoting the adoption of evidence within practice settings. A great deal has been well-disseminated for organizations to use to promote the implementation of evidence. However, despite these advances in implementation science, the application of this knowledge is not routinely used among clinical teams (Tucker et al., 2021, p. 76). This lack of application of findings from the field of IS contributes to the lag and/or inability to implement best practices that persists in healthcare settings.

The language of research and process improvement have been infused into healthcare organizations' atmosphere for centuries and decades, respectively, and are well known to many clinicians and leaders. Once again, however, the language of EBP (including implementation science [IS] and innovation) are new or unknown to many. As a result, implementation science and innovation language have not been fully translated into conversations in real-world clinical settings, contributing to the slow pace of their adoption. Increasing leaders' and clinicians' awareness and knowledge of standardized implementation language and nomenclature would improve communication among evidence users within and across settings. Employing common language related to the use of evidence would promote accurate dissemination of evidence-based work and enhance capacity to assess the effectiveness of evidence-related strategies across multiple settings and situations, thus building evidence-based practice and improving outcomes on a large, global scale.

# LEADERSHIP COMPETENCIES FOR EVIDENCE-BASED PRACTICE

As previously stated, the current state of healthcare does not show evidence-based practice (EBP) in place throughout all healthcare systems, nor are 90% of all clinical decisions evidence-based as recommended by the Institute of Medicine

(IOM, 2007). Many reasons exist as to why this is still the case (e.g., lack of time, expertise, and support), but today's nurse leaders, equipped with advanced education and expertise on imparting evidence into practice at all levels in the organization, are removing these barriers. They are doing so by ensuring the application of scientific evidence, effective use of relevant data, and requiring improved performance standards in all clinical settings through the critical allocation of adequate resources, including the protected time needed for their application. These leaders support staff in the development of evidence-based guidelines such as those used to address management of pain when treating older cancer patients (e.g., Cancer Pain Practice Index [CPPI]) or the translations of evidence into practice (TRIP) for palliative care and other clinical treatment protocols. Minimizing or removing the barriers of time, resources, and inadequate knowledge is critical for evidence-based practice, innovation, and performance improvement to synergistically inform healthcare operations and clinical decisions. Only then can the professed value for using evidence by leaders and staff result in improved patient care outcomes.

Many strategies are available for leaders to utilize to promote the use of evidence, and an important one is the use of competencies to guide performance expectations related to EBP. *Competencies* reflect the expected and measurable level of performance in nursing, including knowledge, skills, abilities, and judgment based on current science that is required to perform effectively and facilitate high-quality, safe nursing care (ANA, 2010; Dunn et al., 2000; Melnyk et al., 2014). In 2014, Melnyk et al. conducted a Delphi study and developed a set of competencies specific to EBP for RNs and APNs to assist healthcare organizations in ensuring that clinicians were delivering the highest quality, safest, evidence-based care. This work resulted in 24 EBP competencies: 13 for practicing nurses and 11 additional competencies for advanced practice nurses (Figure 16.4).

**Evidence-based practice competencies for practicing registered professional nurses**

1. Questions clinical practices for the purpose of improving the quality of care.

2. Describes clinical problems using internal evidence.* (internal evidence* = evidence generated internally within a clinical setting, such as patient assessment data, outcomes management, and quality improvement data)

3. Participates in the formulation of clinical questions using PICOT* format. (*PICOT = Patient population; Intervention or area of interest; Comparison intervention or group; Outcome; Time).

4. Searches for external evidence* to answer focused clinical questions. (external evidence* = evidence generated from research)

5. Participates in critical appraisal of preappraised evidence (such as clinical practice guidelines, evidence-based policies and procedures, and evidence syntheses).

6. Participates in the critical appraisal of published research studies to determine their strength and applicability to clinical practice.

7. Participates in the evaluation and synthesis of a body of evidence gathered to determine its strength and applicability to clinical practice.

8. Collects practice data (e.g., individual patient data, quality improvement data) systematically as internal evidence for clinical decision making in the care of individuals, groups, and populations.

9. Integrates evidence gathered from external and internal sources in order to plan evidence-based practice changes.

10. Implements practice changes based on evidence and clinical expertise and patient preferences to improve care processes and patient outcomes.

11. Evaluates outcomes of evidence-based decisions and practice changes for individuals, groups, and populations to determine best practices.

12. Disseminates best practices supported by evidence to improve quality of care and patient outcomes.

13. Participates in strategies to sustain an evidence-based practice culture.

**Evidence-based practice competencies for practicing advanced practice nurses**
All competencies of practicing registered professional nurses plus:

14. Systematically conducts an exhaustive search for external evidence* to answer clinical questions. (external evidence*: evidence generated from research)

15. Critically appraises relevant preappraised evidence (i.e., clinical guidelines, summaries, synopses, syntheses of relevant external evidence) and primary studies, including evaluation and synthesis.

16. Integrates a body of external evidence from nursing and related fields with internal evidence* in making decisions about patient care. (internal evidence* = evidence generated internally within a clinical setting, such as patient assessment data, outcomes management, and quality improvement data)

17. Leads transdisciplinary teams in applying synthesized evidence to initiate clinical decisions and practice changes to improve the health of individuals, groups, and populations.

18. Generates internal evidence through outcomes management and EBP implementation projects for the purpose of integrating best practices.

19. Measures processes and outcomes of evidence-based clinical decisions.

20. Formulates evidence-based policies and procedures.

21. Participates in the generation of external evidence with other healthcare professionals.

22. Mentors others in evidence-based decision making and the EBP process.

23. Implements strategies to sustain an EBP culture.

24. Communicates best evidence to individuals, groups, colleagues, and policy makers.

*Copyright:* Melnyk, Gallagher-Ford, and Fineout-Overholt (2013).

**FIGURE 16.4**   Evidence-based competencies for practicing registered nurses and advanced practice nurses (Melnyk et al., 2014).

*Note: EBP Competency Scale items from "The Establishment of Evidence-Based Practice Competencies for Practicing Registered Nurses and Advanced Practice Nurses in Real-World Clinical Settings: Proficiencies to Improve Healthcare Quality, Reliability, Patient Outcomes, and Costs.," by B. M. Melnyk et al., 2014,* Worldviews on Evidence-Based Nursing, *11(1), p. 11. Copyright 2014 by Melnyk et al. Reprinted with permission.*

This research team advocated that EBP competencies be incorporated in employee orientation, role accountabilities, performance appraisals, and advancement opportunities. In addition, they and other researchers have identified that leadership is critical to achieving these objectives, but exactly how leaders successfully provide leadership for EBP, create an infrastructure to support it, and promote its use by clinicians had not been well described.

A study done by Caramanica et al. (2022) identified 22 leadership competencies to enable frontline leaders to successfully support clinicians in the use of evidence-based practice in the clinical setting (Figure 16.5).

These EBP competent frontline leaders do not view EBP as a "project," but an expectation that leaders and staff possess the knowledge and skills required in their role responsibilities. Frontline leaders who successfully support the use of evidence foster a spirit of inquiry among clinicians and ask questions such as, "Is this the best way to achieve targeted outcomes?" and, "What evidence supports our thinking and actions in caring for this patient?" In this way, they are co-creating with staff and others a culture that supports applying current scientific evidence obtained through evidence-based practice, research, innovation, or performance improvement. This then leads to desired best practices and innovation, resulting in the achievement of targeted patient care outcomes.

## LEADING EVIDENCE-BASED PRACTICE

1.   Identifies own vital role in enabling evidence-based practice.

2.   Serves as a champion for evidence-based practice projects by readily checking on progress, providing feedback, removing barriers, and offering encouragement.

3.   Develops strong relationships with staff and leaders for the advancement of evidence-based practice.

4.   Prioritizes evidence-based practice projects to align with the organization's goals.

5.   Influences formal organizational policies to enable evidence-based practice.

6.   Facilitates the conduction and implementation of evidence-based practice.

7.   Applies the best evidence to make leadership decisions.

8.   Evaluates the adoption of an evidence-based culture.

## BUILDING INFRASTRUCTURE FOR EVIDENCE-BASED PRACTICE

9.   Assesses readiness for evidence-based practice in the clinical practice environment.

10.   Assesses staff commitment to engaging in evidence-based practice.

11.   Justifies financial resources in support of the evidence-based practice.

12.   Appraises policies, procedures, and standards of practice to ensure these are evidence-based.

13.   Facilitates allocation of multiple resources required to expand evidence-based practice.

## PROMOTING EVIDENCE-BASED PRACTICE

14.   Demonstrates competency in evidence-based practice (knowledge, skill, and attitude).

15.   Promotes the value of evidence-based practice by connecting it to quality, safety, and patient care outcomes.

16.   Provides staff access to education on evidence-based practice.

17. Provides staff access to evidence-based practice experts and mentors.

18. Facilitates staff access to relevant data needed for evidence-based practice.

19. Ensures staff are provided the time needed to participate in evidence-based practice.

20. Holds staff accountable for the integration of evidence-based practice into practice commensurate with their level of clinical expertise/role.

21. Provides meaningful recognition of staff and mentors who engage in evidence-based practice.

22. Promotes the expectation that organizational decisions are made using evidence.

© University of West Georgia, Caramanica, L., & Gallagher-Ford, L.

**FIGURE 16.5**  Nurse managers' leadership competencies to support clinicians in evidence-based practice.

# LEADING EVIDENCE-BASED PRACTICE

The day in nurse leaders' lives is characterized by a myriad of competing priorities that require attention, resulting in an unending list of responsibilities. Thus, nurse leaders who successfully enable the use of evidence by clinicians in the real-world setting do so by transforming how they perform their leadership role responsibilities, not by taking on additional duties. They begin with identifying their vital part in creating a culture that supports and enables evidence and innovation to take hold. Creating a vision for EBP and modeling the way, they demonstrate their role as a key standard-bearer for the use of evidence in all its forms, and that relevant data and solid evidence must also support the enactment of their responsibilities. In their daily work, they observe and evaluate the means and effectiveness through which patient care and services are provided, particularly regarding the extent to which these are supported by evidence. For example, on rounds, these leaders will ask the before-mentioned "spirit of inquiry" questions. While the study conducted by Caramanica et al. (2022) focused on leading the way for EBP, it is realistic to suggest that these and the accompanying behaviors described here support all the other domains included in the use of evidence (research, performance improvement, and innovation) as well.

Nurse leaders who support the use of evidence use their influencing leadership skills to set the expectation for incorporating evidence-based care by successfully establishing strong partnerships throughout the organization. These "fire starters" for using evidence guide the prioritization of such activities that ensure their alignment with organizational priorities, making implementation more likely to be successful. They understand the importance of timing when introducing new evidence and ideas, and they can successfully create opportunities for their introduction by staying close to the practice and empowering those who provide patient care.

As with any major change, resistance should be expected as many "old ways" will need to end, and many "new ways" will need to begin. Emotions will run high as beloved, outdated traditions come to an end, previous "experts" suddenly become novices, and longstanding hierarchical institutions and power grids are challenged and deconstructed. Many organizational structures will need to be reviewed, reimagined, and redesigned to support a new way to solve problems and drive decisions using the best evidence. The current level of evidence for care delivery is not adequate, and this is not acceptable. It is the responsibility of leaders to build the organizational capacity to fully utilize the best evidence to achieve the best outcomes. Achieving the competence (knowledge, skills, and attitudes) to lead this critical work of using evidence needed to assure a better future for healthcare requires active, intentional, personal work for individual leaders. In addition, they will need to set an example for others and establish rigorous expectations they lead.

# BUILDING INFRASTRUCTURE FOR EVIDENCE-BASED PRACTICE

As part of their role in building an infrastructure to support the use of evidence, nurse leaders serve as change agents: creating a compelling reason for the change, employing the use of relevant data to substantiate their concerns, and empowering key stakeholders to create and implement new and better ways to recommend care based on the evidence. Their expertise includes mastery of their political power, such as forming strong partnerships with "owners" of clinical and operational databases that hold pertinent data and information needed by clinicians to ensure they make the best decisions and engage in the highest practice standards. Leaders must empower clinicians with the authority and autonomy to change practice and be allotted adequate time away from their other work to conduct evidence activities. They must be adequately resourced to conduct evidence work (computers, access to databases, librarian support), and implementation infrastructures supporting evidence-based changes must be in place, hardwired, and fully supported by leaders (Gallagher-Ford & Conner, 2020; Schaefer & Welton, 2018). Specific transformational changes to be achieved include:

- The creation of a **department** that houses experts in all four domains to ensure the full use of evidence that is **led** by a leader who supports all domains equitably and adequately

- The requirement that all **policies and procedures** be continuously current and evidence-based

- The creation of and hardwiring of the use of evidence for **organizational operations**

- The provision of adequate **human and financial resources** (including protected time) to support the use of evidence work

- The expectation that all job descriptions will include **competency** in the use of evidence commensurate with role responsibilities.

- The public and timely removal of barriers and resistance so best, evidence-based practice can be achieved

# IMPLICATIONS FOR PRACTICE

The promotion of the use of evidence begins with frontline leaders achieving self-knowledge and skill on what constitutes EBP, and other domains of evidence, as well as how to successfully implement them. Nurse leaders need to start by gaining competence in EBP and the other domains of evidence (knowledge, skill, and a positive attitude) themselves. They must model the use of evidence by integrating evidence into their individual leadership practice decisions; invest in the use of evidence resources, including education, mentors, and protected time for evidence-based work; and build effective infrastructures to support implementation and sustainment of best practice. They enable clinicians to attend workshops to learn the skills necessary for the use and application of evidence, and they ensure the availability of an adequate number of evidence experts to mentor them. In addition, nurse leaders must cultivate a shared value for the use of evidence by clinicians and other key stakeholders with whom they interact, holding them accountable to engage in EBP commensurate with their knowledge, skills, and role responsibilities. These leaders also provide meaningful and continuous rewards and recognition for actively engaging in the use of evidence to ensure sustainability. All of these are essential action items that only leaders can do.

Once a road map (organizational model) is selected to guide the transformational journey, a good place to start is a thorough examination of the organization's current approach to solving problems. How does the organization respond when a "problem" (sentinel event, near miss, never event) occurs? For many organizations, the answer is "call a meeting," one that includes key stakeholders and decision-makers. At that meeting, there is usually a review of the event(s) and the associated data, followed by a robust brainstorming session to "pitch" ideas (or *countermeasures* as they are referred to in LEAN language). An action plan is formulated by the end of a meeting, and that plan is placed on a fast track for rollout in the following days or weeks. What are the chances that the action plan, based on a single brainstorming session involving the people who work in the place where the problem is happening, is the right plan (i.e., includes the strategies that have been demonstrated repeatedly to effectively solve the problem when tested rigorously/scientifically)? The chances are zero, as the people in that room do not know the answer, and the only way to come to know what the best strategies are for solving the problem and to develop the best action plan is to access and use evidence. The current and ineffective problem-solving approach of meeting, brainstorming, and "trying something" based on local/internal opinions is no longer adequate, ethical, or acceptable. Because an effective and efficient methodological approach (EBP) is available and attainable (one that will lead the organization to the best/leading solution, i.e., the right answer that will fix the problem), it is the responsibility of leaders to build the organizational capacity to utilize this far better approach. Pivoting to this methodologically superior approach means that, when there is a problem, the leader will call for an evidence-based team or mentor rather than a meeting with stakeholders first. The EBP team or mentor uses the steps of EBP (from the EBP practice model already in place) and brings the right answer back to the leader. The leader then calls the stakeholder meeting, and the stakeholders' job is to lead and assure the timely implementation of the evidence-based change needed. Their expert brainstorming days are over, and their expert best practice champion days begin! This example highlights the type of fundamental change that leaders need to undertake to transform their organization into the one that can effectively provide evidence-based care to drive the best outcomes.

# SUMMARY

In summary, nursing leadership, at all levels, is an essential factor in the establishment and sustainability of healthcare enterprises where clinicians use evidence in 90% of their decisions and ensure the delivery of safe, quality care and services.

Only when the use of evidence is the standard of practice will the Quadruple Aim in healthcare be achieved (improving quality and safety of the patient care experience, enhancing the health of populations, reducing the cost of healthcare, and improving the work-life of clinicians; Berwick et al., 2008; Bodenheimer & Sinsky, 2014).

Nurse leaders who achieve competence in using evidence will make effective decisions, and their actions will result in the attainment of targeted outcomes. Furthermore, by setting the example as evidence-based leaders, they will model the way, thus creating future leaders who will ensure the sustainability of evidence-based care. This, in turn, will provide the necessary platform upon which global health is possible.

# REFLECTIVE QUESTIONS

1. What happens when leaders and clinicians conduct their roles without using the best evidence to inform their thinking and actions?

2. Given what you learned from this chapter; how can healthcare systems better support their leaders and clinicians in the application of best evidence for their decisions and practice?

3. What would you identify as the first three actions that need to be taken by nurse managers so that they can effectively influence clinicians to use evidence-based practice in the clinical setting?

4. What gets in the way of your own use of best evidence in your daily practice, and what steps can you take to remove these barriers?

5. What would quality, safe care look like if best evidence and processes were used consistently by leaders and staff?

# NARRATIVE

In 2014, the department of nursing at Memorial Sloan Kettering (MSK), an ANCC Magnet designated and NCI designated comprehensive cancer center underwent organizational changes at the executive nursing level. The Senior Vice President and Chief Nursing Officer (SVP CNO) reorganized the divisions of nursing practice, quality, and education under the newly created office of the Deputy Chief Nursing Officer (DCNO). One of the deliverables the DCNO was given was to create, launch, and sustain an evidence-based practice (EBP) infrastructure across the nursing enterprise. As an internationally recognized oncology nursing service, these leaders believed that applying evidence to nursing care delivery would ensure MSK's leadership position in oncology nursing practice. Using a high-reliability framework, the DCNO set out to strengthen the department's approach to EBP. Leadership commitment was foundational to the full actualization of the vision and to ensure sustained EBP competency for every nurse across the care continuum. A partnership with the Helene Fuld Health Trust National Institute for Evidence-based Practice (EBP) was put in motion to leverage an innovative, deliberate, and customized college-level EBP immersion for the nursing enterprise at MSK. At the outset, a pivotal decision was made by the DCNO: all nursing leadership, inclusive of CNO, DCNO, Nursing Directors, Nurse Leaders, CNSs, Nursing Professional Development Specialist's, and Quality Management Nurses, would be required to attend the first EBP immersion together as a cohort. This ensured all of the nursing leadership was learning the method simultaneously, which would mitigate any skepticism and roadblocks to successful EBP adoption. Without leadership engagement and buy-in, the DCNO believed immersion across the enterprise would be futile. Because all nursing leadership was required to participate in the immersion, a safety net was created in the event one level of leadership failed to buy into the enculturation. This unique approach fostered collegial relationships, broke down existing silos, strengthened the department, and built a unique EBP capacity with the goal of preparing all MSK nurses in an established EBP methodology, building EBP competence, and making evidence-based decision-making the standard practice across the nursing enterprise.

Additional deliberate strategies were required to ensure the adoption of EBP at MSK. Recognizing Clinical Nurse Specialists as EBP experts and early adopters, structural changes were necessary to actualize the full vision. In January 2017, the CNS reporting structure was centralized to strengthen, support, and sustain a spirit and culture of inquiry across the care continuum. The vision for EBP enculturation included a call to validate existing policies, procedures, and standards of care and challenge the "Memorial Way" to ensure the existing nursing practice was up to date and in alignment with the evidence and best practice. Collaboration with the well-established and expert team from the Fuld Institute was pivotal to bringing EBP structures and processes to every chairside, bedside, and tableside across the care continuum.

The EBP immersions consisted of a standard curriculum provided by the EBP Institute's faculty and facilitation of implementation by Fuld expert mentors. Multiple cohorts attended the immersion program, with each subsequent cohort strategically assembled to move EBP expertise beyond the leadership cadre by thoughtfully including academic and alliance partners, staff nurses, and Interdisciplinary colleagues. All participants were assigned to one of three unique learning tracks in the program: mentor, leader, or academic. Post immersion, each cohort met with a Fuld EBP expert for follow-up and boosters every three months for 15 months. These sessions were focused on feedback, direction, and support. During this same time, EBP terminology and methods were introduced across the department and incorporated into shared governance bylaws and promotional and staff development processes. MSK librarians developed resources for writing PICO questions and offered courses on evidence searching and reference management. Cohort groups presented their 15 month-long work at a peer symposium/celebration. EBP initiative presentations included clinical inquiry, PICO questions, critical appraisal of the body of evidence conducted, synthesis tables, and evidence-based recommendations for practice or administrative changes to be implemented. Many recommendations have been fully implemented and sustained, and whenever appropriate, measurements of clinical outcomes, value, and returns on investments have been reported.

The strategy of **leadership engagement first** promoted the enculturation of EBP institution-wide and led to measurable outcomes on challenging clinical/institutional initiatives such as falls, handoff, mindfulness, inpatient discharge, palliative care, opioid addiction in the oncology patient, extravasations, etc. To date, more than 60 EBP initiatives have emerged. A measured increase in knowledge of EBP was appreciated because of the intensive immersion. Surveys of knowledge and skill acquisition and attitude about EBP demonstrated a significant change from baseline. A second, unpredicted outcome was that the immersion sparked interest from participants in returning to advanced degree programs.

MSK nursing leadership now utilizes a systematic process for translating evidence into practice. Capitalizing on this new skill set has led to confirmation of existing best practice/policy as well as to bringing novel EBP interventions forward to address universal, ongoing, and problematic clinical issues. The initial leadership immersion became the foundation for embedding EBP into the culture of MSK. Leadership has demonstrated a sustained commitment to the EBP process as mentors, facilitators, and advocates, ultimately impacting patient care in such a positive and meaningful way.

What do you think are the most important leadership actions in this exemplar?

# AUTHOR BIOGRAPHIES

**Lynn Gallagher-Ford PhD, RN, NE-BC, DPFNAP, FAAN/Evidence-based Practice (CH),** is the Chief Operating Officer at the Helene Fuld National Trust Institute for Evidence-based Practice in Nursing and Healthcare at the Ohio State University College of Nursing. Her work is dedicated to research, education, and consultation focused on the integration, and sustainability of evidence-based practice in both academic and clinical settings. Her publications include co-authorship of the textbook *Implementing the EBP Competencies in Healthcare* as well as several landmark studies including the Delphi study that established EBP competencies for practicing RNs and APNs, and "The State of Evidence-Based Practice in US Nurses: Critical Implications for Nurse Leaders and Educators." She is the associate editor of the column; "Implementing and Sustaining EBP in Real World Healthcare Settings" in *Worldviews on Evidence-Based Nursing*. She is a Distinguished Practitioner and Fellow in the National Academies of Practice and a Fellow in the American Academy of Nursing.

**Laura Caramanica, PhD, RN, CNE, CNEP, FACHE, FAAN,** Graduate Program Director & Professor, University of West Georgia, Carrollton, Georgia, has extensive knowledge in evidence-based practice having studied, instructed, and published on this topic for over 25 years. Caramanica is the Graduate Program Director & Professor at the Tanner Health System School of Nursing, University of West Georgia, Carrolton, Georgia. She is an active member of several professional organizations and is currently a board member of the Association for Leadership Science in Nursing as Vice President for (Educational) Programs (ALSN, 2020–2022) and formerly the boards of American Organization of Nurse Leaders (AONL, President, 2012) and the Connecticut Nurses Association (CNA, Secretary & Treasure, 1980s). She is a Fellow in the Academy of Nursing and the Association of Health Care Executives and holds certification in nursing leadership from AONL and ANA. Caramanica served as Chief Nursing Officer in several healthcare systems for 30 years, whereby she instituted several innovative programs for leaders and staff on EBP.

# REFERENCES

Ackerman, M., Porter-O'Grady, T., & Melnyk, B. (2018). Innovation-based practice (IBP) versus evidence-based practice (EBP): A new perspective that assesses and differentiates evidence and innovation. *Worldviews on Evidence-Based Nursing, 15*(3), 159–160. doi: 10.1111/wvn.12292.

American Nurses Association. (2010). *Nursing scope of practice standards.* https://www.nursingworld.org/practice-policy/scope-of-practice

Berwick, D., Nolan, T., & Whittington J. (2008). The triple aim: Care, health, and cost. *Health Affairs, 27*(3), 759–769. https://doi.org/10.1377/hlthaff.27.3.759

Bodenheimer, T., & Sinsky, C. (2014). From triple to quadruple aim: Care of the patient requires care of the provider. *The Annals of Family Medicine, 12*(6), 573–576. doi: https://doi.org/10.1370/afm.1713

Buckwalter, K. C., Cullen, L., Hanrahan, K., Kleiber, C., McCarthy, A. M., Rakel, B., Steelman, V., Tripp-Reimer, T., & Tucker, S., (2017). Iowa model of evidence-based practice: Revisions and validation. *Worldviews on Evidence-Based Nursing, 14*(3), 175–182.

Caramanica, L., Gallagher-Ford, L., Idleman, L., Mindrila, D., Richter, S., & Thomas, B. K. (2022). Establishment of nurse manager leadership competencies to support clinicians in evidence-based practice. *Journal of Nursing Administration, 52*(1), 27–34. doi: 10.1097/NNA.0000000000001099

Dang, D., & Dearholt, S. (2017). *Johns Hopkins nursing evidence-based practice: Model and guidelines* (3rd ed.). Sigma Theta Tau International.

Davidson, S., Weberg, D., Porter-O'Grady, T., & Malloch, K. (2017). *Leadership for evidence-based innovation in nursing and health professions.* Jones & Bartlett Learning.

Dunn K., Wallace, E. Z., & Leipzig, R. M. (2000). A dissemination model for teaching evidence-based medicine. *Academic Medicine, 75*(5), 525–526. doi: 10.1097/00001888-200005000-00048

Fineout-Overholt, E., & Melnyk, B. M. (2006). *Organizational culture and readiness for system-wide implementation of EBP (OCR-SIEP) scale.* ARCC LLC Publishing.

Gale, B. V., & Schaffer, M. A. (2009). Organizational readiness for evidence-based practice. *Journal of Nursing Administration, 39*(2), 91–97. doi: 10.1097/NNA.0b013e318195a48d

Gallagher-Ford, L., & Connor, L. (2020). Transforming healthcare to evidence-based healthcare: A failure of leadership. *The Journal of Nursing Administration, 50*(5), 248–250.

Gallagher-Ford, L., Kohsin, B., & Brozyna, B. (2021). *Models to support the integration and synergies of research EBP, innovation and process improvement* [Manuscript in preparation]. College of Nursing, The Ohio State University.

Gorsuch, C. R. P. F., Gallagher-Ford, L., Koshy T. B., Melnyk, B. M., & Connor, L. (2020). Impact of a formal educational skill building program based on the ARCC Model to enhance evidence based practice competency in nurse teams. *Worldviews on Evidence Based Nursing, 17*(4), 258–268.

Greiner, A., & Knebel, E. (Eds.). (2003). *Health professions education: A bridge to quality.* National Academies Press. https://www.ncbi.nlm.nih.gov/books/NBK221528/

Harding K., Porter, J., Horne-Thompson A., Donley E., & Taylor N. (2014). Not enough time or a low priority? Barriers to evidence-based practice for allied health clinicians. *Journal of Continuing Education in the Health Professions, 34*(4), 224–231. https://doi: 10.1002/chp.21255

Harvey, G., & Kitson, A. (2016). PARIHS revisited: from heuristic to integrated framework for the successful implementation of knowledge into practice. *Implementation Science, 11*(33). https://doi.org/10.1186/s13012-016-0398-2

Helfrich, C., Li, Y., Sharp, N., & Sales, A. E. (2009). Organizational readiness to change assessment (ORCA): Development of an instrument based on the Promoting Action on Research in Health Services (PARIHS) framework. *Implementation Science, 4*(38). https://doi.org/10.1186/1748-5908-4-38

Institute of Medicine. (2007). Appendix C: IOM roundtable on evidence-based medicine roster and background. In IOM (2007) *Evidence-based medicine and the changing nature of health care: IOM annual meeting summary.* https://www.ncbi.nlm.nih.gov/books/NBK52822/

Levin, R. F., Fineout-Overholt, E., Melnyk, B. M., Barnes, M., & Vetter, M. J. (2011). Fostering evidence-based practice to improve nurse and cost outcomes in a community health setting: A pilot test of the advancing research and clinical practice through close collaboration model. *Nursing Administration Quarterly, 35*(1), 21–33. doi: 10.1097/NAQ.0b013e31820320ff

Melnyk, B. M., & Fineout-Overholt, E. (2019). *Evidence-based practice in nursing and healthcare. A guide to best practice* (4th ed.). Wolters Kluwer.

Melnyk, B. M., Fineout-Overholt, E., Gallagher-Ford, L., & Kaplan, L. (2012). The state of evidence-based practice in U.S. nurses: Critical implications for nurse leaders and educators. *Journal of Nursing Administration, 42*(9), 410–417.

Melnyk, B. M., Fineout-Overholt, E., Giggleman, M., & Choy, K. (2017). A test of the ARCC© model improves implementation of evidence-based practice, healthcare culture, and patient outcomes. *Worldviews on Evidence-Based Nursing, 14*(1), 5–9. https://doi.org/10.1111/wvn.12188

Melnyk, B. M., Gallagher-Ford, L., Long, L. E., & Fineout-Overholt, E. (2014). The establishment of evidence-based practice competencies for practicing registered nurses and advanced practice nurses in real-world clinical settings: Proficiencies to improve healthcare quality, reliability, patient outcomes, and costs. *Worldviews on Evidence-Based Nursing, 11*(1), 5–15. https://doi.org/10.1111/wvn.12021

Melnyk, B. M., Gallagher-Ford, L., Thomas, B. K., Troseth, M., Wyngarden, K., & Szalacha, L. (2016). A study of chief nurse executives indicates low prioritization of evidence-based practice and shortcomings in hospital performance metrics across the United States. *Worldviews on Evidence-Based Nursing, 13*(1), 6–14. https://doi.org/10.1111/wvn.12133

Melnyk, B. M., Gallagher-Ford, L., Zellefrow, C., Tucker, S., Thomas, B., Sinnott, L. T., & Tan, A. (2018). The first U.S. study on nurses' evidence-based practice competencies indicates major deficits that threaten healthcare quality, safety, and patient outcomes. *Worldviews on Evidence-Based Nursing, 15*(1), 16–25.

Melnyk, B. M., & Morrison-Beedy, D. (Eds.). (2018). *Intervention research and evidence-based quality improvement: Designing, conducting, analyzing, and funding.* Springer Publishing Company.

Merriam-Webster. (n.d.) *Readiness.* In Merriam-Webster.com dictionary. https://www.merriam-webster.com/dictionary/readiness

Morrar, R. (2014). Innovation and services: A literature review. *Technology, Management Review, 4*(4), 6–14.

Pittman J., Cohee, A., Storey, S., LaMothe, J., Gilbert, J., Bakoyanns, G., Ofner, S., & Newhouse, R. (2019). A multisite health system survey to assess organizational context to support evidence-based practice. *Worldviews on Evidence-Based Nursing, 16*(4), 271–280.

Porter-O'Grady, T., & Malloch, K. (2017). Evidence-based practice and the innovation paradigm: A model for the continuum of practice excellence. In S. Davidson, D. Weberg, T. Porter-O'Grady, & K. Malloch (Eds.), *Leadership for evidence-based innovation in nursing and health professions.* Jones & Barrett Learning.

Schaefer J., & Welton J. (2018). Evidence based practice readiness: A concept analysis. *Journal of Nursing Management, 26*(6), 621–629. doi: 10.1111/jonm.12599.

Speroni, K. G., McLaughlin, M. K., & Friesen, M. A. (2020). Use of evidence-based practice models and research findings in magnet-designated hospitals across the United States: National survey results. *Worldviews on Evidence-Based Nursing, 17*(2), 98–107. https://doi-org.proxy.lib.ohio-state.edu/10.1111/wvn.12428

Tucker, S., McNett, M., Mazurek Melnyk, B., Hanrahan, K., Hunter, S. C., Kim, B., Cullen, L., & Kitson, A. (2021). Implementation science: Application of evidence-based practice models to improve healthcare quality. *Worldviews on Evidence-Based Nursing, 18*(2), 76–84. https://doi.org/10.1111/wvn.12495

Valimaki, T., Partanen, P., & Haggman-Laitila, A. (2020). An integrated review of interventions for enhancing leadership in the implementation of evidence-based nursing. *Worldviews on Evidence-Based Nursing, 15*(6), 424–431.

Wallen, G. R., Mitchell, S. A., Melnyk, B., Fineout-Overholt, E., Miller-Davis, C., Yates, J., & Hastings, C. (2010). Implementing evidence-based practice: Effectiveness of a structured multifaceted mentorship programme. *Journal of Advanced Nursing, 66*(12), 2761–2771.

Wensing, M., & Grol, R. (2019). Knowledge translation in health: How implementation science could contribute more. *BMC Medicine, 17*(88), 1–6.

Westerlund, A., Sundberg, L., & Nilsen, P. (2019). Implementation of implementation science knowledge: The research-practice gap paradox. *Worldviews on Evidence Based Nursing, 16*(5), 332–334. doi: 10.1111/wvn.12403

Woo, B., Lee, J., & Tam, W. (2017). The impact of the advanced practice nursing role on quality of care, clinical outcomes, patient satisfaction, and cost in the emergency and critical care settings: A systematic review. *Human Resources for Health, 15*(63). https://doi.org/10.1186/s12960-017-0237-9

Wu, Y., Brettle, A., Zhou, C., Ou, J., Wang, Y., & Wang, S. (2018). Do educational interventions aimed at nurses to support the implementation of evidence-based practice improve patient outcomes? A systematic review. *Nurse Education Today*, *70*, 109–114. https://doi.org/10.1016/j.nedt.2018.08.026

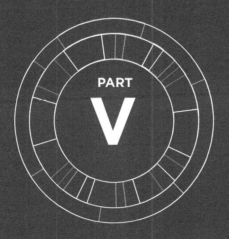

# ENVISION THE FUTURE OF HEALTHCARE LEADERSHIP

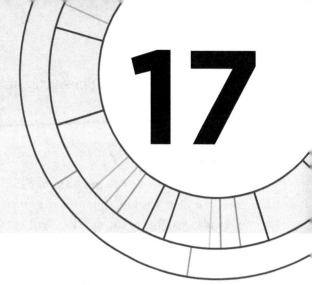

# WISDOM LEADERSHIP: A DEVELOPMENTAL JOURNEY

Daniel J. Pesut, PhD, RN, FAAN

## LEARNING OBJECTIVES

After completing this chapter, the reader should be able to:

- Define the nature of wisdom leadership to inform personal and professional leadership development

- Describe stages of adult cognitive development to inform teaching and learning of wisdom leadership capacities

- Differentiate between horizontal and vertical leadership development to appreciate the significance of leadership development strategies, activities, and methods

- Describe strategies and tools for the development of wisdom leadership capacities to support career development and wisdom capacity building in healthcare organizations

- Explore references and resources to learn more about the development of wisdom leadership capacities

# OVERVIEW

The purposes of this chapter are to define the nature of wisdom leadership and describe how wisdom develops over time. Adult cognitive development theory provides insights in the development of wisdom leadership capacities. Essential concepts for teaching wisdom are highlighted. Strategies and techniques for developing wisdom capacities in healthcare organizations are discussed. Resources and references to support continued exploration of concepts, principles, and practices of wisdom leadership are provided.

Leadership is a developmental journey. Over the course of the journey some leaders develop wisdom, and some do not. What are the "differences that make a difference" between and among leaders who develop wisdom capacities and those who do not?

# WISDOM LEADERSHIP: A DEVELOPMENTAL JOURNEY

Wisdom leadership and wisdom capacities are necessary for leading transformative change in complex organizations. Margaret Plews-Ogan and Gene Beyt (2014) describe the nature of wisdom leadership in academic health science centers and share insights about essential wisdom capacities. Leaders who cultivate and develop these capacities are more likely to be perceived as wise rather than foolish. Wisdom capacities include the ability to reflect, forgive, and be humble, trustworthy, compassionate, relationship oriented, and positive. Wisdom capacities also include the ability to appreciate and apply systems thinking and derive meaning from the analysis and evaluation of competing values and complexity dynamics.

*"One of the greatest gifts we can give to another generation is our experience, our wisdom."*

–Desmond Tutu

Wisdom is an essential concept and element of professional nursing practice as defined in the recently revised scope and standards of professional practice published by the American Nurses Association (2021). *Wisdom* is the ability to transform data into information to produce knowledge that promotes learning to guide evidence-based practice in a culture of inquiry, critical thinking, and research. Matney et al. (2011, 2016) describe *wisdom* as the application of experience, intelligence, creativity, and knowledge, mediated by values, to achieve a common good. This definition links wisdom to performance and nursing practice and supports the idea that wisdom ought to be tied to actions applying knowledge, skills, and abilities. As Fontaine et al. (2014) note:

> Breakthrough change requires social entrepreneurs learn how to align their Wisdom, Understanding and Knowledge. Our goal as leaders is to align *what* we do, *how* we do it, and *who we are*. Wisdom is essential but too often missing in modern leadership. Leading from the soul of our deepest awareness and core values will tap into transformative power to deliver lasting results. (p. 102)

Wise leaders ask different questions, seek multiple perspectives, and see and think in systems (Berger, 2020; Kaipa & Radjou, 2013). Kaipa and Radjou (2013) define *wise leadership* as leveraging intelligence for the greater good by balancing action with reflection, introspection, and ethical clarity. They suggest wise leaders have perspective, are big picture action-oriented thinkers who are clear about their role, employ vision logic, and are driven to serve others. Wise leaders shift from a narrow focus on operation and strategy to an integrated perspective. Wise leaders respond to external events with discernment, flexibility, and authenticity. Wise leaders welcome ambiguity and seek to understand obstacles. They strive to discern what works for themselves and the greater good of an organization or society at large. Wise leaders think about their thinking and develop creative metacognitive skills. Wise leaders know what they know and what they do not know as well as the limits of knowing (Sternberg, 1998, 2003, 2004; Sternberg & Jordan, 2019). Christopher Petersen and Martin Seligman (2004) note that the virtue of wisdom is supported by character strengths that include creativity, curiosity, love of learning, judgment, and perspective. Wise leaders move people to action; activate relationships, networks, and social connections; and manage their energy to maintain resilience (Allison-Napolitano & Pesut, 2015).

# THE BALANCE THEORY OF WISDOM

Robert Sternberg (2004) created the Balance Theory of Wisdom. Sternberg defines *wisdom* as the application of intelligence, creativity, and knowledge to the common good by balancing and mediating the values of self, others, and institutional interests over the long and short terms in service of adapting, shaping, and selecting environments. The functional consequences of this definition suggest that wise people have exceptional insight into human development and life matters, look for deeper meaning, tolerate ambiguity, have compassion, are other- and purpose-focused, and recognize the limits of knowledge. Additionally, Sternberg (1998) identifies the following wisdom capacities:

- *Reasoning ability*: Wise leaders possess a logical mind, good critical thinking skills, and the ability to put old information and theories together in new ways. Wise leaders recognize similarities, differences, and reason clearly, making distinctions between ideas and things.

- *Sagacity*: Wise leaders understand people, display concern for others, consider advice, are perpetually learning, know themselves, are fair, listen to all sides of an issue, and admit to making mistakes.

- Wise leaders learn from ideas and the environment and other people's mistakes. They are *perceptive* and attach importance to ideas.

- Wise leaders possess *good judgment*. They are sensible and think before acting or making decisions, take the long view, are clear thinkers, and they think and reflect before speaking.

- Wise leaders use information, age, experience, and lessons learned from the past to inform and influence decision-making and action.

- Wise leaders have *perspicacity*. They can see through things with intuition and offer solutions on the side of truth and justice as they interpret and understand their environment.

Wise reasoning involves a constellation of practices that include developmental awareness and complexity processing. Wise reasoning involves recognition of uncertainty and change, intellectual humility, and seeking and integrating different perspectives (Grossman et. al 2016). Baltes and Smith (1990) propose an everyday definition of *wisdom* as "good judgment about important but uncertain matters in life" (p. 95). Their theoretical definition is "expert knowledge involving good judgment and advice in the domain fundamental pragmatics of life" (p. 95). The functional consequences of this definition suggest that wise people, as a result of their own experiences over time, have exceptional insight into human development and life matters. Birren and Fisher (1990) observe that one can study component processes of wisdom, including the development of wisdom, the traits of a wise person, and products and processes of wisdom. They note wisdom is an emergent property of an individual's inward and external responses to life experiences. A wise person has learned to balance three aspects of behavior: cognition, affect, and volition. A wise person weighs the knowns and unknowns, resists overwhelming emotion while maintaining interest, and carefully chooses when and where to act (Birren & Fisher, 1990).

# PSYCHOLOGICAL DEVELOPMENT AND WISDOM LEADERSHIP

An emerging body of knowledge and research suggests adult cognitive development continues over one's life span. Robert Kegan's (1982) classic work, *The Evolving Self: Problem and Process in Human Development*, proposes adults grow, mature, and evolve through several states and cognitive developmental stages as they grapple with making sense of complex situations and experiences. Kegan (1998) defined at least three stages of adult development: the *socialized mind,* the *self-authoring mind,* and the *self-transforming mind.* People who have evolved to the self-transforming mind are often deemed wise. Other scholars have advanced Kegan's developmental theories and suggest that it is possible to evolve meaning making and leadership practice through intentions, effort, and experience.

For example, Suzanne Cook-Greuter's (2004) research documents a parallel cognitive developmental pattern and stage progression in adults. She describes and defines eight stages of cognitive development. Her research suggests that people evolve from pre-conventional patterns of thinking characterized by impulsivity to self-protection and conforming to conventional thinking patterns that lead to self-awareness and conscientiousness. Some people continue to evolve, through the stages of autonomy and individuality, and enter the domain of post-conventional thinking. In the post-conventional phase, some people evolve to higher orders of awareness, knowing, unity thinking, and wisdom reasoning.

Researchers Joiner and Josephs (2006) argue wise and successful leaders master four types of agility related to self, context, stakeholders, and creativity. The skills of self-awareness, developmental motivation, purpose, situational awareness, stakeholder understanding, power, connected awareness, and reflective judgment support the development of wisdom leadership as people grow, develop, and mature through the cognitive developmental ages of expert, achiever, catalyst, co-creator, and synergist.

David Rooke and William Torbert (2005) document a similar progressive path in which leaders mature over time and develop different action logics. David Rooke co-founded Harthill Consulting (https://www.harthill.co.uk) in 1985. David, with the team at Harthill, developed the Leadership Development Profile (LDP), an instrument used in assessing "constructivist development" in leaders. People develop and progress from being impulsive to opportunistic to diplomatic. As they continue to evolve, they develop expert and achiever action logics. Beyond achiever, people progress and realize their individualist perspective for meaning making and action logics defined at the higher-level stages of development defined at the strategists, alchemists, and ironists stage. In general, later stages of cognitive development support the realization of leadership agility and wisdom capacities.

# WISDOM: THE PRODUCT OF VERTICAL LEADERSHIP DEVELOPMENT

Adult development through time is correlated with greater understanding and insight about the complexities of dealing with people, purpose, process, and competing values. Nic Petrie (2011, 2014) makes the distinctions between horizontal and vertical leadership development. Horizontal leadership development involves the acquisition and use of information (e.g., data analytics), skills (e.g., conflict resolution), and competencies (e.g., strategic planning techniques) essential for performance-based managers and supervisors. In contrast, vertical leadership development helps people acquire more intricate and advanced ways of thinking and perspective taking. Wisdom is a function of vertical leadership development and sense making derived from managing the complexities of lived experiences and the ability to gain multiple perspectives regarding self, others, and greater social contexts.

Petrie (2015) suggest three primary conditions trigger or activate vertical development of leaders: 1) a heat experience, 2) colliding perspectives, and 3) elevated sense making. These same three conditions support the development of wisdom capacities. *Heat experiences* are complex situations encountered by leaders where habitual ways of thinking and sense making do not work and are inadequate. Such disorienting dilemmas stimulate the search for new and better ways to comprehend the situation. *Colliding perspectives* emerge as leaders encounter people with different worldviews and mental models that challenge a leader's perspective. *Elevated sense making* is necessary to help leaders evolve, transcend, and include earlier developmental ways of thinking and reasoning with more developed worldviews to make sense of complex, uncertain, and volatile situations. Frequently, elevated sense making is assisted with the help of a coach, mentor, or peer support group. Think back to the definitions and descriptions and essential capacities of wisdom described earlier in the chapter. Wisdom capacities are formed through vertical leadership challenges, experiences, and practices. Wisdom leadership and vertical leadership development necessitate agility, mindfulness, and inner work as well as identity, reputation, and legacy management (Johns, 2016; Pesut, 2001, 2008, 2015; Pesut & Thompson, 2018).

Petric (2015) explains the "how to" of vertical leadership development in a Center for Creative Leadership White Paper that describes 15 approaches to promote vertical leadership development. He also notes the essential ingredients for vertical leadership development in organizations are a risk-taking culture, cultivation of a systems thinking mindset, attention to deliberative dialogue, organizational learning, peer coaching, polarity management, and skills in framing and reframing situations. Leaders committed to lifelong learning and professional development work through heat experiences and colliding perspectives. They seek out coaches, peers, and mentors to exercise elevated sense-making skills. Leaders who are successful negotiating heat experiences and colliding perspectives with elevated sense-making skills are likely to develop wisdom that they can pass on to next-generation leaders (Linderman et al., 2015). So how might we activate the vertical development and wisdom capacities of people with whom we work? What are some practical methods and tools one can use to develop wisdom capacities? What mentoring strategies support the development of wisdom throughout a career? Is it possible to teach wisdom?

# CREATING WISDOM LEADERSHIP CAPACITIES

There are several resources that promote teaching and learning of wisdom capacities. For example, the University of Chicago operates the Center for Practical Wisdom (https://wisdomcenter.uchicago.edu/about). The mission of the Center is to deepen scientific understanding of wisdom and the role that wisdom plays in decision-making and everyday life choices. The Center connects scientists, scholars, educators, and students internationally who are interested in studying and understanding wisdom. The Center provides guidance and support for learning about wisdom research, instigates wisdom research, and disseminates the findings of the research. The Center works to increase public interest in wisdom, advocates for enhancing personal wisdom, and curates resources to help people and institutions become wiser. The Center is engaged in research to explore and understand how individuals develop wisdom and the conditions and circumstances in which people are most likely to make wise decisions.

The Teaching for Wisdom Project (Sternberg et al., 2007) is another program that fosters the development, teaching, and learning of wisdom capacities. Sternberg and his colleagues have outlined six pedagogical procedures that teachers can use to teach students how to think rather than what to think. The principles include:

1. Encourage students to read classic works and reflect on the wisdom of the sages

2. Engage students in discussion about what they have read and how lessons learned can be applied in their own lives

3. Challenge students to think about their own values and how their values influence their thinking and reasoning

4. Encourage students to consider the role of critical, creative, and practical thinking when confronted with challenges and dilemmas

5. Encourage students to weigh the good and bad outcomes of a course of action with a greater good in mind

6. Role model wise thinking for students as they propose problems, raise questions, and tackle complex dilemmas and situations

Recall the work of Margaret Plews-Ogan and Gene Beyt (2014) who authored the book *Wisdom Leadership: Leading Positive Change in Academic Health Centers.* Dr. Beyt collated several practical tools and suggestions to promote the development of wisdom capacities at the individual, team and group, and organizational level. Table 17.1 outlines what he believes are practical methods and tools to develop wisdom capacities.

For each of the wisdom capacities—meaning, reflection, forgiveness, humility, trust, compassion, relationality, positiveness, and understanding of complexity—he suggests strategies and tactics that are useful for individuals, groups, teams, and organizations. At the individual level, life goals, purpose, and values inform and influence meaning making. Through self-assessment, reflective writing, and mindfulness-based activities, people can develop compassion and humility as well as trust and forgiveness. Leading with humble inquiry supports relationality and discernment of positive intentions. Using a system thinking mindset, people see themselves as part of a system in time and context with attention to complexity processing.

At the group or team level, the activation of group reflection at team meetings supports sharing and insights related to personal stories and lived experiences in context. Group peer support and team mentoring, coupled with active listening and empathy, help create compassion, forgiveness, humility, and trust. Interpersonal coordination and the initiation of family-centered rounds build the capacity for relationality. Adopt the Appreciative Inquiry 4-(D) cycle of improvement:

- **Discovery:** Identify and appreciate what works.

- **Dream:** Imagine what might be.

- **Design:** Develop systems and structures leveraging the best of what was and what might be.

- **Destiny:** Implement or deliver the proposed design.

Use complexity-inspired approaches to change such as Liberating Structures and Appreciative Inquiry to support engagement, interaction, and the development of wisdom capacities (Moody et al., 2007; Pesut, 2018).

**TABLE 17.1** Practical Methods and Tools to Develop Wisdom Capacities

| WISDOM CAPACITIES | TOOLS FOR INDIVIDUALS | TOOLS FOR GROUPS AND TEAMS | TOOLS FOR ORGANIZATIONS |
|---|---|---|---|
| Meaning | Integrate with life goal; Carry the "good question" | Group reflections at team meetings | Patient-centeredness for all organizational initiatives |
| Reflection | Self-assessments, reflective writing, and mindfulness activities | Personal disclosure tools, symbolic objects, family of origin stories | Appreciative interview, inquiry tools and training programs |
| Forgiveness, Humility, Trust | Disruptor program, disclosure, apology | Group peer support, mentoring for team members | Professionalism programs, peer support and education, trusted advisory program |
| Compassion | Awareness, role modeling, "Doing-Seeing-Being" | Activating empathy, advance listening, "the pause" | Compassionate care and empathetic leadership training program |
| Relationality | Relational leadership, "leading with humble inquiry" | Relational coordination, family-centered rounds | Relational co-production, patients as partners |
| Positiveness | Intentional positivity. "Positive Intentions" (diary, identifying, reflecting, using), post-traumatic growth | Inquiry balanced with self-advocacy, positive mood, gossip, talk and the 4-(D) cycle of improvement: Discovery, Dream, Design, Destiny | Programs in appreciative practice (Appreciative Inquiry, check ins, intent, flip/frame, active positive response, gratitude, co-creation) |
| Understanding of Complexity | Adopt view of living systems (self-organizing, adaptable, flexible, emergent, resilient)<br><br>Causation and attribution | Naturally, creative conversation, therapeutic relationships, storytelling, positive deviance approaches | Programs recognizing the "memory of the whole"<br><br>Teams to get work done, "It takes a village" |

At the organization level, vision, purpose, and mission, grounded in core values, support and enhance meaning and contribution. Appreciative Inquiry training and development programs that inspire and educate staff will build capacities for compassionate care and relational co-production in service of health-related missions and visions. Mindfulness and Appreciative Inquiry support the creation of a positive work environment in the context of complexity.

# IMPLICATIONS FOR PRACTICE: A WISDOM LEADERSHIP CASE STUDY

Angela Barron McBride is a living legend of the American Academy of Nursing and has mentored many people during her academic career. She has passed on her advice about the growth and development of nursing leaders in her award-winning book *The Growth and Development of Nurse Leaders* (McBride, 2019). In the second edition of her book, she shares personal and professional insights and stories, coupled with practical advice about how to succeed in a leadership role and how best to mentor others over the stages of a career. She describes the personal qualities required of a good leader, the value of attaining self-knowledge, sustaining career optimism in the face of failure, orchestrating a career, achieving organizational goals, effective communication, the importance of strategic vision, and the journey toward wisdom. Her book is a case study of wisdom leadership in action. She writes about the personal side of leadership, leadership as achieving organizational goals, and the transformational aspects of leadership. She notes the central task of leadership is to "inspire and catalyze others to achieve shared goals and institutional mission in an environment where the context and meanings are evolving, thus the constant need to design new ways of achieving long held values" (McBride, 2019, p. xxii).

At the beginning of this chapter, the quote from Desmond Tutu was intended to set the frame and direction of this work. "One of the greatest gifts we can give to another generation is our experience, our wisdom." Mentoring is a gift to next-generation leaders. McBride is renowned for her documentation of mentoring strategies needed at each of five career stages. The stages, developmental tasks, means, and role of the mentor at each stage are outlined in Table 17.2.

McBride outlines five stages of a career: preparation, independent contributions, development of home setting, development of the field (healthcare), and the gadfly (wise person) period of a career. At each stage, mentors play a significant role in helping a mentee to achieve the developmental tasks associated with each stage of a career. The means by which professionals develop over and through time are consistent with the Balance Theory of Wisdom described earlier in this chapter.

Recall Sternberg's (2004) definition of wisdom as the application of intelligence, creativity, and knowledge to the common good by balancing and mediating the values of self, others, and institutional interests over the long and short terms in service of adapting, shaping, and selecting environments. As one analyzes the developmental task and means for mentoring at each career stage in the McBride model, one can discern how the career stage, means, and mentoring role is a map for the development of wisdom capacities. Learning values, developing critical and clinical inquiry skills, working interdependently, and balancing individual interests and institutional interests (home setting) as one pays attention to present day issues and challenges creates a vision for the future for all strategies and tactics that lead to the development of wisdom. Throughout a career, individuals adapt, shape, and select environments. And when a person reaches that gadfly/wise person period of their career, wisdom influence continues without institutional obligations or constraints. McBride is a case study example of wisdom leadership in action. Information from her biography as Emerita Dean of Indiana University School of Nursing explains her wisdom development journey.

**TABLE 17.2**   Career Stages and Mentoring Needed at Each Stage to Support Wisdom Capacities

| STAGE | DEVELOPMEN-TAL TASK | MEANS | MENTOR ROLE |
|---|---|---|---|
| Preparation | Learning values, knowledge, and clinical inquiry skills essential to a practice profession and healthcare | Analysis and evaluation of personal strengths, values, and contributions<br><br>Formal education, socialization experiences, licensure, certifications, membership in professional organizations<br><br>Strategies for stress management | Model values and practices<br><br>Encourage problem-solving<br><br>Help set short- and long-term goals<br><br>Guide to experiences that build competencies and expand vision<br><br>Welcome to the profession and identity as a fledgling healthcare leader |
| Independent Contributions | Moving from fledgling to competence, while working independently and interdependently with others | Deal with the inevitable gap between ideals learned and realities of work setting<br><br>Ensure that personal practice reflects best practice<br><br>Develop ability to think, synthesize, and critically act<br><br>Build teams<br><br>Develop collegial networks<br><br>Participate in governance<br><br>Mentor less experienced and less educated | Help navigate inner workings of institution and profession<br><br>Open doors of opportunity<br><br>Direct to resources<br><br>Facilitate networking<br><br>Keep focus on meeting professional and institution success benchmarks<br><br>Provide feedback to improve practice, teaching, and research |

| | | | |
|---|---|---|---|
| Development of Home Setting | Build home setting's image, resources, and infrastructure while moving personally and professionally from competence to expertise | Assume responsibility for programs<br><br>Engage in strategic planning<br><br>Head quality improvement efforts<br><br>Develop junior colleagues<br><br>Assume major roles in discipline-specific organizations | Help individual learn to juggle multiple projects and responsibilities<br><br>Provide feedback regarding strategy and tactics<br><br>Suggest possible "next steps"<br><br>Help person make best use of others |
| Development of Field/ Healthcare | Shape future of healthcare and field/specialty by exercising power of authority and creating a vision for the future | Consult in area of expertise<br><br>Serve as advisor to local, regional, national, and/or international efforts and organizations<br><br>Set agenda for the future<br><br>Assume major roles in international organizations | Provide tips on effective board behavior<br><br>Recommend for discipline-specific and interprofessional opportunities<br><br>Sponsor for honors |
| The Gadfly (Wise Person Period) | Continue to shape healthcare and field when no longer constrained by institutional obligations | Coach current generation of leaders<br><br>Take on special projects that require high-level integrative abilities<br><br>Speak and write provocatively to challenge new thinking | Help in envisioning post "retirement" opportunities<br><br>Recommend for special projects |

Dr. McBride was influenced by the women's movement of the 1960s because it shed new light on what constituted women's health. "Gynecology as plumbing" became supplanted by innovative ideas about "GYN-ecology as the interaction between women and their environments." She was influenced by Simone de Beauvoir's classic *The Second Sex* (1971), in which she argued that women were the perpetual "other," with men's behavior assumed to be normative. McBride grew up in a world that regularly described the father as the head of the family and the mother as the heart, and de Beauvoir's critique got her to wondering how children could be expected to integrate the head and heart in their own lives if the adults were not modeling such behavior. That led McBride (1973) to write the first well-regarded book on motherhood considering the women's movement, entitled *The Growth and Development of Mothers*, which was named one of the best books of 1973 by both *The New York Times* and the *American Journal of Nursing*. Her critique of either/or thinking also caused her to have new thoughts about women always having responsibility for maintenance activities while men were expected to be change agents. Those thoughts steered her to champion nursing research when she was the first Associate Dean for Research at IUSON and later the National Advisory Council for both the National Institute of Mental Health and NIH's Office of Women's Health Research. When she became Dean (1991–2003), she put Indiana University School of Nursing on the map nationally by building areas of nursing excellence in web-based and interactive learning, behavioral oncology, quality of life in chronic illness, and healthy families/healthy communities. It was interesting to experience her wisdom leadership capacities as a member of her executive administrative council.

As a Department Chair at Indiana University (1997–2005), the author would participate in administrative and executive committee meetings chaired by McBride. Often there would be complicated and complex issues that the group would encounter. One of McBride's strategies would be to describe the issue and then extend an invitation to those in the meeting to help her think about the issue because her decision was "not fully cooked." She would elicit ideas, suggestions, and opinions from all the people at the meeting, and as each person offered a suggestion, the complexities and elevated sense making of the group became more systematic, comprehensive, inclusive, and meaningful. By the end of the meeting, her invitation for complexity processing resulted in wise decisions and action strategies.

She has held prominent leadership posts, including President of Sigma Theta Tau International and the American Academy of Nursing. She served on the board of Indiana University Health, an 18-network hospital, and chairs its committee on quality and patient safety, and directed the annual leadership conference for the National Hartford Center of Gerontological Nursing Excellence. She has served on advisory boards for the National Institute of Mental Health and the National Institutes of Health's Office of Research on Women's Health, and the Robert Wood Johnson Nurse Faculty Scholars Program. McBride began to discern how nurses could exert leadership in medicine-dominated and male-dominated settings and wound up writing *The Growth and Development of Nurse Leaders* (2011, 2019). McBride has role modeled wisdom leadership throughout her career. As part of that wisdom, she has promoted leadership and nursing and lobbies others to take nurse leaders seriously, including nurses themselves.

# SUMMARY

The purpose of this chapter was to define the nature of wisdom leadership. Adult cognitive development theory provides insights on how wisdom develops over and through time. People grow and mature and often must develop new action logics to make sense of complex and complicated challenges. Wise leaders ask different questions, seek out multiple perspectives, and see and think in systems. Principles and procedures for teaching wisdom were identified. Strategies and techniques for developing wisdom capacities in healthcare organizations were discussed. Stages in a career were identified, and the role of a mentor in helping mentees be successful were illustrated.

As noted in the beginning, leadership is a developmental journey. Over the course of the journey, some leaders develop wisdom. Leaders who do develop wisdom are more likely to embrace and role model the Balance Theory of Wisdom and operate at a post-conventional stage of cognitive development. That is, they use intelligence, creativity, and knowledge in service to a greater good. They are mindful of their own values and the values of others. They think and act with the long- and short-term perspectives in mind. They adapt, shape, and select environments that serve professional and institutional missions and interests. Wisdom is a product of vertical leadership development and knowledge achieved because of mastering "heat experiences," embracing colliding perspectives, and engaging with others in elevated sense-making activities. Mentoring matters on the developmental wisdom journey.

# REFLECTIVE QUESTIONS

1. What did you appreciate about the discussion of wisdom leadership presented in this chapter?

2. How did ideas and material presented influence your thinking and feeling?

3. What if any commitments to action will you make because of reading this chapter?

4. How might you apply the Balance Theory of Wisdom to a leadership issue you are currently trying to influence and manage?

5. What aspects of the Balance Theory of Wisdom definition are you dealing with successfully? What needs more attention?

6. As you reflect on the adult cognitive developmental stages presented in this work, what is your personal assessment of your current stage of development?

7. In your own words, how do you explain the differences between horizontal and vertical leadership development?

8. Read and reflect on Nic Petrie's 2015 article, "The How to of Vertical Leadership Development" (https://s3.amazonaws.com/kajabi-store-fronts-production/sites/1193/themes/1903840/downloads/XwpFxnoQUmeOfyLVdXif_Nick_Petrie_CCL_2015_The_How_of_Vertical_Development_Part_II.pdf )

9.  Which of the 15 approaches Petrie suggests are of interest to you and relevant to your leadership development plans?

10. What are strategies one can use to teach wisdom or develop wisdom capacities with students, peers, and/or colleagues?

# AUTHOR BIOGRAPHY

**Daniel J. Pesut, PhD, RN, FAAN,** Emeritus Professor, University of Minnesota School of Nursing and Emeritus Katherine R. and C. Walton Lillehei Chair of Nursing Leadership at University of Minnesota, is a nurse educator, academic, researcher, consultant, and coach. He served as the Director of the Katharine J. Densford International Center for Nursing Leadership from 2012 until his retirement in 2021. Pesut earned a PhD in Nursing from the University of Michigan, a master's degree in Psychiatric Mental Health Nursing from the University of Texas Health Science Center in San Antonio, Texas, and BS degree in Nursing from Northern Illinois University, DeKalb, Illinois. He is past President (2003–2005) of the Honor Society of Nursing, Sigma Theta Tau International. He is a Fellow in the American Academy of Nursing. He is the recipient of numerous awards including the Honor Society of Nursing, Sigma Theta Tau International Edith Moore Copeland Founder's Award for Creativity. He is an Honorary Member of the Global Academy of Holistic Nursing.

# REFERENCES

Allison-Napolitano, E., & Pesut, D. J. (2015). *Bounce forward: The extraordinary resilience of nurse leadership.* American Nurses Association.

American Nurses Association. (2021). *Nursing: Scope and standards of practice* (4th ed.). Author.

Baltes, P., & Smith, J. (1990). Towards a psychology of wisdom and its ontogenesis. In R. Sternberg (Ed.), *Wisdom: Its nature, origins, and development* (pp. 87–120). Cambridge University Press.

Berger, J. G. (2020). Changing on the job. Stanford University Press.

Birren, J. E., & Fisher, L. M. (1990) The elements of wisdom: Overview and integration. In R. J. Sternberg (Ed.), *Wisdom: Its nature, origins, and development* (pp. 317–332). Cambridge University Press.

Cook Greuter, S. R. (2004). Making the case for a developmental perspective. *Industrial and Commercial Training, 36*(7), 275–281. doi: 10.1108/00197850410563902

de Beauvoir, S. (1971). *The second sex.* Alfred A Knopf.

Fontaine, D. K., Rushton, C. H., Sharma, M., Plews-Ogan, M., & Beyt, E. (2014). Cultivating compassion and empathy. In M. Plews-Ogan & E. Beyt (Eds.), *Wisdom leadership in academic health care centers: Leading positive change* (pp. 92–110). Radcliffe Publishing.

Grossmann, I., Gerlach, T. M., & Denissen, J. J. (2016). Wise reasoning in the face of everyday life challenges. *Social Psychological and Personality Science, 7*(7), 611–622.

Johns, C. (2016). *Mindful leadership: A guide for the health care professions.* Palgrave Macmillan.

Joiner, W. B., & Josephs, S. A. (2006). *Leadership agility: Five levels of mastery for anticipating and initiating change.* John Wiley & Sons.

Kaipa, P., & Radjou, N. (2013). *From smart to wise: Acting and leading with wisdom.* Jossey-Bass.

Kegan, R. (1982). *The evolving self.* Harvard University Press.

Kegan, R. (1998). *In over our heads: The mental demands of modern life.* Harvard University Press.

Kegan, R., & Lahey, L. L. (1984). Adult leadership and adult development: A constructivist view. In B. Kellerman, *Leadership: Multidisciplinary perspectives* (199–230). Pearson.

Linderman, A., Pesut, D., & Disch, J. (2015). Sense making and knowledge transfer: Capturing the knowledge and wisdom of nursing leaders. *Journal of professional Nursing, 31*(4), 290–297.

Matney, S. A., Avant, K., & Staggers, N. (2016). Toward an understanding of wisdom in nursing. *The Online Journal of Issues in Nursing, 21*(1), 9.

Matney, S. A., Brewster, P. J., Sward, K. A., Cloyes, K. G., & Staggers, N. (2011). Philosophical approaches to the nursing informatics data-information-knowledge-wisdom framework. *Advances in Nursing Science, 34*(1), 6–18.

McBride, A. B. (1973). *The growth and development of mothers.* Harper & Row.

McBride, A. B. (2011). *The growth and development of nurse leaders.* Springer Publishing Company.

McBride, A. B. (2014). Leadership and the journey toward wisdom. In M. Plews-Ogan & E. Beyt (Eds.), *Wisdom leadership in academic health care centers: Leading positive change* (pp. 193–210). Radcliffe Publishing.

McBride, A. B. (Ed.). (2019). *The growth and development of nurse leaders.* Springer Publishing Company.

Moody, R. C., Horton-Deutsch, S., & Pesut, D. J. (2007). Appreciative inquiry for leading in complex systems: Supporting the transformation of academic nursing culture. *Journal of Nursing Education, 46*(7), 319–324.

Pesut, D. J. (2001). Healing into the future: Recreating the profession of nursing through inner work. In N. Chaska (Ed.), *The nursing profession: Tomorrow and beyond* (pp. 853–865). Sage Publications, Inc.

Pesut, D. J. (2008). The wisdom of renewal. *American Nurse Today, 3*(7), 34–36.

Pesut, D. J. (2015). Avoiding derailment: Leadership strategies for identity, reputation, and legacy management. In *Leadership & nursing contemporary perspectives* (pp. 251–261). Churchill Livingston, Elsevier.

Pesut, D. J. (2018). Media review: The surprising power of liberating structures. *Interdisciplinary Journal of Partnership Studies, 3*(1).

Pesut, D. J., & Thompson, S. A. (2018). Nursing leadership in academic nursing: The wisdom of development and the development of wisdom. *Journal of Professional Nursing, 34*(2), 122–127.

Peterson, C., & Seligman, M. (2004). *Character strengths and virtues: A handbook and classification.* American Psychological Association/Oxford University Press.

Petrie, N. (2011). *Future trends in leadership development* [White paper]. Center for Creative Leadership. https://leanconstruction.org/media/learning_laboratory/Leadership/Future_Trends_in_Leadership_Development.pdf

Petrie, N. (2014). *Vertical leadership development – part 1: Developing leaders for a complex world* [White paper]. Center for Creative Leadership. https://antoinette555.files.wordpress.com/2015/10/nick-petrie-vertical-leadership-part1.pdf

Petrie, N. (2015). *The how-to of vertical leadership development – part 2: 30 experts, 3 conditions, and 15 approaches.* Center for Creative Leadership. https://www.stageshift.coach/resource_redirect/downloads/sites/1193/themes/1903840/downloads/XwpFxnoQUmeOfyLVdXif_Nick_Petrie_CCL_2015_The_How_of_Vertical_Development_Part_II.pdf

Plews-Ogan, M., & Beyt, G. (Eds.). (2014). *Wisdom leadership in academic health science centers: Leading positive change*. Radcliffe Publishing.

Rooke, D., & Torbert, W. R. (2005). Seven transformations of leadership. *Harvard Business Review, 83*(4), 66–76.

Sternberg, R. J. (1998). A balance theory of wisdom. *Review of General Psychology, 2*(4), 347–365.

Sternberg, R. J. (2003). *Wisdom, intelligence, and creativity synthesized*. Cambridge University Press.

Sternberg, R. J. (2004). Words to the wise about wisdom. *Human Development, 47*(5), 286–289.

Sternberg, R. J., & Jordan, J. (Eds.). (2019). *The Cambridge handbook of wisdom*. Cambridge University Press.

Sternberg, R. J., Reznitskaya, A., & Jarvin, L. (2007). Teaching for wisdom: What matters is not just what students know, but how they use it. *London Review of Education, 5*(2), 143–158.

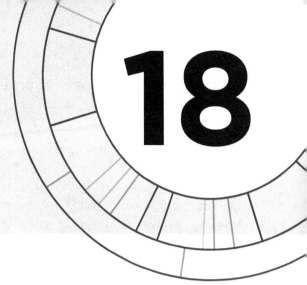

# 18

# DIVERSITY, EQUITY, AND INCLUSION IN EDUCATION AND HEALTH SYSTEMS

Lucy Mkandawire-Valhmu, PhD, RN
Kaboni Whitney Gondwe, PhD, RN
Jennifer J. Doering, PhD, RN
Jeneile Luebke, PhD, RN,
Peggy L. Chinn, PhD, DSc(Hon), RN, FAAN

---

## LEARNING OBJECTIVES

After completing this chapter, you will:

- Understand the concepts of diversity, equity, and inclusion in education

- Explicate ways to address barriers in nursing education for American Indian nurses

- Explain the role of administrators in nursing education to improve how schools promote diversity, equity, and inclusion

- Describe the situations of diversity, equity, and inclusion in healthcare, including immigrant health and nurse migration

---

# OVERVIEW

Healthcare inequity that leads to disparate health outcomes for Black, Indigenous, and all people of color (BIPOC) is a central concern of nursing as a profession. Yet, the nursing profession is a part of the broader society and is also a microcosm of it (Nardi et al., 2020). The discrimination, racism and stereotyping that abounds in the US and Western societies more generally also exists in nursing practice and nursing academia. Virginia Adams, in a brief published in the *American Journal of Nursing*, argues why Black lives matter by speaking to the discrimination she faced as both a practicing nurse as well as a nurse academic (Adams, 2021).

One way in which racism, discrimination, and inequity reflect in nursing is our inability as a profession to recruit and retain BIPOC students and to reflect the diversity of our broader society. Equal opportunity and educational access for BIPOC students are often furthered by the structure of the nursing academic environment. BIPOC students are often expected to adjust and to adapt to a mainstream White academic environment where they may experience racism and discrimination from faculty and peers (Ackermann-Barger & Hummel, 2015). Our pedagogical approach for nursing students must change if we are to create an equitable academic environment conducive to the learning of all our students, especially BIPOC students who have ordinarily experienced exclusion, yet are vital to creating a nursing workforce that is truly reflective of our diverse society.

# DIVERSITY, EQUITY, AND INCLUSION IN EDUCATION

For BIPOC students, their experiences of racism within the broader society are anticipated in a majority White college or school of nursing. Mainstream ideologies and stereotypes rooted in White privilege consciously or unconsciously inform how we interact in nursing academia as faculty with our students or among students as peers. One such ideology is how poor health outcomes that have resulted from a legacy of colonialism and slavery are often stereotypically interpreted as cultural, with BIPOC people blamed for their health experiences. Doran et al. (2019) point out that in relation to the Indigenous people of Australia specifically, "The health inequities of Australian Indigenous people arise from human rights failures, not from Aboriginal culture" (p. 166). This is not the prevailing understanding in mainstream society.

White et al. (2020) identified mistrust of White faculty as a key theme in their qualitative study that focused on African American nurses' reflections of nursing schools. Prevailing stereotypes of African Americans in a broader society informed this mistrust. In this study, African American nurses believed that White faculty were unaware of how their various stereotypical and racist behaviors affected their academic success.

As nurse educators, we need to recognize that our BIPOC students are expected to enter into a predominantly White space every day of their learning in a college or school of nursing. This predominantly White space is seen and accepted as normative and is a space that is easier for White students to navigate than it is for BIPOC students to navigate. In this space, BIPOC students sit next to and around peers and interact with faculty whose life experiences may be vastly different from their own; peers and faculty who may bring to the space harmful, racist ideologies that have implications on learning and success. One attribute for not retaining BIPOC nursing students is thought to be the White academic nursing environment and furthered by a Eurocentric curriculum that does not foster the success of BIPOC students (Bell, 2020; Endo, 2020). The cultural orientation of many ethnic minority populations is collectivistic and values cooperation and the well-being of the collective, whereas European-American culture focuses more on the individual. This fundamental difference has implications for the kind of academic space and climate that is created, which affects the success of BIPOC students as they are required to conform to a different philosophical paradigm shift to succeed.

Given the segregated nature of some of our urban metropolitan environments, White students often enter nursing school without interacting with peers who identify differently in terms of their racial identity or even life experiences. For example, Milwaukee, where a number of the co-authors of this chapter are located, is considered one of the most segregated cities in the United States (Rosenblatt & Cossyleon, 2018). It has extreme inequalities in education, health, and social well-being for approximately one-third of the population who identify as African American. A large cross-sectional study conducted by Kaya et al. (2021) with nursing students showed that students with friends of different cultural backgrounds were more culturally sensitive and less ethnocentric than students without friends of different cultural backgrounds. In a segregated metropolitan area, most mainstream White students have not had meaningful personal interactions with people of different racial identities when they enter nursing school.

As faculty members teaching nursing students in this hyper-segregated metropolitan environment, we have had classroom experiences where students have expressed concerns in the presence of their BIPOC peers about going to clinical settings that are located in the "ghetto." In some instances, BIPOC students have openly verbalized how difficult it is to hear about such concerns from their peers, often racialized and prejudicial concerns. These experiences are consistent with the nursing literature, which shows that even though healthcare students are often motivated to treat ethnic minority groups fairly, they sometimes exhibit unconscious stereotyping in their encounters with ethnic minorities (Barber et al., 2020). Racial prejudice is considered an institutional barrier to the recruitment, retention, and, ultimately, success of BIPOC students. Other barriers that affect the academic climate include faculty attitudes and inadequacies in meeting the needs of BIPOC students.

A limited understanding of the history of colonialism and the resultant life experiences among White students often leads to stereotyping. Learning about diversity and equity is often part of many nursing curricula. Many colleges and schools of nursing have intentionally incorporated health disparities and implicit bias, for example, into the curricula. But the learning of White students often occurs at the expense of BIPOC students who have to witness this learning in whatever form it takes throughout their nursing studies. Suppose stereotypical comments are made during learning. In that case, growth may occur for mainstream students, but this happens while hurting BIPOC students and creating an environment that is not conducive to their own learning. The normative culture of the White academic space needs to be contested because it upholds racism and inequity (Wylie et al., 2021). The unsafe and unequal learning space created makes it challenging for BIPOC students to succeed, especially in college. Resultant social isolation leads BIPOC students, especially in their first year of college, to drop out. Data show that African American male students, for example, need to identify and be part of an academic institution where they will find the support and nurture that would enable them to achieve academic success and to integrate socially (Hilton & Bonner, 2017).

Ethnic minority nurses are key to addressing health disparities among ethnic minority populations in the United States. They have an in-depth understanding of the populations they identify with and their capacity to provide culturally relevant and culturally safe care and help us all understand how to do the same (Bell, 2020; Endo, 2020). Providing underserved populations with culturally knowledgeable professionals is expected to help shift health inequities by tapping into the population's preference for caregivers viewed as more reliable, trustworthy, and accessible (Alsan et al., 2018). Ethnic minority nurses could help bridge the gap in providing culturally safe nursing care, thus improving health outcomes for minority populations. But unequal access to educational opportunities in nursing academia has led to our inability to recruit and retain BIPOC students into the nursing profession. In particular, the nursing profession does not draw or ensure the academic success of African American students (White et al., 2020). The literature emphasizes the important role that nurse educators play in instilling confidence, enhancing personal determination, and motivating and encouraging BIPOC nursing students to succeed and maintain enthusiasm for the profession of nursing.

Our inability to speak up about these racist realities and the institutional racism inherent in nursing academia leads to the silencing of our BIPOC students as nursing faculty have essentially refused to acknowledge their lived experiences (Zanchetta et al., 2021). It is time for all nurse educators to recognize and speak up on the reality of racism and how it affects our ability to recruit BIPOC students and enable them to succeed in nursing academia. Australian authors, Sherwood et al. (2020), identify this, based on the words of Indigenous elders, as returning to the fire and speaking into the silence. Nardi ct al. (2020) argue for the need for change involving anti-racist work in nursing academia that is transformative and sustainable. These authors also say that this is a change that we have to desire and make every effort to attain.

Given the inequitable academic environment that we have described, nursing faculty need to revisit the current way in which we all approach teaching and learning and academic spaces. There is a need for a deliberate development of interventions that would enhance the success of BIPOC students. A key recommendation made by Nardi et al. (2020) is developing critical self-awareness among nurses in leadership positions concerning racism. These authors point out how conversations and dialogue need to occur regarding critical but often uncomfortable topics about power, privilege, and institutional racism. Reflexivity helps us recognize and acknowledge who we are, where we are situated in the hierarchical structures, and our role in moving towards a more equitable society. Another intervention proposed by Garcia et al. (2021) is incorporating listening sessions or creating a safe space where BIPOC students can have their experiences validated and be assured that every effort is being made to remove obstacles for their learning and success.

# NURSING EDUCATION FOR AMERICAN INDIAN NURSES

Underrepresented populations, such as American Indians and Alaska Natives (i.e., Native American or Indigenous—the original inhabitants of North America), suffer disproportionately from health disparities and inequities compared to the general population of the United States (Indian Health Service, 2019). Recognizing and addressing these health disparities is of utmost importance. The Healthy People 2030 Framework highlights the elimination of disparities as a national priority for the next decade (US Department of Health and Human Services [DHHS], 2021). Disparities in education due to opportunity gaps further exacerbate health disparities as few students can successfully graduate with the requirements to enter competitively and make it through nursing school. The ensuing lack of representation has implications for trust between communities and healthcare professionals and the healthcare establishment they are apart from. Ultimately, this affects healthcare access and health outcomes for populations already situated on the margins of society.

Racial/ethnic minorities are historically and currently underrepresented in the nursing profession. According to a 2018 national sample survey of registered nurses conducted by the US DHHS, underrepresented registered nurses (RNs) represent 26.7% of the RN workforce in the US. The majority of the RN workforce in the US is comprised of 73.3% White/Caucasian and only 0.3% American Indian/Alaskan Native. Other underrepresented groups include 7.8% Black/African American; 5.2% Asian; 10.2% Hispanic/Latino; 0.6% Hawaiian Native/Pacific Islander; 1.7% two or more races, and 1% "other." In some states in the US, the lack of diversity among nurses is dire. For example, in Wisconsin, 6% of RNs identify as being from diverse racial/ethnic backgrounds, and only 0.4% of RNs in Wisconsin identify as American Indian/Alaska Native (Zahner et al., 2019). Overall, Wisconsin is similar to most states in the US, with the nursing workforce diversity well below the national benchmark of 25% (Zahner et al., 2019).

The American Association of Colleges of Nursing (2017) stresses that lacking diverse nursing faculties can tremendously impact academic nursing infrastructure and students' success. There are many barriers to completing undergraduate and graduate nursing programs for American Indians and other underrepresented students. For American Indians, geographic distance from family and community or moving from small, close-knit tribal communities to large, unsupportive, and unfamiliar urban environments can contribute to feelings of isolation. There may also be experiences with racism and discrimination within predominantly White institutions (Jochman et al., 2019). *Historical trauma*, also referred to as *historical loss*, refers to unresolved grief that is cumulative and perpetuates through Indigenous generations from the loss of ancestral homelands, language, and culture due to colonization (Tucker et al., 2016).

One strategy for addressing health disparities as recommended by the US DHHS (2015) is thus to increase the diversity of the healthcare workforce. American Indian nurses are a critical component to healthcare delivery for American Indian people throughout the United States. Approximately 60% of nurses working across Indian Health Service (IHS) clinics and hospitals in tribal communities in the US identify as American Indian (Brockie et al., 2021). In some states, such as Wisconsin, only 10% of nurses providing services at tribal health facilities identify as American Indian (Great Lakes Inter-Tribal Council [GLITC], 2011), while almost 100% of patients are American Indian/Alaska Native. The federal government has failed to adequately fund the IHS system, with funding covering only 60% of the healthcare needs of eligible American Indians, further compounding health disparities, poor health outcomes, and premature death (IHS, 2019). In urban areas, the IHS funding disparities are much worse. Overall, approximately 70% of American Indians live in urban areas today due to federal relocation policies, losing access to tribally affiliated healthcare services (Casselman, 2016). American Indians may also be reluctant to seek care from mainstream healthcare facilities due to a lack of trust in non-Native healthcare providers or healthcare facilities where services are often not culturally relevant (Deer, 2015).

# UNDERREPRESENTATION OF AMERICAN INDIAN FACULTY

The lack of diversity among practicing nurses is also reflected in nursing academia. Despite efforts to increase the diversity and amount of doctoral-prepared nurses, there is an especially severe shortage of PhD-prepared nurses, specifically among

PhD-prepared nurses from underrepresented backgrounds (Salerno et al., 2018). Evidence shows that underrepresented PhD-prepared nurses are well-positioned to address health disparities through their research efforts and teaching and mentoring other minority students, and they contribute to nursing curricula that are sensitive to the needs of BIPOC patients and communities. Significant barriers, however, exist for schools of nursing that seek to recruit and retain minority nursing faculty. According to the 2017 National Nursing Workforce Survey, 1.1% of all nurses hold a PhD in nursing. For American Indians, the percentage of PhD prepared nurses is much smaller. To date, there are approximately 35 doctoral-prepared American Indian nurses (including both DNP and PhD degrees) in the US, with even fewer American Indian nurses pursuing roles in academia or research (Brockie et al., 2021).

The ability of academic institutions and programs to retain faculty is a crucial component for success and to remain competitive. Many qualified doctoral-prepared ethnic minorities, including American Indians, have avoided a career in academia, further compounding faculty shortages. Evidence from the literature supports that underrepresented individuals in faculty positions frequently do not remain in academic settings for the long term due to perceived racism or lack of support (Mkandawire-Valhmu et al., 2010). Therefore, higher education institutions must ensure that the commitment to recruiting and retaining a diverse faculty and student body, including Indigenous faculty, is the highest priority.

The recruitment and retention of American Indian nursing students within graduate nursing programs is crucial in advancing nurse leadership opportunities and also dependent upon representation by PhD-prepared American Indian nurses. The presence of ethnic minority and underrepresented nurse faculty within academic institutions ensures the continued support and mentorship needed to bolster student success within their courses and programs and nurture and guide future underrepresented faculty (Davis et al., 2021). Underrepresented students may feel challenged when trying to imagine themselves in professional and leadership roles within nursing without the ability to see and work alongside role models who look like themselves.

It is also imperative that American Indian nurse researchers research American Indian people, led in collaboration with tribal communities to promote health equity and restore trust between academic institutions and tribal nations resulting from oppressive research practices. Additionally, American Indian–led research creates opportunities for American Indian graduate students to be involved in research efforts under the supportive guidance and mentorship of American Indian faculty. American Indian faculty would also have greater opportunities for success in Indigenizing curricula, attaining tenure, and leading successful research and academic careers.

American Indian nurses are uniquely positioned to directly address health disparities while leading change through their presence in academic and leadership roles. In research, the use of Indigenous-specific methodologies and frameworks contributes to developing culturally informed and meaningful approaches to Indigenous-specific health research (Snow et al., 2016). Indigenous-specific methodologies and frameworks in research consider the history of objectification through oppressive practices in the provision of healthcare to American Indians and how it affects trust and even healthcare access within tribal communities (Snow et al., 2016). American Indian researchers who focus their research on their people continue to infuse their unique respective beliefs, knowledge, values, and customs into the research process, leading to culturally sensitive and meaningful studies that benefit their communities while advancing science that addresses health disparities and improves health outcomes.

# PROMOTING DIVERSITY IN NURSING EDUCATION ADMINISTRATION

It is no secret that some of the Whitest spaces in nursing are in the ranks of the administrative leadership of nursing schools. The call for the diversification of nursing to better reflect the population nurses serve has been acknowledged for decades within many nursing schools' statements of mission, vision, and values (American Academy of Colleges of Nursing [AACN], 2017). Yet, meaningful progress collectively as a profession has been unacceptably slow and often performative (Bell, 2020). The racial reckoning and pandemic of 2020 have resulted in renewed awareness and efforts to engage in racial justice and equity action in nursing schools. Given, however, that so many nursing school administrators are White (along with primarily cisgender and female-identified), some are asking: What is the role of administrative leaders in nursing higher education to engage in racial justice and equity work? How does one begin? How are those efforts received if work has started, and how does one know whether efforts are effective? If you have a position in academic leadership in nursing, have you asked these questions of yourself and your role in your institution? If you teach in a nursing school, have you asked this question of your administrative leadership?

It is time to seriously question and dismantle White dominance in higher education and nursing (Bell, 2020). Nursing's (White) response to its complicity in racial injustice and upholding systemic oppression has ranged from hesitancy to outright resistance (Weitzel et al., 2020). Nursing is often acutely uncomfortable with turning the gaze on itself and questioning bias or racism within heralded disciplinary narratives of care, caring, advocacy, and social justice, to name a few. Similarly, discourse about the nursing metaparadigm of Person, Health, Environment, and Nursing often lacks identity and difference considerations (Chinn & Kraemer, 2018; Smith & Liehr, 2018) and is not commonly discussed using intersectional or decolonizing lenses (Weitzel et al., 2020). Whether intentional or not, discourses about such important disciplinary concepts are often whitewashed or identify as colorblind or neutral, all of which are harmful to students, nurses, and the people we care for who identify as BIPOC. The structures of nursing curricula, higher education in general, and healthcare are also structurally racist and harmful (Barber et al., 2020). The American Academy of Colleges of Nursing (AACN) recently came out with the *Re-Envisioned Essentials*, which will shape the discipline's future for years to come (AACN, 2021). The revised *Essentials* take an important step forward by indicating that nursing needs to shift academic cultures within higher education to:

...address structural racism, systemic inequity, and discrimination
in how nurses are prepared. Nurse educators are called to critically
evaluate policies, processes, curricula, and structures for homogeneity,
classism, color-blindness, and non-inclusive environments. (AACN,
2021, p. 39)

Toolkits are being developed to provide nursing schools with advice about how
to modify curricula across all levels of preparation, from professional entry to
practice to advanced practice. Still, administrators would be remiss to approach
this effort using common approaches for revising curricula. Achieving the afore-
mentioned "culture shift" will require that wholly new approaches are developed
and resources are deployed.

Nurse educators and administrators in higher education vary widely in their
awareness, experience, and fluency to engage in conversations about race, racism,
Whiteness, colonialism, identity, and difference. There currently is no "floor"
or standard that every nurse, nurse educator, or education administrator has as
a baseline competency to engage in conversations about these topics, much less
teach such concepts, develop anti-racist pedagogies, or develop equity science
methods and frameworks (Hogan et al., 2018). This may seem daunting, yet our
challenge is also our opportunity, and nursing has risen to the challenge countless
times in our profession's past. While racial concerns may be especially important
within the United States, beyond the US, nurse educators, administers, and leaders
across the world also have the opportunity and obligation to advance questions
about privilege and representation within schools, healthcare systems, and countries, however this presents within regional and local contexts. Contesting privilege in all its forms is a hallmark of ethical practice and stands in service of the
ultimate goal of nursing care that meets patients' unique needs and contexts.

In nursing, we have weathered many challenges and acknowledge the difficult
and foundational work that our nursing forbearers carried out against incredible
gender and professional biases to achieve outcomes such as entry into the academy, the establishment of nursing doctoral education, recognition as a separate

knowledge discipline, and autonomy and control in the regulation of practice in states (Chinn & Kramer, 2018). Understanding the contributions of the many nurse scholars, scientists, and administrators who led and shaped that work through a historical lens suggests they did the best they could at the time, given the constraints they faced. That being said, it does not diminish our profession to critique that work for what is often missing: the voices of BIPOC individuals.

# DIVERSITY, EQUITY, AND INCLUSION IN HEALTHCARE

Diversity, equity, and inclusion (DEI) in healthcare is a concept central to the work of nurses and nurse leaders. It not only affects our work in nursing education, as we have described above, but it also has implications for nursing practice. As nurses and nurse leaders, we are champions for change and can help frame the DEI discussions in the various settings in which we work (Johnson-Mallard et al., 2019). The 2020 Year of the Nurse showed us the essential role we all play in shaping healthcare and supporting one another in delivering healthcare services. We can use our influence to shape the context in which care is provided and to create safe spaces for our patients, fellow nurses, and the communities we serve. The COVID-19 pandemic has taught everyone that it is time to seriously reflect on the issues surrounding global health, race, and justice. This pandemic was global, and a spike in one part of the world served to threaten the safety and well-being of every human being on this planet. People around the world endured the COVID-19 pandemic in the midst of global protests over the death of George Floyd (Hill et al., 2020) and ongoing concerns about police brutality towards Black Americans and other forms of structural racism. Activists also raised the alarm about discrimination against Asian Americans and Pacific Islanders (AAPI; Abrams, 2021) and heightened awareness of the history of racism and discrimination towards the AAPI community.

# HISTORY OF STRUCTURAL RACISM

The history of structural racism in North America began with the maltreatment of Indigenous and Black people who experienced genocide, enslavement, and a system that was deliberately created to uphold racial oppression (Bailey et al., 2021). These systems of racial oppression have impacted BIPOC people for centuries and have ultimately affected their health outcomes. At the writing of this manuscript, hundreds of unmarked graves of children have been discovered, with the first discovery in British Columbia at the Kamloops Indian Residential School and the more recent discovery made by the Cowessess Nation at the Marieval Indian Residential School in Saskatchewan. These discoveries are a stark reminder of how racial oppression manifests, the unspeakable harm and suffering it causes, and its reverberating effects on future generations impacted. The healthcare system is a microcosm of the broader society where racism and discrimination have been created and continue to exist. Racism and discrimination continue to greatly impact the US healthcare system, leading to disparate and poorer health outcomes for BIPOC people (National Academies of Sciences Engineering and Medicine, 2017). Understanding institutional racism begins with recognizing the systemic effects of laws, policies, and practices privileging some racial groups while marginalizing or oppressing other racial groups (Williams et al., 2019). Epidemiological evidence has shown that segregated individuals are at risk of adverse health outcomes over the life course (Williams et al., 2019). When caring for marginalized populations, it is important to understand the factors that exacerbate poor health outcomes and advocate for the well-being of populations most adversely affected by racism and discrimination.

# RACISM IN HEALTHCARE

Medical racism and discrimination are increasingly key topics of discussion. Racism and discrimination within a healthcare setting may occur at the hands of healthcare providers towards their patients, resulting in mistrust in patient-provider relationships (Jaiswal, 2019). BIPOC patients have expressed experiencing discrimination compared to White patients. Medical mistrust, perceived racism in healthcare, and everyday experiences of racism have been shown to delay seeking preventative services among African American men (Powell et al., 2019). Black women are also most likely to die in childbirth. The literature indicates Black women feel unheard when they seek healthcare services (Adebayo et al, 2019; Owens & Fett, 2019). This too has implications for maternal morbidity and mortality. Centering the voices of BIPOC patients is important in addressing adverse health outcomes, improving trust with our patients, and encouraging all to seek care early.

## IMMIGRANT HEALTH

We cannot talk of discrimination without also mentioning the challenges migrant populations face in our healthcare system. Globally, the population of migrants, refugees, and displaced persons (MRDPs) is growing rapidly. In the US, the immigrant population has quadrupled over the past 60 years, with immigrants now accounting for 14% of the population, an equivalent of 45 million people (Budiman et al., 2020). MRDPs constitute one of the most vulnerable populations globally (International Council of Nurses, 2018) that continue to face barriers in accessing healthcare in the receiving or host nations. As migrants settle in a new place, they experience stress associated with assimilating into a different society, which exposes them to the emotional strain of adapting, in addition to experiences of discrimination—a state known as *acculturative stress* (Liem et al., 2021). The health status of migrants thus declines with continued or longer presence in the US (Martin et al., 2018). The sociopolitical environment and the demands of acculturation provoke a great deal of stress that adversely affects the health outcomes of migrant populations (Olukotun et al., 2019). Accessing healthcare is also challenging among migrant patients because they face barriers such as legal obstacles, discrimination, fear, communication problems, financial issues, stigma, and lack of health resources.

# NURSE MIGRATION AND DISCRIMINATION AGAINST BIPOC NURSES

Another form of discrimination is that faced by BIPOC and migrant nurses. Black nurses in the US have faced discrimination within the profession. In 1908, when the American Nurses Association (ANA) refused to admit Black nurses, Martha Minerva Franklin and her colleagues founded the National Association of Colored Graduate Nurses (NACGN; Caldwell & Pirani, 2020). With time, the ANA began to admit Black nurses and today, the President of the ANA, Dr. Ernest Grant, is a Black man. Still, there is work to be done to ensure that there is equitable representation across all sectors of nursing leadership that is reflective of the diversity of the communities that nurses serve Apart from the need for representation at leadership levels, most healthcare institutions allow patients the right to refuse care from a nurse or healthcare professional who are non-White on the basis of racial or ethnic identity. This further marginalizes non-White nurses, including Black nurses, reinforcing their invisibility in the healthcare system (Caldwell & Pirani, 2020). The lack of support towards BIPOC nurses may affect retention as well as representation in the healthcare system, a representation that is crucial to addressing health inequities.

The migration of nurses across the globe has been a topic of ethical concern as nurses migrate from their home countries in search of better opportunities. The nursing brain drain has largely impacted poorer states such as those in sub-Saharan Africa and Southeast Asia, causing unequal distribution of nurses and midwives globally and affecting the quality of care in the most affected countries (Peters et al., 2020). Marginalization, inequality, and discrimination have been reported by migrant nurses (Pung & Goh, 2017; Semu, 2020). Discrimination occurs through interactions with employers as well as patients (Semu, 2020). African nurses have also expressed that they are rarely assigned to the units of their preference and that male nurses are favored over female nurses and rise faster in the hierarchy (Semu, 2020). African nurses also face structural racism where they have experienced deskilling, being assigned to tasks requiring less education and experience, excessive monitoring, pay inequity, and linguistic barriers (Semu, 2020). African nurses expressed that they felt they were being judged based on their racial identity and accent. They lacked support from managers, peers, and supervisors, who often gave them unfair treatment and stereotyped them. They are also rejected by patients (Semu, 2020). This phenomenon, defined as *racist bullying*, refers to the racially motivated discrimination experiences faced by migrant nurses of color.

# IMPLICATIONS FOR PRACTICE

To promote a safe environment for diverse faculty and students, White or non-diverse faculty should refrain from the notion of "colorblindness." This includes beliefs such as "treating everyone the same" or avoiding challenging dialogue around issues of history, race, oppression, and politics. Rather, it is time for nursing faculty to demonstrate the significance of learning how to navigate charged or sensitive topics openly and safely with students in the classroom and with faculty and colleagues (Crooks et al., 2021) and actively resist tokenizing American Indian or other faculty of color.

American Indian and other BIPOC faculty and scholars frequently experience tokenism when they have been requested to represent their entire racial/ethnic group because few or no other faculty do so. This has resulted in larger workloads or higher expectations and standards for achieving tenure and promotion (Blackstock, 2020; Carr, 2020; Crooks et al., 2021). Tokenism among faculty of color results in increased stress and mental health concerns contributing to health disparities (Crooks et al., 2021; Matthews et al., 2020).

Lastly, there is a critical need to consider how the process of promotion and tenure may perpetuate oppression through the hindrance of promotion for BIPOC faculty through institutional bias. For example, many BIPOC scholars prioritize addressing health disparities within their research, which may not be considered a priority topic in the eyes of grant funders or administration. Additionally, many underrepresented scholars carry out their research using community-engaged and community-based research methods. These research methods require tremendous amounts of time and energy for scholars, particularly in the early planning stages of a study, but are necessary to address health disparities and inequities and establish trust within communities (Ginther et al., 2016; Hoppe et al., 2019). This time and energy are often not recognized by administration or tenure committees, which may inhibit promotion. One way to recognize this critically important work is to appreciate and count the time spent in the early stages of community-engaged scholarship as productivity within their tenure or promotion case (Crooks et al., 2021).

# MOVING FORWARD: RECKONING WITH RACISM IN PRACTICE

The path ahead to overcome the challenges in inequities and disparities is clear—nurses as individuals and nursing as a profession must find ways to address racism to achieve justice and equity. The first step, which this chapter presents, is to acknowledge the problem, name it, and examine the challenges we face in achieving the ends we seek. From this acknowledgment, we can form effective ways to address the challenges and create new realities. Since the public murder of George Floyd in the United States, people worldwide have faced the realities of racism in ways never before possible, and many programs and projects have been developed to increase awareness of implicit bias, to increase diversity, and to work toward inclusion and equity.

However, the fact remains that addressing the reality of racism is a long road, and it is incumbent on each person, each organization, to join in this journey. The currently ongoing project "Overdue Reckoning on Racism in Nursing" (NurseManifest, 2021) is an example of an innovative approach that can be used as a model to open, honest discussion and change the typical ways individuals from different racial identities in nursing interact with one another. This project centers the voices of nurses of color, bringing together (virtually) nurses of color and White nurses to examine the realities of racism in nursing and envision ways of overcoming the challenges with a bold anti-racist stance. The "Principles of Reckoning" that guide the discussions are as follows (NurseManifest, 2021):

- We claim the courage to join together through the experience of building our anti-racist capacity nursing.

- We cherish the contributions and honor the voices of Black, Indigenous, Latinx, and other nurses of color and yield the floor to their voices throughout our time together.

- We recognize that we cannot move forward without a deep understanding of Black, Indigenous, Latinx, and other nurses of color experiences with racism.

- The insights and recommendations of Black, Indigenous, Latinx, and other nurses of color are vital to ground our thinking and guide our actions.

- We pledge to listen deeply and with respect to any and all expressions of anger, rage, despair, and grief arising from racism.

- We commit to healing those harmed by racism.

- We commit to challenging, resisting, and ending the voices and actions that sustain White privilege.

- We seek to nurture authentic anti-racist awareness.

- We will inspire and nurture action as we boldly claim an anti-racist identity for nursing.

Each time a group gathers on Zoom for an "overdue" discussion, these principles are read out loud, taking a few moments to center our intentions and commitments for our discussion together. During the initial series of discussions in the fall of 2020, about 40 nurses of color and 50 White nurses logged in each week.

The ongoing sessions range from a couple of dozen to about 50 participants. Being in a group that consisted of a substantial proportion of nurses of color was a new experience for everyone. For nurses of color, having the time and space to speak in a context where people are listening was a novel and a welcomed opportunity. The host of the discussions, Lucinda Canty, set the stage for each discussion by speaking to her own perspective as a Black nurse. For White nurses, remaining silent to listen to the voices of nurses of color was not only a new experience; it brought up a new awareness of White privilege—how the dominance of the "White voice" sustains racism.

# SUMMARY

This one simple premise—that the authentic voices of people of color are vital—is key to moving forward. It is time to acknowledge the reality of harm caused by racism. Without this recognition and action to take a firm anti-racist stance, efforts to achieve diversity, inclusion, and equity are futile. All of the challenges we address in this chapter are significant issues and challenges that must be faced to build a better future. In doing so, nurses of all racial identities can come together, recognizing that how we conduct ourselves in our day-to-day interactions provides a microcosm of the large social dynamics that sustain the inequities of racism. By taking bold steps to change our own interactions and relationships with one another, we build a foundation to make meaningful changes in the systems around us.

# REFLECTIVE QUESTIONS

1.  Name one way in which racism, discrimination, and inequity reflect in nursing.

2.  How can we create safe academic environments to recruit and retain American Indian and other students of color into graduate nursing programs to diversify nursing leadership roles?

3.  How can we remove barriers to promotion and tenure for American Indian and other scholars of color within academic institutions?

4.  How do you foster an inclusive environment for patients and nurses of color in your unit, and what is the role of nurse leaders in promoting inclusive environments?

5.  What is the role of administrative leaders in nursing higher education to engage in racial justice and equity work?

---

# NARRATIVE

Rachel is a registered nurse on a medical-surgical unit who identifies as African American/Black. At the beginning of her shift, Rachel is assigned to a 55-year-old White male patient. During her routine assessments, the patient asked if Rachel could call the nurse to the room. Rachel explained that she is a registered nurse and she has the necessary training to manage the patient's condition. The patient became upset and asked Rachel to call her supervisor.

You are a nurse manager on a medical-surgical unit. When you enter the room, the patient says: "I do not want a Black nurse. I would prefer to have a White nurse. I am not sure if she knows what she is doing." Rachel also verbalizes to you that she feels discriminated against based on her race despite her competence to carry out the assigned tasks.

How do you respond to this encounter?

---

# AUTHOR BIOGRAPHIES

**Lucy Mkandawire-Valhmu, PhD, RN,** Associate Professor, University of Wisconsin-Milwaukee College of Nursing, is a feminist scholar with her research and scholarship centering on advancing nursing science to improve health outcomes for marginalized women and mentoring future nurse scientists in doing the same. Her theoretical and analytic contributions provide the tools and insight necessary for the nursing profession to play a leading role in addressing the most important health needs of women globally. Mkandawire-Valhmu's scholarship helps raise awareness among nurses of how race, class, and gender intersect to impact women's health, and centers the work of nurses in addressing the disparate health outcomes experienced by marginalized populations of women. She is the author of *Cultural Safety, Healthcare, and Vulnerable Populations: A Critical Theoretical Perspective*, a text that seeks to assist students of the healthcare professions in developing awareness about the realities of health disparities, the historical context that informs them, and their role in becoming culturally safe providers.

**Kaboni Whitney Gondwe, PhD, RN,** Assistant Professor, University of Wisconsin-Milwaukee College of Nursing, Medical College of Wisconsin, Clinical Translational Science Institute, is originally from Malawi, and in this book, she draws her experience as both an immigrant and Black nurse in the US. Her research focuses on maternal and child health, and she is currently working on maternal mental health and mother-infant relationship in Malawi and the United States. Gondwe has published literature on effects of mental health, migration, and racial discrimination for women. She holds a PhD in Nursing and Doctoral Certificate in Global Health from Duke University, Master of Science in Nursing Administration and Nursing Education from Ohio University, and Certificate in Midwifery and BSN from the University of Malawi, Kamuzu College of Nursing.

**Jennifer J. Doering, PhD, RN,** Associate Dean for Academic Affairs and Associate Professor, University of Wisconsin-Milwaukee College of Nursing, earned an undergraduate degree in nursing from the University of Minnesota in Minneapolis and master's and doctoral degrees from the University of Arizona in Tucson. Doering's research centers around promoting health equity in vulnerable mothers and infants by studying how to improve sleep, fatigue, and mental health in pregnant and parenting women. Doering also studies infant sleep environments, including reasons where and how parents decide to place their babies to sleep, unintentional bedsharing, and infant sleep products. Doering teaches the philosophy of science and knowledge development to budding nurse scholars.

**Jeneile Luebke PhD, RN,** is a post-doctoral nurse research fellow at University of Wisconsin-Madison. She in an enrolled member of Bad River Band of Lake Superior Chippewa Indians. She received her BS and MS in Nursing from UW-Madison and her PhD in Nursing at UW-Milwaukee. Her doctoral dissertation, completed in spring 2020, centers Indigenous women's voices by better understanding the individual lived experiences with intimate partner violence in urban areas of Wisconsin through in-depth qualitative interviews. This data highlights the need for survivor-led and culturally safe interventions to provide survivors with the care and resources that they need and deserve. Her areas of research and expertise include gender-based violence against Indigenous women and community-engaged research using an Indigenous feminist framework. Her current work focuses on the impacts of gender-based violence on the health and well-being of Indigenous women and addressing barriers to accessing culturally specific care.

**Peggy L. Chinn, PhD, DSc(Hon), RN, FAAN,** Editor, Professor Emerita, University of Connecticut, is founding Editor of *Advances in Nursing Science* and author of books and journal articles on nursing theory, feminism and nursing, the art of nursing, and nursing education. She is co-founder of NurseManifest (www.nursemanifest.com), a project to inspire and empower grassroots action by nurses to shape the future of nursing and healthcare based on nursing's fundamental values. She is a co-founder and web manager of Nursology.net, established in September 2018. Her theory of cooperative group process, *Peace and Power*, is grounded in critical feminist theory and nursing philosophy, and is recognized as a model for critical research methods, teaching and learning, community-based practice, and political activism. Her most recent activist project, "Overdue Reckoning on Racism in Nursing" (https://nursemanifest.com/2020/08/17/overdue-reckoning-on-racism-in-nursing), brings together nurses of color and White nurses to engage in "truth and reconciliation" as a path to meaningful systemic change.

# REFERENCES

Abrams, Z. (2021). The mental health impact of anti-Asian racism. *American Psychological Association, 52*(5), 22. https://www.apa.org/monitor/2021/07/impact-anti-asian-racism

Ackerman-Barger, K., & Hummel, F. (2015). Critical race theory as a lens for exploring inclusion and equity in nursing education. *The Journal of Theory Construction & Testing, 19*(2), 39–46.

Adams, V. W. (2021). Because black lives did not matter. *The American Journal of Nursing, 121*(1), 11. https://doi.org/10.1097/01.NAJ.0000731608.19853.14

Adebayo, C. T., Walker, K., Hawkins, M., Olukotun, O., Shaw, L., Sahlstein Parcell, E., Dressel, A., Luft, H., Mkandawire-Valhmu, L. (2019). Race and Blackness: A thematic review of communication challenges confronting the Black community within the United States health care system. *Journal of Transcultural Nursing*. Advance online publication. https://doi.org/10.1177/1043659619889111

Alsan, M., Garrick, O., & Graziani, G. (2019). Does diversity matter for health? Experimental evidence from Oakland. *The American Economic Review, 109*(12), 4071–4111. https://doi.org/10.1257/aer.20181446

American Association of Colleges of Nursing. (2017, Mar 20). *AACN position statement: Diversity, inclusion, and equity in academic nursing.* https://www.aacnnursing.org/Portals/42/News/Position-Statements/Diversity-Inclusion.pdf

American Association of Colleges of Nursing. (2021). *Re-Envisioned essentials: A roadmap for the transformation of nursing education.* https://www.aacnnursing.org/Portals/42/AcademicNursing/pdf/Essentials-2021.pdf

Bailey, Z. D., Feldman, J. M., & Bassett, M. T. (2021). How structural racism works - Racist policies as a root cause of U.S. Racial Health Inequities. *The New England Journal of Medicine, 384*(8), 768–773. https://doi.org/10.1056/NEJMms2025396

Barber, P. H., Hayes, T. B., Johnson, T. L., Marquez-Magana, L., & 10, 2. s. (2020). Systemic racism in higher education. *Science (American Association for the Advancement of Science), 369*(6510), 1440–1441. https://doi.org/10.1126/science.abd7140

Bell, B. (2020). White dominance in nursing education: A target for anti-racist efforts. *Nursing Inquiry, 28,* e12379. https://doi.org/10.1111/nin.12379

Blackstock, U. (2020). *Why Black doctors like me are leaving faculty positions in academic medical centers.* STAT.

Brockie, T., Clark, T. C., Best, O., Power, T., Bourque Bearskin, L., Kurtz, Lowe, J., Wilson, D. (2021). Indigenous social exclusion to inclusion: Case studies on Indigenous nursing leadership in four high income countries. *Journal of Clinical Nursing,* (March), 1–15. https://doi.org/10.1111/jocn.15801

Budiman, A., Tamir, C., Mora, L., & Noe-Bustamante, L. (2020, August 20, 2020). *Facts on US immigrants, 2018: Statistical portrait of the foreign-born population in the United States.* Pew Research Center. https://www.pewresearch.org/hispanic/2020/08/20/facts-on-u-s-immigrants-previous-years-data/

Caldwell, M., & Pirani, F. (2020, July 2). Racism against Black nurses is a historic problem that still exists today. *The Atlanta Journal-Consitution.* https://www.ajc.com/news/racism-against-black-nurses-historic-problem-that-still-exists-today/WXgpiNAYHIuIKnoZRdZnxI/

Carr, R. M. (2020). Reflections of a Black woman physician scientist. *The Journal of Clinical Investigation, 130*(11), https://doi.org/10.1172/JCI144525

Casselman, A. L. (2016). *Injustice in Indian country: Jurisdiction, American law, and sexual violence against native women.* Peter Lang.

Chinn, P. L., & Kramer, M. A. (2018). *Knowledge development in nursing* (10th ed.). Mosby.

Crooks, N., Smith, A., & Lofton, S. (2021). Building bridges and capacity for Black, Indigenous, and scholars of color in the era of COVID-19 and Black Lives Matter. *Nursing Outlook, 0,* 1–11. https://doi.org/10.1016/j.outlook.2021.03.022

Davis, T. M., Jones, M. K., Settles, I. H., & Russell, P. G. (2021). Barriers to the successful mentoring of faculty of color. *Journal of Career Development.* https://doi.org/10.1177/08948453211013375

Deer, S. (2015). *The beginning and end of rape: Confronting sexual violence in native America.* University of Minnesota Press.

Doran, F., Wrigley, B., & Lewis, S. (2019). Exploring cultural safety with nurse academics. Research findings suggest time to "step up". *Contemporary Nurse, 55*(2-3), 156–170.

Endo, R. (2020). Retaining and supporting faculty who are Black, Indigenous, and people of color: The promise of a multi-leveled mentoring-partnership model. *Multicultural Perspectives (Mahwah, N.J.), 22*(4), 169-177. https://doi.org/10.1080/15210960.2020.1845178

Garcia, J.T., VandeVusse, L., Simandl, G., Johnson, A.N., Mu, Q, & Dahlman, J. (2021). Diverse students collaborating to address social determinants of health using listening sessions. *Journal of Professional Nursing, 37,* 451–458. https://doi.org/10.1016/j.profnurs.2020.04.011

Ginther, D. K., Kahn, S., & Schaffer, W. T. (2016). Gender, race/ethnicity, and National Institutes of Health R01research awards: Is there evidence of a double bind for women of color? *Academic Medicine: Journal of the Association of American Medical Colleges, 91*(8), 1098. https://doi.org/10.1097/ACM.0000000000001278

Great Lakes Inter-Tribal Council, Inc. (2011). "Increasing cultural congruence among nurses in Wisconsin," Grant Proposal to the Wisconsin Partnership Program. University of Wisconsin-Madison; Awarded 2012.

Hill, E., Tiefenthäler, A., Triebert, C., Jordan, D., Willis, H., & Stein, R. (2020, May 31). How George Floyd was killed in police custody. *The New York Times.* https://www.nytimes.com/2020/05/31/us/george-floyd-investigation.html

Hilton, A. A., & Bonner, F. A. (2017). Today's urban black male: The importance of finding the right college to realize maximum success. *Urban Education (Beverly Hills, Calif.), 52*(9), 1051–1056. https://doi.org/10.1177/0042085915620652

Hogan, V., Rowley, D. L., White, S. B., Faustin, Y. (2018). *Maternal Child Health Journal 22*(2), 147–153. https://doi.org/10.1007/s10995-017-2411-z

Hoppe, T. A., Litovitz, A., Willis, K. A., Meseroll, R. A., Perkins, M. J., Hutchins, B. I., Davis, A. F., Lauer, M. S., Valantine, H. A., & Anderson, J. M. (2019). Topic choice contributes to the lower rate of NIH awards to African-American/Black scientists. *Science Advances, 5*(10), eaaw7238. https://doi.org/10.1126/sciadv.aaw7238

Indian Health Service. (2019) *Fact sheets: Disparities.* https://www.ihs.gov/newsroom/factsheets/disparities/

International Council of Nurses. (2018). *Health of migrants, refugees and displaced persons.* https://www.icn.ch/sites/default/files/inline-files/ICN%20PS%20Health%20of%20migrants%2C%20refugees%20and%20displaced%20persons.pdf

Jaiswal, J. (2019). Whose responsibility is it to dismantle medical mistrust? future directions for researchers and health care providers. *Behavioral Medicine (Washington, D.C.), 45*(2), 188–196. https://doi.org/10.1080/08964289.2019.1630357

Jochman, J. C., Cheadle, J. E., Goosby, B. J., Tomaso, C., Kozikowski, C., & Nelson, T. (2019). Mental health outcomes of discrimination among college students on a predominately white campus: A prospective study. *Socius: Sociological Research for a Dynamic World, 5.* https://doi.org/10.1177/2378023119842728

Johnson-Mallard, V., Jones, R., Coffman, M., Gauda, J., Deming, K., Pacheco, M., & Campbell, J. (2019). The Robert Wood Johnson nurse faculty scholars diversity and inclusion research. *Health Equity, 3*(1), 297–303. https://doi.org/10.1089/heq.2019.0026

Kaya, Y., Arslan, S., Erbas, A., Yasar, B.N., Küçükkelepçe, G.E. (2021). The effect of ethnocentrism and moral sensitivity on intercultural sensitivity in nursing students, descriptive cross-sectional research study. *Nursing Education Today, 100*, 1–7. https://doi.org/10.1016/j.nedt.2021.104867

Liem, A., Renzaho, A. M. N., Hannam, K., Lam, A. I. F., & Hall, B. J. (2021). Acculturative stress and coping among migrant workers: A global mixed-methods systematic review. *Applied Psychology: Health and Well-Being, 13*(3) 491–517. https://doi.org/10.1111/aphw.12271

Martin, C. L., Haan, M. N., Fernandez-Rhodes, L., Lee, A., & Aiello, A. E. (2018). Association Between Immigration History and Inflammatory Marker Profiles Among Older Adult Mexican Americans. *Biodemography and Social Biology, 64*(1), 30–42. https://doi.org/10.1080/19485565.2018.1449631

Matthews, A. K., Allen-Meares, P., Watson, K., Crooks, N., Smith, A., Hart, A., Estrella, M. L., & Kim, S. (2020). The use of strategies from the social sciences to inform pipeline development programs for underrepresented minority faculty and students in the health sciences. *Journal of Clinical and Translational Science, 5*(1), 1–21. https://doi.org/10.1017/cts.2020.566

Mkandawire-Valhmu, L., Kako, P. M., & Stevens, P. E. (2010). Mentoring women faculty of color in nursing academia: Creating an environment that supports scholarly growth and retention. *Nursing Outlook, 58*(3), 135–141. https://doi.org/10.1016/j.outlook.2010.02.001

Nardi, D., Waite, R., Nowak, M., Hatcher, B., Hines-Martin, V., & Stacciarini, J.R. (2020). Achieving health equity through eradicating structural racism in the United States: A call to action for nursing leadership. *Journal of Nursing Scholarship, 52*(6), 696–704. https://doi.org/10.1111/jnu.12602

National Academies of Sciences, Engineering, and Medicine (2017). *Communities in action: Pathways to health equity*. The National Academies Press. https://doi.org/10.17226/24624

NurseManifest. (2021). Overdue reckoning on racism in nursing. https://nursemanifest.com/ongoing-overdue-reckoning-on-racism-in-nursing/

Olukotun, O., Gondwe, K., & Mkandawire-Valhmu, L. (2019). The Mental health implications of living in the shadows: The lived experience and coping strategies of undocumented African migrant women. *Behavioural Sciences, 9*(12). https://doi.org/10.3390/bs9120127

Owens, D. C., & Fett, S. M. (2019). Black maternal and infant health: Historical legacies of slavery. *American Journal of Public Health (1971), 109*(10), 1342–1345. https://doi.org/10.2105/AJPH.2019.305243

Peters, A., Palomo, R., & Pittet, D. (2020). The great nursing brain drain and its effects on patient safety. *Antimicrob Resist Infect Control, 9*(1), 57. https://doi.org/10.1186/s13756-020-00719-4

Powell, W., Richmond, J., Mohottige, D., Yen, I., Joslyn, A., & Corbie-Smith, G. (2019). Medical mistrust, racism, and delays in preventive health screening among African-American men. *Behavioral Medicine (Washington, D.C.), 45*(2), 102–117. https://doi.org/10.1080/08964289.2019.1585327

Pung, L., & Goh, Y. (2017). Challenges faced by international nurses when migrating: An integrative literature review. *International Nursing Review, 64*(1), 146–165. https://doi.org/10.1111/inr.12306

Rosenblatt, P., & Cossyleon, J. E. (2018). Pushing the boundaries: Searching for housing in the most segregated metropolis in America: Pushing the boundaries. *City & Community, 17*(1), 87–108. https://doi.org/10.1111/cico.12288

Salerno, J. P., Gonzalez-Guarda, R., & Hooshmand, M. (2018). Increasing the pipeline and diversity of doctorally prepared nurses: description and preliminary evaluation of a health disparities summer research program. *Public Health Nursing, 34*(5), 493–499. https://doi.org/10.1111/phn.12341

Semu, L. L. (2020). The Intersectionality of Race and Trajectories of African Women into the Nursing Career in the United States. *Behavioral Sciences, 10*(4). https://doi.org/10.3390/bs10040069

Sherwood, J., West, R., & Geia, L. (2020). "Taking our blindfolds off": Acknowledging the vision of First Nations peoples for nursing and midwifery. *Australian Journal of Advanced Nursing, 38*(1), 1–5. https://doi.org/10.37464/2020.381.413

Smith, M. J., & Liehr, P. R. (2018). *Middle range theory for nursing* (4th ed). Springer.

Snow, K. C., Hays, D. G., Caliwagan, G., Ford, D. J., Mariotti, D., Mwendwa, J. M., & Scott, W. E. (2016). Guiding principles for indigenous research practices. *Action Research (London, England), 14*(4), 357–375. https://doi.org/10.1177/1476750315622542

Tucker, R. P., Wingate, L. R. & O'Keefe, V. M. (2016). Historical loss thinking and symptoms of depression are influenced by ethnic experience in American Indian college students. *Cultural Diversity and Ethnic Minority Psychology, 22*(3), 350–358.

US Department of Health and Human Services. (2013). *HHS action plan to reduce racial and ethnic disparities. A nation free of health and health care disparities.* http://minorityhealth.hhs.gov/npa/files/Plans/HHS/HHS_Plan_complete.pdf

US Department of Health and Human Services. (2021). *Healthy People 2030 framework.* https://health.gov/healthypeople/about/healthy-people-2030-framework

Weitzel, J., Luebke, J., Wesp, L., Graf, M. D. C., Ruiz, A., Dressel, A., & Mkandawire-Valhmu, L. (2020). *ANS: Advances in Nursing Science 43*(2), 102–113. doi: 10.1097/ANS.0000000000000290

White, B. J., Mentag, N. M., & Kaunda, B. R. (2020). African American nurses describe experiences of mistrust and trust while in nursing school. *Nursing Education Perspectives, 41*(3), 157–162. https://doi.org/10.1097/01.NEP.0000000000000606

Williams, D. R., Lawrence, J. A., & Davis, B. A. (2019). Racism and health: Evidence and needed research. *Annual Review of Public Health, 40*(1), 105–125. https://doi.org/10.1146/annurev-publhealth-040218-043750

Wylie, L., McConkey, S., Corrado, A. M. (2021). It's a journey not a check box: Indigenous cultural safety from training to transformation. *International Journal of Indigenous Health, 16*(1), 314–332. https://doi.org/10.32799/ijih.v16i1.33240

Zahner, S., Pinekenstein, B., Kowalkowski, J., Henriques, J., & Brzozowski, S. (2019). *Wisconsin 2018 RN workforce survey.* Wisconsin Center for Nursing, Inc.

Zanchetta, M. S., Cognet, M., Rahman, R., Byam, A., Carlier, P., Foubert, C., Lagersie, Z., & Espindola, R. F. (2021). Blindness, deafness, silence and invisibility that shields racism in nursing education-practice in multicultural hubs of immigration. *Journal of Professional Nursing, 37*, 467–476. https://doi.org/10.1016/j.profnurs.2020.06.012

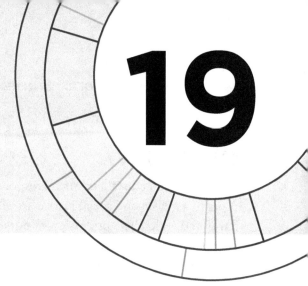

# 19

# TRANSFORMING HEALTH POLICY

AnnMarie Lee Walton, PhD, MPH, RN, OCN, CHES, FAAN
Chandra L. Speight, PhD, RN, NP-C, CNE
Ernest J. Grant, PhD, RN, FAAN
Ena M. Williams, MBA/MSM, RN, CENP
Dennis A. Taylor, DNP, PhD, ACNP-BC, NEA-BC, FCCM

## LEARNING OBJECTIVES

After completing this chapter, you should be able to understand:

- Policy formulation

- Nurses' power individually and collectively in shaping policy

- The roles and responsibilities of the nurse in shaping policy

# OVERVIEW

Nurses have an ethical and social responsibility to advocate for their patients. The roots of activism and social justice are embedded in professional practice standards and ethics. The profession of nursing is a social contract with society and demands professional responsibility. Across settings, nurses spend the most time with patients and thus understand the barriers to access, financial resources, and time that patients face. There is so much that nurses can do to impact and shape policy.

This chapter introduces the history of nurse advocates in policy change and transformation. It then explains the policymaking process, emphasizing how nurses can access each stage—agenda setting, policy formulation, decision-making, policy implementation, and policy evaluation. It discusses nurses' roles, responsibilities, and power individually and collectively in shaping policy. It also considers the power that nurses can yield by contributing to evidence and/or emphasizing healthcare as a human right. It reviews historical efforts by nurse advocates in the US as an exemplar of the impact of nurses on policy. Priorities set forth by the ANA are enumerated, along with clear calls to action for nurses at the local, national, and international levels.

# HISTORY OF U.S. NURSE POLICY ADVOCATES

Nurses have a rich history and record of accomplishment in achieving advances in healthcare. Professional nursing organizations began to form between 1893 and 1912. Their interests first revolved around the issues confronting the profession but later expanded to include social and political reforms affecting society. Organizations first organized around the highly political issue of state registration. Until 1903, when the first state nurse registration acts were passed, anyone could use the title "nurse." Although the early registration acts varied in their protection of the public from inadequately prepared nurses, they signified the political efforts of organized nursing. Since nursing leaders did not yet have the right to vote, support for this legislation was gained through letter-writing campaigns, personal visits to the legislatures, professional journals, and support of the public press.

There are many examples of nurses who have initiated social reform and healthcare advocacy. The history of the modern nursing movement in the US, which began in 1873, is the story of a group of women who responded to the changing role of women in society. They advocated a new profession for women and better healthcare for the public. In forging the nursing profession in this modern period, nurses had to enter the political arena to gain legitimate authority over their education and practice.

The American Nurses Association (ANA) and the National League for Nursing exerted their political expertise to overcome inferior nursing practices. They formed the National Organization for Public Health Nursing (NOPHN) in 1912. This organization's members joined with other civic-minded citizens to improve the health of those living in the US. While nursing organizations were forming, the campaign for women's voting rights, or *suffrage*, was underway. For nurses, suffrage meant gaining a political voice in laws regulating practice, education, and health. Professional nursing organizations provided the medium for nurses to share common experiences and thus find a collective voice. Once these organizations established themselves as viable associations, nurses expanded their horizons to include broader women's issues, including suffrage, in their political agenda.

The following are just a few examples of how nursing has impacted social issues:

- The 1935 Social Security Act: Nurses were asked to review the Act prior to implementation. They also testified before Congress as to the impact this legislation would have on patients and the elderly.

- The 1946 Mental Health Act: Mental health nurses were involved as content experts and contributed to the language of the Act.

- The 1964 Civil Rights Act: Black nurses were interviewed and gave numerous examples of discrimination and racism.

- The 1965 Medicare Act: Nurses were asked to testify before Congress as to the impact of poor healthcare on the elderly in the United States.

- The 1990 Americans with Disabilities Act: Several nurses were involved in legal cases that formed the backbone of the Act.

- The 2010 Affordable Care Act: Nurses provided significant input to the details of this piece of legislation.

Professional nursing organizations have also advocated for and achieved policy reform that protects members of the profession. Some examples include:

- The Federal Needlestick Safety and Prevention Act (2000)

- Mandated Nurse to Patient Staffing Ratios (California 2003)

- Elimination of Mandatory Overtime (2008)

- Increased Scope of Practice and Full Practice Authority for Advanced Practice Nurses (CARES Act 2020)

Below explains the policymaking process, emphasizing how nurses can access each stage: agenda setting, policy formulation, decision-making, policy implementation, and policy evaluation.

# THE POLICYMAKING PROCESS

Governments across the globe enact policies that affect registered nurses and impact their work environments, scope of practice, and overall ability to provide patient care. Though factors including regime type and electoral system shape the specifics of a nation's policymaking process, policymaking can be understood using a five-phase model: agenda setting, policy formulation, decision-making, policy implementation, and policy evaluation (Janda et al., 2017). A general description of the policymaking process follows. However, readers should note that policymaking processes are not necessarily linear, phases do not always happen in sequence, and phases are often not discrete.

## AGENDA SETTING

*Agenda setting* occurs when a problem or issue comes to the attention of policymakers. Many theories have been proposed to understand the agenda-setting process. Kingdon's (2010) multiple streams theory describes the policymaking arena as three streams: problems or issues flow in one stream, solutions or policies flow in a second stream, and political conditions flow in a third stream. When the streams flow independently, the political arena is stagnant, and few policy solutions are considered. When forces cause the streams to merge, a window of opportunity is created, which pushes issues on the political agenda and initiates the policymaking process. Such forces include natural disasters, social crises like the opioid epidemic, technological advances, scientific discoveries, and the emergence of new diseases. Individual politicians, political parties, interest groups, trade unions, bureaucrats, and other political actors also work to bring the streams together to create agenda-setting opportunities for issues important to them.

Punctuated equilibrium theory (Baumgartner & Jones, 2009) provides another model to describe agenda setting. The model recognizes that policymaking processes are often characterized by long periods of stagnation around a particular problem when few policy solutions are debated or enacted. This stagnant period is interrupted by rapid bursts of transformation when issues are catapulted to the policy agenda, and rapid policy formulation commences. For example, the terrorist attack in the US on September 11, 2001, ended a period of policy stagnation surrounding anti-terrorism legislation and sparked the rapid introduction and passage of bills related to terrorism prevention and airline safety. Globally, the COVID-19 pandemic has similarly brought issues concerning infectious disease and pandemic preparedness to policy agendas.

# POLICY FORMULATION

*Policy formulation* follows the agenda-setting process. Once legislators recognize a problem as worthy of a political solution, they begin formulating potential policies. Legislators draft policies themselves or work from drafts submitted to them by executive leaders, bureaucrats, think tanks, interest groups, trade unions, or other political actors (Janda et al., 2017). Questions legislators consider when formulating policy include: what are the specific policy goals and the potential costs and benefits of the proposed policy solution, what stakeholders are involved, and who stands to benefit or lose? These debates are typically informed by a myriad of political actors, including the mass media, interest groups, community organizations, think tanks, influential individuals, executive leaders, bureaucrats, and the legislators' constituents. In tightly closed authoritarian or semi-authoritarian nations, legislators largely rubber-stamp policies generated by the executive branch (Alemán & Navia, 2016). In sum, during the policy formulation period, issues that have reached the political agenda are further framed, and a policy solution is developed.

# DECISION-MAKING

A nation's type of legislative system, type of electoral system, level of centralization, and level of democratization dictate decision-making processes. In the US, a decentralized federal democracy, policy decisions are made at local, state, and national levels with some variation at each level (Janda et al., 2017). At the national level, proposed legislation (a bill) must first be considered separately by the US House and the US Senate. A conference committee must resolve differences between the House and Senate bills, and both the House and the Senate must pass the bill. Legislation can be signed into law or vetoed by the president. A president's veto can be overridden by a two-thirds majority in the House and Senate. In rare instances, presidents can "pocket-veto" legislation by not acting on the legislation if Congress goes out of session within 10 days of the president receiving the bill. In other political contexts, decisions may be made by parliaments or other institutions unique to the nation.

# POLICY IMPLEMENTATION

*Policy implementation* is the process by which a policy is executed. Often, policies passed by legislative bodies are vague, providing implementing agencies significant discretion in exactly how policies will be enacted (Janda et al., 2017). Less commonly, policies are highly prescriptive, allowing little leeway in policy implementation. Policies are usually vague enough that the policy implementation period extends the policy formulation period because the details of implementation shape the policies themselves. In most political systems, bureaucrats formulate the legally binding rules and regulations that accompany any given policy. The extent of bureaucratic discretion in policy implementation and the ability of other political actors to influence the process varies based on the nation's political culture, how democratic the nation is, the relative strength of its bureaucratic institutions, and the nature of the policy itself. Bureaucrats often have opportunities to make policy-related rules to favor their organizations' interests. Stakeholders often have additional opportunities to persuade bureaucrats to implement policies in ways favorable to their interests. Courts are sometimes involved in the implementation process and are responsible for ensuring proposed rules and regulations do not violate groups' or citizens' rights. In the US, at the national level, bureaucrats are required to publish draft rules and regulations and provide time for public input.

# POLICY EVALUATION

*Policy evaluation* constitutes the final stage of the policymaking process and often prompts a cyclical return to the agenda setting and/or policy formulation phase. Legislators, bureaucrats, interest groups, trade unions, think tanks, academics, and political parties evaluate whether a policy is meeting its projected goals, what unintended consequences (good or bad) may have emerged, and how the policy could be modified to be more effective (Janda et al., 2017).

# POLICYMAKING LEVELS

*Policymaking* happens at multiple levels depending on a particular nation's system of government. In the US, a federalized democracy, power is divided among local, state, and national governments. Many policies that affect public health, healthcare professionals, and healthcare delivery are made at the local and state level (Janda et al., 2017). For example, restaurant menu labeling laws in the United States were initially enacted at local and state levels (Block, 2018). New York City, Seattle, and Philadelphia were among the first municipalities to require restaurants to post calorie information in 2008, 2009, and 2010, respectively. Variability between and within local and state laws frustrated restaurant industry representatives, who lobbied the national government to pass restaurant labeling laws that would override state laws. After a lengthy rulemaking process, national calorie labeling regulations were passed in 2010 but only implemented in 2018.

# ACCESSING THE POLICYMAKING PROCESS

Globally, the importance of nurse involvement in all stages of the policymaking process is increasingly recognized. The International Council of Nurses (ICN, 2021a, para. 1), representing over 130 nurse organizations including the American Nurses Association (ANA), the Chinese Nursing Association, the Brazilian Conselho Federal de Enfermagem, the National Association of Nigeria Nurses and Midwives, and the Persatuan Perawat Nasional Indonesia, states "ensuring that nurses have a voice in the development and implementation of health policy is fundamental to ensuring these policies are effective and meet the real needs of patients, families, and communities around the world." Yet, the extent to which nurses can access policymaking processes depends on variables such as how open or democratic the political system is and whether nurses have a formal government role. While this section focuses on the role of domestic nurse actors on individual political systems' policies, nurses increasingly work in transnational groups to affect domestic policies and policies of organizations like the European Union and the Association of Southeast Asian Nations (Kunaviktikul et al., 2019; World Health Organization [WHO], 2020).

Registered nurses in most countries form groups to represent nursing interests in the policymaking process. In highly democratic nations like Canada and Australia, such groups have strong access to the policymaking process. In authoritarian nations like China and Saudi Arabia, access to policymaking is limited to non-existent. Yet, in highly democratic nations, the relative influence of government officials on political outcomes like policy formulation is small, while in more authoritarian regimes, the relative influence of government officials on policy formulation is significant (Risse-Kappen, 1995). Thus, when groups in more authoritarian regimes are able to access government officials, they are more likely to impact policy formulation because the officials accessed have greater policy influence. Relatedly, regimes tending toward authoritarianism are often better equipped to address issues with policy solutions than countries with strong participatory democracy because policy can be formulated quickly (Bunyavejchewin & Sirichuanjun, 2021). Yet, citizens in such regimes are more vulnerable to policies that conceal crises and protect ruling interests at the expense of the public good. Overall, the political context in which registered nurses access policymaking affects their scope of access and potential outcomes.

Another variable affecting access is whether the government has an official nursing officer. New Zealand created the first Government Chief Nursing Officer post in the late 1800s (ICN, 2020). Many nations currently have official government nursing officers. For example, England, Scotland, Ireland, and Wales have a government-appointed Chief Nursing Officer responsible for formulating and implementing a national nursing strategy. Over 70% of WHO member nations report having a government senior nursing officer. Yet, the ICN warns the scope of these officers' power and influence varies significantly. Indeed, in some nations, the senior nursing officer is not required to be a registered nurse or midwife. Despite these caveats, the government chief nursing officer role provides nursing groups an official point of government access, and having such a position is associated with stronger regulation of nurse working conditions and education (WHO, 2020). The US has no such governmental nursing position.

# AGENDA SETTING

Nurses can access the policymaking process by influencing the policy agenda and ensuring legislators and executives address issues of importance to nursing. Nurses work alone and in groups to create or seize windows of opportunity. Depending on the nature of the issue, the relative openness of the political context, and the country's political culture, nurses and nursing groups might work within established government channels to effect change, or engage in grassroots activities or coercive strategies to push issues onto the political agenda. In the US, the ANA builds relationships with elected officials to influence the policy agenda and advocate for the organization's policy priorities (ANA, n.d.-a)

# POLICY FORMULATION

Nurses play a role in policy formulation. In highly democratic nations where citizens and groups have a robust decision-making process, nurse groups typically use established channels to influence policy formulation. Nurse interest groups form relationships with elected officials and urge their members to contact officials to persuade them to consider and pass legislation supporting nursing interests. The American Association of Nurse Practitioners (n.d.), for example, maintains an advocacy center to educate nurse practitioner members on nurse practitioner–related policy. The organization provides policy email updates and prompts nurse practitioners to contact their representatives and express support or opposition to potential policies. Particularly in nations where the government administers healthcare, nursing groups negotiate directly with government leaders. In Canada's decentralized parliamentary democracy, unions representing Quebec's nurses negotiated with provincial legislators for a bill that would decrease staff to patient ratios and increase nurse salaries (La Presse Canadienne, 2021). In more centralized and less democratic nations, nurse groups may need to use coercive measures to influence policy. In Poland, for example, nurses went on strike in opposition to a government-proposed nurse pay increase (*The First News*, 2021). The proposed raise did not meet the demands of nurse labor unions, so they staged a one-day strike and threatened additional strikes if demands for higher wages were not met.

# DECISION-MAKING

The decision-making process is dictated almost solely by the specific rules a nation has adopted about passing policy. Tactics used by nursing interest groups to get issues onto the political agenda and shape the policy formulation process also work in decision-making. For example, in the US, when a nursing organization donates funds to a politician's campaign, the organization often gains influence over how that politician votes on nursing-related issues. Nursing interest groups in the US use grassroots letter writing and phone call campaigns at all levels of government to pressure legislators to vote for or against policies of importance to the nurse organization. In North Carolina, for example, the North Carolina Nurses Association (n.d.) encourages members to contact their legislators about pending legislation, including the North Carolina SAVE Act, which would grant nurse practitioners full-practice authority and remove barriers to healthcare access in the state. Members are encouraged to contact their state legislators and attend legislative sessions to encourage legislators to vote in favor of the SAVE Act.

# POLICY IMPLEMENTATION

Policy implementation provides additional opportunities for nursing groups to influence policy. In the US, bureaucrat-led agencies play a strong role in policy implementation and seek public guidance on policy-related rules and regulations. Each agency must publish potential rules for public comment. The ANA (n.d.-a) monitors multiple federal agencies, including the Agency for Health Research and Quality, the Centers for Medicare and Medicaid Services, the Department of Health and Human Services, the Department of Veteran's Affairs, and the Drug Enforcement Agency. The ANA reviews potential rules for areas of concern and submits comments to the agencies. The ANA describes its role in commenting on draft rules and regulations as one of the most active areas of ANA participation in the policymaking process. For example, the ANA recently submitted comments to the Centers for Medicare and Medicaid Services on several proposed rules related to nursing policy and patient access to care (Hatmaker, 2020). The ANA urged continued reimbursement for audio-only telehealth, noting that millions of older adults do not have access to smartphones or other internet devices needed for video telehealth. The ANA also urged the removal of federal barriers to advanced practice nurse supervision requirements for diagnostic testing.

## POLICY EVALUATION

The policy evaluation process allows nurse groups to follow policy implementation, determine whether and how the policies have met goals, identify unintended consequences, and advocate for policy revision. For example, in New Zealand, the New Zealand Nurses Association found shortcomings when evaluating the government's pandemic response policy, specifically related to the care of those living in aged residential care facilities ("NZNO," 2020). The ANA (n.d.-b) was instrumental in evaluating the impact of federal laws limiting nurse practitioners' ability to prescribe buprenorphine for substance use disorder and encouraging federal lawmakers to extend prescribing privileges to all advanced practice registered nurses in order to increase access to substance use disorder treatment.

## POLICY, POLITICS, AND POWER IN NURSING

Nurses must recognize their collective strength and authority to influence policy and healthcare. Nurses have always used their power to advocate on behalf of their patients; however, to shape the nursing profession, nurses must actively influence policy and lead change. Such leadership requires understanding health policy content, the policymaking process and context, and the stakeholders and their interests. Nurses see, hear, and know how policy affects patients and communities (Salvage & White, 2019), are guided by a moral compass, and simultaneously see the big picture and the consequences on a micro level. While policy and politics determine health and nursing practice, nurses often carry out decisions made by others and sometimes have little say in them, although they are increasingly knowledgeable and skilled. In settings where policy decisions are made—parliaments, governments, and boardrooms—nurse leaders are often neither heard nor heeded. This is starting to change. The global Nursing Now Challenge is working with the International Council of Nurses, and the World Health Organization, to create and strengthen strategic nursing leadership, as modelled by the International Council of Nurses' Global Nursing Leadership Institute. A new window of opportunity is opening, with the bicentennial of Florence Nightingale's birth in 2020. Now is the moment!

Because nurses are the largest global health workforce and often the only healthcare providers available, they are uniquely positioned to interface between the health system, the community, and policymakers. Few nurses, however, recognize the importance of using their collective voice to advocate on behalf of workplace or regulatory policies. There are approximately 23 million nurses and midwives globally, with 4.2 million registered nurses currently practicing in the US, yet only 4% serve on boards of hospitals, municipal organizations, or elected offices (Nurses on Boards Coalition, 2018). Given this small amount of participation at the decision-making table, one can't help but wonder: what would happen if nurses realized the power they have to change health and healthcare?

Academic progression within any nursing program must focus on the student's successful comprehension of the nurse-client relationship, and health policy may not necessarily be included in the curriculum. Strategic and policy leadership development is also missing from most nursing programs (Salvage & White, 2019). Consequently, one of the many factors that may contribute to nurses not being involved in policy (within or outside of the workplace setting) is their lack of knowledge of what policy is and the confidence that they have the skills to influence it (Taft & Nanna, 2008). Educational institutions must prepare nurses as policy influencers and policymakers at all levels of educational preparation (Rasheed et al., 2020).

Political activity is another way for nurses to influence policy. Whether policies will influence their ability to practice or ensure patients have better healthcare outcomes, nurses must understand and participate in the policymaking process. Many nurses think of themselves only as nurses and not as policy influencers. Some nurses may think there is and should be a divide between healthcare and politics and thus overlook the influence policy has on health outcomes. Nurses should ask themselves, "Who do we want making the decisions about workplace safety standards and professional occupational and environmental health nursing practice standards?" By becoming actively involved in the policymaking process, nurses will be able to influence policy development. Brokaw (2016) notes that nurses have a moral and professional obligation to be engaged in legislation that impacts their patients. By doing so, nurses are ultimately advocating on behalf of their patients. Although some nurses may feel that they may not have the time, energy, or knowledge to influence policy, they must be encouraged to think just the opposite.

National nursing organizations offer an important avenue for nurses to participate, lead, and collaborate on issues that affect health and healthcare. This can be accomplished by nurses using their individual and collective power to influence policy and politics at the local and national levels. Nurses are uniquely positioned to contribute to health policy and politics because of their knowledge and experience acquired in the work environment. For example, a nurse may choose to join a professional organization's advocacy efforts that may focus on particular health or healthcare-related topic. The benefit of this collaboration is that the nurse is not working alone but with a group that has a similar objective, a well-thought-out strategy, and available resources such as lobbyists, grassroots programs, and a political action committee (PAC) to achieve the end goal.

Nurses may also choose to influence policy by writing letters either for print/social media or to their elected officials. When doing so, the nurse should be sure to point out the pros or cons of biased reporting of the proposed policy. In such communications, there should also be a concerted effort to address the vulnerable populations targeted by such a policy, as well as the policy's economic, social, and environmental impacts. The nurse may also choose to volunteer to serve as a healthcare consultant or lend testimony to a regulatory legislative committee. Such testimony would allow the nurse to provide the latest evidence-based practice to support their position. They may also use this as an opportunity to regularly communicate with their elected officials.

Nursing institutions and regulatory bodies should prepare and encourage nurses to work as policymakers rather than implementers and advocate for the rightful place of nurses at policymaking forums (Rasheed et al., 2020). Nurses cannot be on the periphery of decision-making tables but must use public policy as a tool for change (Long, 2009). For example, the Nurses on Boards Coalition successfully placed over 10,000 nurses on various boards across the US by 2020 (Nurses on Boards Coalition, 2018). More nurses need to be encouraged to serve on boards and take the lead on policy initiatives. Nurses must let their willingness to serve to be known and take bold steps to nominate themselves.

As the nursing profession continues to be an essential component of health and healthcare, there is a global need for nurses to recognize, develop, and exercise their skills in policy, politics, and power. Partnering with global organizations can help empower nurses to become savvy in the art of global policy initiatives. The recent declaration by the World Health Organization (WHO) of 2020 as the "International Year of the Nurse and Midwife" is a perfect example of a global call for nurses to take on leadership roles, influence policy, and lead change. In *The State of the World's Nursing 2020* report, the WHO (2020) calls for countries to enable nurses to take on leadership roles to improve nursing care, nurse education, and health overall. In addition to calling for an increase in the nursing workforce and safe working environments, the report also called for the establishment of leadership positions, including a government chief nurse (or equivalent), and for support of leadership development among young nurses (WHO, 2020). This recommendation recognizes the critical role nurses play in policy development to improve global health.

The Nursing Now Challenge is a global campaign to improve the world's health by raising the status and profile of nursing. The campaign aims to help develop the next generation of young nurses and midwives as leaders, practitioners, and advocates in health by working with their employers (Bayliss-Pratt et al., 2020). One suggested activity is for employers to initiate a rolling program whereby a number of young nurses and midwives are given seats on the board of an organization to gain knowledge and experience with leadership at the executive decision-making level. A second suggestion is for nurses to be paired with nurse leaders or executives of a national nursing organization. There is also a suggestion for the employer to arrange a special visit or internship with a member of the local or national government or a health official to learn about the policymaking process.

# INDIVIDUAL AND COLLECTIVE POWER IN SHAPING POLICY

Power is one of the most important but least clear concepts in political science. In public policy, the question of power arises in questions like, "Who is in charge? Who are the policymakers? Who is *thought* to be in charge, and who is *actually* in charge?" These questions prompt consideration of institutions, individuals, and informal sources of influence. Power can be used for legitimate or harmful purposes to achieve common goods or marginalize a group's interest (Cairney, 2020). Power can be held by individuals or groups and can emanate from elected or appointed office (formal power) or influence (informal power). Both types of power may control resources, including money and people (Higbea & Cline, 2021). Power can also be both the capacity for action (the potential to act) as well as the exercise of power (visible, measurable; Cairney, 2020).

Power can be obtained from a variety of sources. It is worth exploring where power comes from to understand how to enhance that power and to appreciate that although an individual may exert one or more types of power, when networks, groups, and coalitions work together, they can exert many sources of power (see Chapter 4 for more about power). White (2016) organized and summarized power sources as follows:

- *Legitimate or positional power*: derived from a belief that one has the right to power (e.g., Chief Nursing Officer)

- *Reward power*: based on the ability to compensate another (e.g., the power a nurse manager has to conduct an annual evaluation that impacts pay raises)

- *Expert power*: based on knowledge, skills, abilities versus positional power (e.g., nurses become experts in healthcare and the patient experience)

- *Referent power*: association with a leader who commands a high level of respect (e.g., when a celebrity champions a cause for a nursing organization)

- *Coercive power*: the ability to punish that is based on fear (e.g., threatening to have someone fired for speaking out against an injustice)

- *Information power*: when one individual/group has special information that another person/group wants (e.g., access to data that would promote a cause/agenda)

- *Connection power*: held by those who have close or extensive connections to powerful others (e.g., a nurse knows influential politicians)

- *Persuasion power*: the ability to influence or convince others to agree with a position (e.g., persuading a legislator to sponsor legislation)

- *Empowerment*: comes from any of the above shared among the group (e.g., when nurses together use consensus to guide decision-making)

# POWER IN A GLOBAL HEALTH CONTEXT

Considering power individually, organizationally, and globally illustrates how power asymmetries shape health inequities. In a 2014 report by the *Lancet*, the University of Oslo Commission on Global Governance for Health defined the term *global political determinants of health* as norms, policies, and practices that arise from global interactions among entities (Ottersen et al., 2014). The global perspective embedded in this definition captures the impact of global inequities on social determinants of health. When considering health inequities globally, the concept of healthcare as a human right emerges and can be used to challenge policies that compromise a human's right to healthcare (Gore & Parker, 2019). This is a viewpoint often not expressed in the US context.

Examining health and healthcare on a global scale offers other lessons. In India, practitioners of traditional medicine exercise power within a biomedical system. Local health tradition practitioners have referent power, derived from their associations with doctors, lawyers, and government officials; they also have expert power and are invited to speak about conditions and treatments; they collectively organize, which fosters empowerment; and they have a moral imperative for service (Nambiar & Mishra, 2019). This example illustrates how many sources of power exist for a group that has a relatively subordinate position in the biomedical system and indicates how these power sources can be leveraged to achieve a goal.

Furthermore, a study of interest groups, in this case medical specialists in India and Niger, sought policy solutions focused on curative rather than population health even though they acknowledged the need for improvements at the health system level. These groups of professionals were small and fragmented compared to groups in high-income countries but were able to dominate discussions during stakeholder meetings, resist proposals to extend rural health using non-clinical workers, use their networks to access regulatory committees, and arrange training to promote their policy interests (Dalglish et al., 2019). There is so much applicability of these concepts to the US domestic landscape, and sometimes these global examples seem more objective.

Finally, international non-governmental organizations (INGOs) can engage in political advocacy and national policy processes on behalf of donors. Ipas in Malawi and Marie Stopes International in South Sudan, both funded by the UK Department for International Development, were able to influence reproductive health policies in two countries with highly conservative reproductive health policies. INGOs emphasized their role in providing technical advice on human rights, evidence, and guidelines while also brokering alliances, mobilizing expert power and financial resources, and shaping public policy options (Storeng et al., 2019). The work of donor-funded INGOs is rarely analyzed as political and yet is highly powerful.

Individual nurses and nursing organizations can exercise their power by advocating for human rights, can work within a system that may not value nursing, can organize, and can serve as expert educators and shape policy options.

## THE POWER OF EVIDENCE

Evidence-based policymaking is an approach to policymaking that appeals to nurses who are trained to examine the "evidence" prior to making clinical or practice changes. Yet, it is critical to acknowledge that even evidence-based policymaking is potentially biased, as the makers of such policies determine what constitutes knowledge and who is qualified to create knowledge (Cairney, 2020). It is well documented that patterns of social inequality have been framed as the flaws of the unsuccessful and merits of the successful rather than in systemic rules and norms described by people who do not have power (Ahmed, 2017). Moreover, as cited in Cairney (2020), some voices, especially those of women of color, are missing from intellectual history, and ways of knowing (*epistemologies*) like personal or grounded experiences are viewed as less scientific than knowledge generated predominantly by White male European scientists. When nurses are asked to generate evidence to assist in evidence-based policymaking, it is critical that nurses consider what or who may be missing from the body of evidence and why.

Individual nurses can play a strong role in shaping public policy. Ennen (2001) clearly delineated four areas for action. The first is to learn about candidates and vote. The second is to communicate about issues of importance to nursing: get to know local legislators and communicate opinions to legislators and the community by making calls, writing emails and letters, and penning op-eds. The third is to become active in professional organizations, which facilitate collective power. Professional organizations (at the local, national, international, and specialty levels) often have full-time lobbyists; they offer educational opportunities of their own (e.g., Hill Days, The Nurse In Washington Internship, online sessions, and webinars); they give nurses a chance to practice leadership skills; and they influence the media to represent nursing favorably. The fourth way for nurses to exert power both individually and collectively is direct involvement with policies. Nurses can be part of policy analysis, help design policy, use personal networks and connections to garner support for legislation under consideration, and even seek office at the local and national level.

# POLITICAL CHANGE AGENTS

Sometimes just the mere mention of the word "change" can evoke a variety of thoughts and feelings. Change may be viewed as a threat or disruption to one's comfort zone, whether psychological or physiological. Nurses cannot allow policy to remain status quo. Doing so will jeopardize the future of health and healthcare outcomes. Nurses must embrace and lead change. The recently released *Future of Nursing* report stresses that nurses lead in numerous ways within healthcare, both in healthcare organizations and beyond their organizational boundaries (National Academies of Sciences, Engineering, and Medicine, 2021). Nurses must find their voices and become political change agents, whether in their work environment or for society as a whole. Many nurses may believe that it is not within their ability or power to bring about change. However, through well-planned and executed advocacy, nurses *can* make a difference while still respecting the boundaries of professional ethics and workplace policies (Paton, 2020). The process of becoming political change agents starts with nurses refusing to be bystanders and becoming politically savvy and involved when issues regarding health, healthcare, and society itself arise.

For far too long, nurses have remained on the sidelines. While our physician colleagues may be called upon by the media, legislative, and regulatory agencies to provide their expertise or commentary, nurses are usually not sought out to comment on such topics, even though the results of such measures may directly affect nurses' ability to practice or may reduce access to care for the communities they serve. As change agents, nurses should befriend members of the media and volunteer to serve as spokespeople for various health-related topics. Nurses must realize their role as advocates (change agents) for health and the community. Being political change agents means that nurses must recognize and know how proposed policy and politics may affect the community, the social contributors to health, and subsequently, healthcare itself. Nurses must continue to push for a seat at the table where such policies are being discussed and developed and have their voices heard. Remaining silent or rubber-stamping the agenda without questioning the consequences implies acceptance. The nursing profession, health, and healthcare do not benefit from silence. Nurses should also be willing to lend their expertise to policymakers and assist in crafting the legislative healthcare agendas.

Additionally, part of being political change agents means that nurses must become involved with their fellow nurse colleagues and others within their community. The ICN Code of Ethics for Nurses clearly states, "nurses advocate for equity and social justice in resource allocation, access to health care and other social and economic services" (ICN, 2021b, p. 3). Nurses must recognize the need to attend community town hall events, speak up, and ask tough questions on behalf of those who may not recognize or understand the consequence of such proposed policies. They may host community gatherings to discuss, strategize, and develop a plan of action that will mobilize other nurses and members of the community. This helps to heighten community involvement in the political process. It is crucial that the information discussed is accurate and, where possible, backed by the latest evidence-based research and addresses the pros and cons of the proposed change.

A plan of action should be framed to fit the needs of the community and not a personal political agenda. The nurse should take care to actively listen to the comments and suggestions offered by others in the group. They must remember that communication is central to all advocacy—getting the message out there, gaining the support of stakeholders and the public cannot be achieved without a strong communication plan (Paton, 2020). A crucial component while discussing the plan should also include a list of items about which the group may be willing to find a feasible compromise and items that the group will stand firm against.

Finally, being change agents may mean that nurses may consider running for political office. Whereas the thought of such an endeavor may frighten some, others may feel that it is the only way to transform healthcare and achieve change. According to *Becker's Hospital Review*, three nurses currently serve in the US House of Representatives (Masson, 2020). Making the decision to run for political office is not to be taken lightly. Although nurses enjoy the trust of the public, that may be put aside when the decision to run for public office has been made. Pompilio (2018) suggests that in addition to having the motivation and passion, the nurse must also consider their prior experience as a leader and the financial expenses involved in running for office. Nonetheless, the passion and willingness to become a change agent will help the nurse achieve the end goal of supporting legislation that is equitable and just for all.

# IMPLICATIONS FOR PRACTICE: THE PROFESSIONAL NURSE ROLE—TAKING RESPONSIBILITY TO SHAPE POLICY

Nurses have a rich history and record of accomplishment in achieving advances in healthcare. The ANA Code of Ethics states that nurses should advocate for their profession and states that nurses should act individually and collectively through political actions for social change. Provision 9.4 of the ANA Code of Ethics advocates for social reform. International, national, state, and local professional nursing associations and organizations speak for nurses in reshaping healthcare policy, regulations, and legislation. They address issues such as healthcare accessibility, quality, cost, human rights violations, racism, homelessness, hunger, violence, and the stigma of illness.

The ANA's top federal legislative priorities in 2021 are as follows (ANA, n.d.-c):

1.  Health System Transformation

    ANA believes that any attempt to transform the American healthcare system must follow four principles:

    a)  Ensure universal access to a standard package of essential healthcare services for all citizens and residents.

    b)  Optimize primary, community-based and preventive care while supporting the cost-effective use of innovative, technology-driven, acute, hospital-based services.

    c)  Encourage mechanisms to stimulate cost-effective use of healthcare services while minimizing burdens on those who do not have the means to share in costs.

    d)  Ensure a sufficient supply of a skilled workforce dedicated to providing high-quality healthcare services.

2.  Nursing Workforce Development

    Fully-trained nurses are critical to quality and cost-effectiveness. Title VIII programs bolster nursing education from entry-level preparation through graduate study. These programs have helped build the supply and distribution of qualified nurses needed in all healthcare settings for five decades.

3.  Safe Staffing

    ANA continues to advocate for safe staffing approaches that:

    a)  Assure that RNs are not forced to work without orientation in units in which they are not adequately trained or experienced.

    b)  Establish procedures for receiving and investigating complaints.

    c)  Allow for civil monetary penalties for known violations.

    d)  Include whistleblower protections.

    e)  Require public reporting of staffing information.

    A balanced approach to promote the development and implementation of valid, reliable, unit-by-unit nurse staffing plans ensures robust patient safety and optimal health outcomes.

4.  Home Health

    As a result of advocacy efforts to Capitol Hill in 2020, the Home Health Care Planning Improvement Act (S. 296/H.R. 2150) was included in the Coronavirus Aid, Relief, and Economic Security (CARES) Act. Now, nurse practitioners (NPs) and clinical nurse specialists (CNSs) can order home health services for Medicare beneficiaries without physician approval.

5.  Opioid Epidemic

    ANA supports nurses who are facing this crisis head-on through targeted continuing education, backing federal legislation that allows nurses to practice to the full extent of their training and education, providing recommendations to federal agencies on solutions to address access, the scope of practices, and education barriers, and advocating for policies that allow advanced practice registered nurses to prescribe medication-assisted therapy for substance use disorder.

6.  Workplace Violence

    Nurse abuse can be prevented with collaborative approaches. For years, the ANA has led the charge to end nurse abuse, raising awareness about the threats and pushing for administrative and legislative solutions at the federal level, and supporting nurse advocates at the state level. Yet, few healthcare employers have developed suitable plans to prevent workplace violence, putting nurses and others at risk daily just for doing their job. It is of the utmost importance to report abuse against nurses whenever it is safe to do so. Similarly, the ANA continues to advocate for pathways for whistleblowers to come forward to report such abusive actions.

7.  COVID-19

    Healthcare providers, including registered nurses across all healthcare settings, continue to serve on the front lines as the nation responds to the COVID-19 pandemic. The ANA has served as an independent resource and thought leader to nurses, essential workers, states, the public, media, government agencies, Congress, and the prior and current administrations. As a response to the pandemic evolves, so too has the nature of the ANA's work—addressing priority issues from the availability of Personal Protective Equipment (PPE) and decontamination to vaccine rollout and distribution guidance.

# NURSES' POWER TO MAKE CHANGE

As can be seen by reviewing the above topics and issues, nurses have a significant influence on the healthcare policies that affect their own work environments and on issues that impact the patients they care for every day. It is the professional responsibility of the nurse to be engaged and informed as to what these issues are and what can be done at the local, regional, or national level to positively impact the care we provide to patients.

Barriers to involvement and strategies to address them are presented below:

- **Powerlessness:** There is power in numbers. Nurses can approach policy-makers en masse. Nursing represents the largest segment of the healthcare workforce and has a lot of collective power.

- **Lacking a structure to be heard:** Advocate for shared governance structures that allow for listening to and implementing solutions from a wide variety of nurses.

- **Limited leadership opportunities:** Advocate for and support formal and informal leadership development courses and opportunities. Ensure that mentoring programs for aspiring nurse leaders include advocacy and policy skills.

- **HIPAA—fear of breaching confidentiality:** Share deidentified stories to learn and improve work conditions. Narrative can be persuasive.

- **Differing levels of education:** Despite differences in formal education, nurses are all experts in the patient experience and can improve policies and procedures that impact patient care and outcomes.

- **Lack of education in policy development:** Volunteer for unit-based or system-wide committees, councils, or task forces that focus on policy issues. Do the same within professional organizations. Take advantage of free and low-cost educational opportunities by professional nurse associations.

- **Feeling overwhelmed by complex policies and politics:** Consider the history of the policy and if they require revision in the current context.

- **The need for more mentors and leaders to show the way to effective involvement:** Encourage nurses to mentor other nurses in these skills. Find formal and informal opportunities to practice these skills.

If nurses always keep what is in the patient's best interest as their first priority, they cannot fail. Involvement and engagement in health policy are time-consuming and often frustrating. It frequently takes many attempts at change before substantial progress is made. The nurse must keep in mind that policy impact and change is a slow process and not become frustrated by obstacles and contrarian views. Patience, team-building, and support from coalitions are vitally important to major policy change success.

Policy change is not only at the federal level. Policy change at the local or institutional level may be just as impactful for patients as a piece of federal legislation. The most important thing to take away is that *all* nurses can impact health and healthcare policy. It is our responsibility to advocate for our patients and our profession at every opportunity.

## SUMMARY

Nurses are experts in quality, safety, and the patient experience and must engage in all levels of the policymaking process. There is a role for nurses individually and collectively in agenda setting, policy formulation, decision-making, policy implementation, and policy evaluation. Nurses must be taught how to be involved in policy within and outside the workplace to improve health and healthcare. This may include voting, sharing opinions or perspectives on issues by writing letters or contributing op-eds, serving as a resource for legislators, participating in nursing professional organizations, serving on boards and commissions, and running for elected offices. Nurses should be educated to understand power in its many forms and use it for the collective good. Nurses will benefit from learning nursing history and the central role nurses have played in policies of the past. Nurses should be familiar with both the professional code of ethics and the legislative priorities of their professional organizations. If nurses keep the priorities of their patients and profession in focus, they can have a significant impact on policy at the local, national, and international levels.

# REFLECTIVE QUESTIONS

1. Briefly describe the five-phase model of policymaking.

2. How can nurses play a role in each of the five phases of policymaking?

3. Describe policy-related activities that nurses can engage in at the individual level.

4. How do nursing professional organizations participate in the policymaking process?

5. Name and reflect on sources of power that you possess that you may not have been aware of previously.

## NARRATIVE

Nurse and patient advocacy groups in North Carolina (NC) have been calling for the removal of physician supervisory requirements for NC's advanced practice registered nurses (APRNs). NC law currently requires APRNs to have a collaborative practice agreement with a supervising physician. These physicians do not actually "supervise" or even work in the same location as the APRN, and, in many cases, APRNs must pay physicians to serve as their supervisors. NC is one of only a handful of states that continues to require collaborative practice agreements. APRN education and certification have been standardized nationally since the early 1990s, and research indicates APRNs provide safe, effective care. Research also indicates collaborative practice/ supervisory requirements increase the cost of care, decrease access to care, and provide no value to patient care. Yet NC, a rural state where millions of citizens experience significant disparities in healthcare access, continues to restrict APRN practice.

The NC SAVE Act (NC Senate Bill 249/House Bill 277) would remove physician oversight requirements for NC's APRNs. NC State Representative Gale Adcock, who is a nurse practitioner, introduced the SAVE Act to NC's legislature in the 2021 session. The bill has bipartisan support and is also sponsored by the other three registered nurses who serve in NC's legislature, among other legislative members. Groups supporting the legislation include the North Carolina Nurses Association and their PAC, the AARP North Carolina, Americans for Prosperity North Carolina, the March of Dimes, the National Academy of Medicine, and the Rural Center. Business groups including the Convenient

Care Association and Amazon also endorse the bill, citing its potential for improving access to healthcare. Only physician groups oppose the legislation, citing unsubstantiated patient safety concerns.

The NC legislature has considered bills related to APRN supervision several times over the past few years. In past sessions, bills that would have removed APRN practice restrictions died during the legislative session. Nurse and patient advocacy groups hope the bill will be passed this session. The SAVE Act has the bipartisan support of a record number of NC Representatives and Senators. The COVID-19 crisis highlighted the fragility of the state's healthcare system and the importance of increasing healthcare access, particularly in NC's rural regions. Moreover, as part of efforts to increase healthcare access during the COVID-19 crisis, the NC legislature temporarily lifted several restrictions on APRN practice that would be made permanent if the SAVE Act is passed. Lifting these APRN practice restrictions may have illustrated to lawmakers that the restrictions served no purpose but to restrict healthcare access.

# AUTHOR BIOGRAPHIES

**AnnMarie Lee Walton, PhD, MPH, RN, OCN, CHES, FAAN,** is an Assistant Professor at the Duke University School of Nursing, where she teaches health policy and population health courses. She educates future nurse leaders to value and apply their expertise in quality, safety, and the patient experience; to consider social contributors to health; and to lead improvements in health and healthcare in our country. Walton's program of research centers on understanding and minimizing occupational exposure to carcinogens. She has been a leader in developing, advocating for, and implementing a state law focused on safer hazardous drug handling. As a result of that work, Walton was honored as a Breakthrough Leader in Nursing by the Future of Nursing Campaign for Action in 2014 and as the Oncology Nursing Society Health Policy and Advocacy Award winner in 2016. She became a Fellow in the American Academy of Nursing in 2020.

**Chandra L. Speight, PhD, RN, NP-C, CNE,** is an Assistant Professor in the Department of Advanced Nursing Practice and Education in the College of Nursing at East Carolina University. Her research focuses on the overlapping topics of nurse practitioner clinical competence and capacity, healthcare access, and healthcare policy and has been published in *Nursing Forum* and the *Journal of the American Association of Nurse Practitioners*. She has shared her work at the Southern Nursing Research Society Annual Conference, the North Carolina Nurses Association Nurse Practitioner Spring Symposium, the American Nurses Association Quality Conference, and the National Council of State Boards of Nursing Scientific Symposium. In addition to teaching healthcare policy, translational science, and clinical courses to advanced practice nursing students, Speight practices as a family nurse practitioner in eastern North Carolina and focuses on proving care to individuals experiencing healthcare disparities.

**Ernest J. Grant, PhD, RN, FAAN,** is the 36th President of the American Nurses Association (ANA), the nation's largest nursing organization representing the interests of the nation's 4.3 million registered nurses. He is the first man to be elected to the office of president of the American Nurses Association in its 125 years of existence. A distinguished leader, Grant has more than 30 years of nursing experience and is an internationally recognized burn-care and fire-safety expert. He has worked with politicians and nurse leaders to promote nursing advocacy and global life safety initiatives. Grant was selected by the US Celebration of World Standards Day Planning Committee as the 2021 recipient of the prestigious Ronald H. Brown Standards Leadership Award. He is also the 2021 Recipient of the American Academy of Nursing Civitas Award. This award is given to an individual with a history of exceptional dedication in promoting quality care. Grant also serves as adjunct faculty for the UNC-Chapel Hill School of Nursing, where he works with undergraduate and graduate nursing students in the classroom and clinical settings.

**Ena M. Williams, MBA/MSM, RN, CENP,** Senior Vice President and Chief Nursing Officer, Yale New Haven Hospital, is an experienced executive who has worked in a variety of roles, cultures, and healthcare settings throughout her career. Along with her professional experience, Ena has had much experience both leading and engaging in organizations throughout her career that required her to be engaged in the political arena of nursing. Early in her career, she was very active in her professional organizations and served in several capacities that required her to be engaged in advocacy and policy design and development. Ena continues to be active in her community and professional organizations by serving on several boards, chairing task forces to address nursing, healthcare, and local policies. Ena has published in PEER journals and written several book chapters. She has been recognized multiple times by a wide variety of organizations for her work in nursing, healthcare, and the community.

**Dennis A. Taylor, DNP, PhD, ACNP-BC, NEA-BC, FCCM,** Trauma Acute Care Nurse Practitioner, Wake Forest Baptist Health, has over 45 years' experience as an educator, executive, and healthcare clinician. He was educated at Wake Forest University (BA in Biology and Psychology and MBA in Healthcare Administration), Appalachian State University (MEd. in Adult Education and Curriculum Design), Seton Hall University (BSN in Nursing and MSN as an Acute Care Nurse Practitioner) and the University of South Carolina (DNP). Taylor has completed a post-doctoral PhD Fellowship in Pharmacogenomics from the University of Colorado. He has served as Chief Flight Nurse, Assistant Vice President, and Vice President, System Nursing. He currently holds a faculty position in the Department of Academic Nursing at Wake Forest Baptist Health where he teaches in the Doctor of Nursing Practice program and practices clinically as an Acute Care Nurse Practitioner in the Department of Surgery, Trauma Services. Taylor served as Chair of the North Carolina Commission on Advanced Practice Nursing and President of the North Carolina Nurses Association.

# REFERENCES

Ahmed, S. (2017). *Living a Feminist Life*. Duke University Press. doi:10.2307/j.ctv11g9836

Alemán, E., & Navia, P. (2016). Presidential Power, Legislative Rules, and Lawmaking in Chile. In E. Alemán & G. Tsebelis (Eds.), *Legislative institutions and lawmaking in Latin America* (pp. 99–121). Oxford University Press.

American Association of Nurse Practitioners. (n.d.). *Advocacy Center*. https://www.aanp.org/advocacy/advocacy-center

American Nurses Association. (n.d.-a). *Agencies and regulations*. https://www.nursingworld.org/practice-policy/advocacy/federal/agencies-regulations/

American Nurses Association. (n.d.-b). *Opioid epidemic*. RN Action. https://ana.aristotle.com/SitePages/Opioid.Epidemic.aspx

American Nurses Association (n.d.-c). *Federal Issues*. https://www.nursingworld.org/practice-policy/advocacy/federal/

American Nurses Association. (2020). *Nurses serving in Congress*. https://www.nursingworld.org/practice-policy/advocacy/federal/nurses-serving-in-congress/

Baumgartner, F. R., & Jones, B. D. (2009). *Agendas and Instability in American Politics*. University of Chicago Press.

Bayliss-Pratt, L., Daley, M., & Bhattacharya-Craven, A. (2020). Nursing Now 2020: The Nightingale Challenge. *International Nursing Review, 67*(1). https://doi.org/10.1111/inr.12579

Block, J. P. (2018). The Calorie-Labeling Saga - Federal Preemption and Delayed Implementation of Public Health Law. *The New England Journal of Medicine, 379*(2), 103–105. https://doi.org/10.1056/NEJMp1802953

Brokaw, J. J. (2016, September 22). The nursing profession's potential impact on policy and politics. *American Nurse*. https://www.myamericannurse.com/nursing-professions-potential-impact-policy-politics/

Bunyavejchewin, P., & Sirichuanjun, K. (2021). How regime type and governance quality affect policy responses to COVID-19: A preliminary analysis. *Heliyon, 7*(2). https://doi.org/10.1016/j.heliyon.2021.e06349

Cairney, P. (2020). Power and Public Policy. In Cairney, P. (Ed.), *Understanding Public Policy: Theories and Issues*. (2nd ed.). Red Globe Press.

Dalglish, S. L., Sriram, V., Scott, K., & Rodríguez, D. C. (2019). A framework for medical power in two case studies of health policymaking in India and Niger. *Global Public Health: An International Journal for Research, Policy and Practice, 14*(4), 542–554. https://doi.org/10.1080/17441692.2018.1457705

Ennen, K. A. (2001). Shaping the future of practice through political activity: how nurses can influence health care policy. *AAOHN Journal: Official Journal of the American Association of Occupational Health Nurses, 49*(12), 557–569.

*The First News*. (2021, June 7). Disappointed with gov't proposals, Polish nurses go on strike. *The First News*. https://www.thefirstnews.com/article/disappointed-with-govt-proposals-polish-nurses-go-on-strike-22417

Gore, R., & Parker, R. (2019). Analysing power and politics in health policies and systems. *Global Public Health, 14*(4), 481–488. https://doi.org/10.1080/17441692.2019.1575446

Hatmaker, D. (2020, October 5). *American Nurses Association letter to Centers for Medicare and Medicaid Services regarding payment policies under the physician fee schedule.* https://www.nursingworld.org/~4a8723/globalassets/docs/ana/comment-letters/ana-comments-to-cms-2020-10-05.pdf

Higbea, R. J., & Cline, G. (2021). *Government and Policy for U.S. Health Leaders.* Jones & Bartlett Learning.

International Council of Nurses. (2020). *ICN Briefing: Government Chief Nursing Officer (GCNO) positions.* https://www.icn.ch/system/files/documents/2020-01/ICN%20briefing_GCNO_ENG.pdf

International Council of Nurses. (2021a). *Nursing Policy.* https://www.icn.ch/nursing-policy

International Council of Nurses. (2021b). *The ICN Code of Ethics for Nurses,* Revised 2021. https://www.icn.ch/system/files/documents/2020-10/CoE_Version%20for%20Consultation_October%202020_EN.pdf

Janda, K., Berry, J. M., Goldman, J., Schildkraut, D. J., & Manna, P. (2017). *The challenge of democracy. American government in global politics* (14th ed.). Cengage Learning.

Kingdon, J.W. (2010). *Agendas, Alternatives, and Public Policies* (2nd ed.). Pearson

Kunaviktikul, W., Turale, S., Petrini, M. A., Tungpunkom, P., & Avant, K. C. (2019). Experiences from Southeast Asia on nursing education, practice, mobility and influencing policy. *International Nursing Review, 66*(4), 474–481. https://doi.org/10.1111/inr.12556

La Presse Canadienne. (2021, June 16). Quebec nurses union reaches a deal with the provincial government. *The Montreal Gazette.* https://montrealgazette.com/news/local-news/quebec-nurses-union-reaches-deal-with-provincial-government

Masson, G. (2020, November 6). 18 physicians, nurses and other healthcare providers elected to congress. *Becker's Hospital Review.* https://www.beckershospitalreview.com/hospital-management-administration/16-physicians-nurses-and-other-healthcare-providers-elected-to-congress.html

Nambiar, D., & Mishra, A. (2019). 'A light inside a pot': Sites and sources of power emerging from an ethnography of traditional healing in South India. *Global public health, 14*(4), 515–527. https://doi.org/10.1080/17441692.2018.1564349

National Academies of Sciences, Engineering, and Medicine. (2021). *The Future of Nursing 2020-2030: Charting a Path to Achieve Health Equity.* The National Academic Press. https://doi.org/10.17226/25982

North Carolina Nurses Association. (n.d.). *Advocacy: SAVE Act.* https://ncnurses.org/advocacy/legislative/save-act/

Nurses on Boards Coalition. (2018). *Nurses on Boards Coalition.* https://www.nursesonboardscoalition.org/

NZNO on ARC pandemic plan. (2020). *Kai Tiaki Nursing New Zealand, 26*(10), 39.

Ottersen, O., Dasgupta, J., Blouin, C., Buss, P., Chongsuvivaatwong, V., Frenk, J., & Fukuda-Parr, S. (2014). The Lancet-University of Oslo Commission on global governance for health: The political origins of health inequity: Prospects for change. *The Lancet, 383,* 630-667. https://doi.org/10.1016/S0140-6736(13)62407-1

Paton, F. (2020, September 26). Advocacy Guide for Nurses: How to Be a Change Agent. *Nurseslab.* https://nurseslabs.com/advocacy-guide-nurses-change-agent/

Pompilio, E. (2018, October 23). Nurses in Politics. *Elite Learning.* https://www.elitecme.com/resource-center/nursing/nurses-in-politics

Rasheed, S. P., Younas, A., & Mehdi, F. (2020). Challenges, extent of involvement, and the impact of nurses' involvement in politics and policy making in in last two decades: An integrative review. *Journal of Nursing Scholarship, 52*(4), 446–455. https://doi.org/10.1111/jnu.12567

Risse-Kappen, T. (1995). Bringing transnational relations back in: Introduction. In Risse-Kappen, T. (Ed.). *Bringing transnational relations back in: Non-state actors, domestic structures, and international institutions*. Cambridge.

Salvage, J., & White, J. (2019). Nursing leadership and health policy: Everybody's business. *International Nursing Review, 66*(2), 147–150. https://doi.org/10.1111/inr.12523

Storeng, K. T., Palmer, J., Daire, J., & Kloster, M. O. (2019). Behind the scenes: International NGOs' influence on reproductive health policy in Malawi and South Sudan. *Global Public Health: An International Journal for Research, Policy and Practice, 14*(4), 555–569. https://doi.org/10.1080/174416 92.2018.1446545

Taft, S. H., & Nanna, K. M. (2008). What are the sources of health policy that influence nursing practice? *Policy, Politics & Nursing Practice, 9*(4), 274–287. https://doi.org/10.1177/1527154408319287

White, K. M. (2016). Political Analysis and Strategies. In Mason, D. J., Gardner, D. B., Outlaw, F. H., & O'Gandy, E.T. (Eds.), *Policy & Politics in Nursing and Health Care, 8*, pp. 84–86. Elsevier.

World Health Organization. (2020). *State of the world's nursing 2020: Investing in education, jobs and leadership*. World Health Organization. https://apps.who.int/iris/handle/10665/331677

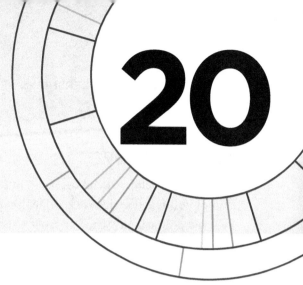

# 20

# LEADERSHIP IN SOCIAL AND POLITICAL DETERMINANTS OF HEALTH

Carey S. Clark, PhD, RN, AHN-BSC RYT, FAAN
Rachel Johnson-Koenke, PhD, LCSW

## LEARNING OBJECTIVES

Upon completion of the chapter, learners will:

- Recognize the relationship between human caring and political advocacy when addressing social and political determinants of health

- Consider the movement to expand social justice to include caring-moral justice in consideration of nurses' caring advocacy role

- Explore the circle of nursing leadership and advocacy efforts through caring, social justice, equity, and inclusion lenses

- Define political and social determinants of health as related to caring and the advocacy role of the nurse

- Identify how power structures influence social policy and shape health for those in power vs. those without power and how this relates to systemic racism in the healthcare arena

# OVERVIEW

This chapter defines social determinants of health in consideration of the definition of political determinants of health and explores the nurse's role in enacting a sacred political advocacy approach. For portions of the population who have been historically disenfranchised and oppressed, mainly Black, Indigenous, and people of color (BIPOC) populations, those who are in power have set up political structures to deny these minoritized groups access to social resources, quality healthcare, and political capital (Braveman, 2014). Historically there have been multiple, often unclear, definitions of terms addressing this systematic inequality (Braveman, 2014). The process of defining the social and political determinants of health (SPDH) has had a significant impact on how large portions of the population access healthcare and their opportunities to improve their quality of life and well-being. In the nursing literature and healthcare workplace, there has been an overemphasis on the individual's responsibility for their health status, instead of understanding and striving to address the larger social context and political structures that impact health (Drevdahl, 2018). This chapter will explore these concepts moving towards understanding the structural and social context of health disparities in nursing leadership roles, political advocacy, and Unitary Caring Science.

This chapter also outlines expanding nursing leadership to consider how the practice of Unitary Caring Science principles can encompass caring, sacred activism, equity, and inclusion. The chapter explores how social justice may move toward including a framework of caring-moral justice for nurses, as caring nurses examine our moral imperative to love our diverse communities and social groups. The chapter defines the social determinants of health, challenges nursing leaders to consider the political determinants of health, and contemplates how people who are in power have made political decisions to disenfranchise certain groups in achieving positive health outcomes and well-being.

As the profession considers nursing leadership, caring-based advocacy is a key aspect of the practice of Unitary Caring Science at a systems level. Therefore, nursing leaders are called to use their power to support healthcare systems in addressing historical and current systematic racism and oppression. There is a social-justice-based ethical imperative for nurses and other healthcare professions to revolutionize our healthcare systems as we infuse the sacred work of caring for the individual, other healthcare professionals, and our communities as the core of the work we do.

# TRADITIONAL SOCIAL AND POLITICAL DETERMINANTS OF HEALTH: DEFINITIONS

The Centers for Disease Control and Prevention (CDC) defined the *social determinants of health* (SDOH) as the conditions in the places where people live, work, learn, and play that impact a range of health risks and outcomes (CDC, 2021). Those circumstances that contribute to health outcomes are shaped by the many resources, including money and power, available at the local, state, and national levels. SDOH are viewed as the reason why we have health inequities within and between countries. These health inequities are viewed as unfair and truly avoidable. When considering the SDOH, the nurse can look at resources expanded toward safe housing, availability of healthy food, available health and human services, and environmental considerations such as toxin exposure. Through this lens, poverty and limited educational opportunities are correlated with poor health outcomes.

*Structural or systemic racism* may be defined as the system of public policies, institutional practices, cultural representations, and other societal norms that work together to create ongoing cycles of racial inequality (The Aspen Institute,

2016). Systemic racism remains under-addressed in the traditional understanding of SDOH. However, systemic/structural racism impacts how resources are provided, and critical race theory may help us uncover the roots of many of our health inequities. A Public Health Critical Race Praxis (Ford & Airhihenbuwa, 2010) can help us examine the contemporary racial phenomenon, identifying and defining the conventions that inadvertently or overtly reinforce social hierarchies. Notably, the model provides tools for striving toward racial equality, ending inequities, and addressing racism in meaningful ways.

# SDOH: HEALTHCARE ACCESS AND QUALITY

This concept refers to people's access to care, focusing on primary care and insurance coverage and *health literacy*, the ability of the population to understand services and their health status (CDC, 2021). Despite efforts like the Affordable Care Act (ACA) to help ensure that all people are covered by health insurance in the United States, at least 10% of the population does not have health insurance, and many people are burdened by the high cost and high deductibles associated with health insurance. Due to associated costs, many people go without coverage and/or forgo preventative visits or chronic care treatments. Factors such as living far from a primary care provider or simply not finding a primary care provider prevent people from accessing care. African Americans' uninsured rate declined with the ACA. However, the uninsured rate for African Americans remains at 9.7%, over twice the rate of Whites, with an uninsured rate of 5.4% (Taylor, 2019).

Healthy People 2030 (United States Department of Health and Human Services [US DHHS], n.d.-a) has a goal set that more people will access care. In 2015, only 8% of adults over age 35 received all of the recommended evidence-based preventative health screenings, and the current goal for 2030 is to increase this number to 10.5%. These minimal increases will have some financial impact but likely will do little to enhance overall health outcomes. No emphasis is placed on discovering the racialization of access to healthcare.

Disparities across the races remain, as African Americans spend far more on healthcare while having less access. While the average American spends 11% of their income on healthcare (premiums, doctors' visits, copays, pharmaceuticals), for African Americans, the number skyrockets to 20% of their income on these expenses (Taylor, 2019). Furthermore, the lack of Medicaid expansion, provider shortages, and health disparities are evident in the southern states' unique patterns and impact African Americans disproportionately (Taylor, 2019).

## SDOH: EDUCATION

People who attain higher levels of education will be much more likely to live longer and experience greater health (CDC, 2021; US DHHS, n.d.-b). Children with disabilities, those from low-income families, and those facing social and racial discrimination are more likely to drop out of high school and not attend college, thereby reducing their chances of attaining well-paying jobs while increasing their risks for depression, heart disease, and diabetes. Healthy People 2030 (US DHHS, n.d.-b) also recognized that the stress of living in poverty could negatively impact the brain development of young people.

Healthy People 2030 (US DHHS, n.d.-b) acknowledged that 84.1 % of students attending public high schools graduated with a four-year diploma, and the goal for 2030 includes increasing this to 90.7%. Taking a longer view, we note that 90% of African Americans ages 25-29 have completed high school, and college graduation rates have grown. While income gains have been made, African Americans still earn less than their White counterparts and are far more likely to live in poverty (Taylor, 2019). An emphasis with Healthy People 2030 is placed on vocational training, alternative schools, social-emotional skills training, and counseling. Other vital objectives in this area include identifying children who have experienced trauma, supporting them in accessing health services and increasing the proportion of trauma-informed early childhood, elementary, and secondary school settings. Neither of these objectives has baseline data available. Notably, there is no emphasis on addressing funding of public education and related racialization issues around education and income in the Healthy People 2030 document.

## SDOH: SOCIAL AND COMMUNITY CONTEXT

With SDOH, an emphasis is placed on people getting the social and community support they need; in particular, having positive relationships may help to reduce the impact of SDOH, particularly those that may be beyond the person's control (e.g., neighborhood climate, discrimination, poverty; CDC, 2021). Healthy People 2030 (US DHHS, n.d.-c) makes it clear that people who have a parent in jail or have been bullied or discriminated against must get community support to improve health and well-being. This objective includes reducing the number of children with an incarcerated parent and increasing the proportion of adolescents who have a trusted adult with whom they can talk. To undertake this effort, we must begin to examine the structural racism that has led to the mass incarceration of BIPOC populations.

Having an incarcerated parent is just one stressor that many African Americans endure. We must consider how higher rates of poverty, low-paying jobs, food insecurity, unsafe housing, and racism contribute to the toxic stress states of African Americans (Taylor, 2019). Until we deal with the myriad structural racism-based complexities that create toxic stress for minorities in America, inequities will abound.

## SDOH: ECONOMIC STABILITY

Another goal for Healthy People 2030 (US DHHS, n.d.-d) is to help people earn steady incomes to meet their healthcare needs. People with disabilities or injuries, along with the 10% of the population who live in poverty, often cannot afford healthy foods, healthcare, or housing. Objectives under this goal include reducing the numbers of people living in poverty and increasing the proportion of children who live with at least one working parent; in 2017, 77% of children ages 17 and under lived with at least one employed parent full time, while the goal for 2030 is to increase these numbers to 85.1% (US DHHS, n.d.-d).

## SDOH: NEIGHBORHOOD AND BUILT ENVIRONMENT

The neighborhood where one lives determines access to quality housing, transportation, and availability of healthy foods, clean water sources, and good air quality. Safety and crime are also considered with the neighborhood environment (CDC, 2021). In the United States, many lower-income people from BIPOC populations live in neighborhoods with high rates of violence, unsafe air or water, and many other safety risk factors. An example of Healthy People 2030 objective in this area is to increase access to safe drinking water from 90.2% in 2018 to 92.1% in 2030 (US DHHS, n.d.-e).

## MOVING TOWARD POLITICAL DETERMINANTS OF HEALTH

Examining health and healthcare outcomes through a political lens requires nurses to analyze how different constellations, processes, institutions, competing interests, and ideologies shape people's health given the political systems and cultures across the governing bodies where they live (Kickbusch, 2015). Health remains a political issue due to uneven distribution, the need for political action to impact health determinants and create change, and health being a human rights and citizenship issue (Kickbusch, 2015). Our governmental policies and politics are the critical drivers that created the current social environment and climate and may be viewed as the upstream issues leading to the downstream realities of SDOH (Dawes, 2020).

Good health of citizens is critical to the state functioning properly, and the health of citizens is directly related to the globalization of trade, commerce, foreign policy, economies, and security. Ideally, public health research would have a greater focus on building a body of evidence around how political actions and ideologies impact healthcare outcomes. Indeed, all healthcare providers likely need more training around the importance of building advocacy and political analysis skills (Kickbusch, 2015). Taylor (2019) states that we must address racism, bias, and structural racism to create health equity and ensure that all providers, personnel, and staff are adequately trained and supported to address and eliminate bias in healthcare systems. We must use social support systems, community providers, and patient-centered approaches as we create and use evidence-based approaches to ending racism in our healthcare systems. Accountability efforts might link these issues to payment to ensure healthcare systems take true strides needed to enact these efforts.

# SOCIAL AND POLITICAL DETERMINANTS OF HEALTH: STIGMA

Viens (2019) reminds us that the social environment makes living a healthy lifestyle challenging to sustain over time; therefore, action and funding to address SDOH become a shared responsibility between the state and the people. There is also a personal moral understanding of SDOH. Far too often, people are told to take self-responsibility to create lifestyle changes versus making actual changes in policy, practices, and funding conducive to changing the SDOH for any given population. One of the issues with looking at social and political determinants of health (SPDH) is that stigma is a concern. Following are some evidence-based examples of how stigma is related to the SPDH.

## OBESITY

While more than one-third of Americans are obese, most people believe that obesity is caused by a person's behavior versus considering social and environmental factors (e.g., fast food availability, lack of safe spaces to exercise, large portions, and food deserts). There is also a lack of public support for creating effective policy addressing the many SPDH factors contributing to obesity in America (Young et al., 2016). Young et al. (2016) found that how messaging around obesity is perceived correlates with political ideology; in theory, greater consideration of SPDH may lead to less stigma around obesity once people understand the complexity of this health condition. Our policymakers may find that focusing on obesity as a complex issue considering the SPDH versus individual blame may lead to the development of policies that support the health of communities.

## UNHEALTHY ENVIRONMENTS AND POLITICAL POWER

A researcher found that in the Mississippi Delta—which is the most impoverished region of the United States, being the unhealthiest region in the most harmful state—systemic racism within the political system impacts the ability to create meaningful change around healthcare systems and healthcare outcomes (Jones, 2019). While the World Health Organization (Reich, 2019) recognizes that healthy choices are impossible to make when one lives in poverty and lacks financial resources, education, safe housing, and the ability to exercise safely, little research has been funded and conducted to explore how public policy, political processes, cultural values, and political power impact healthcare outcomes.

In the Mississippi Delta area, the state's rejection of Medicaid expansion related to the Affordable Care Act has had a devastating impact on the health and well-being of its residents. Additionally, less spending on students residing in the region's educational system and severe gaps in public infrastructure such as those related to transportation all impact the health of its residents (Jones, 2019). Simply calling for action and increased political emphasis reflects a fundamental misunderstanding of the true obstacles nurses face toward achieving health equity for populations while also denying nurses our opportunity to form caring-unitary partnerships with those we serve. To create true change when examining SPDH, the nurse needs to integrate policy, political science, and health research approaches to address the needs of the people (Jones, 2019) while utilizing a guiding framework of Unitary Caring Science.

Dawes (2018) states that now is the time to act. In 25 years, racial and ethnic minorities will be the majority population with a resultant predicted rise in obesity, chronic diseases, and growth of both vulnerable and aging populations. It is not a singular factor that has driven health inequities, but rather a complexity of law and policy's impact on the SPDH, coupled with the system's failure to place a lens on equity. Although the Affordable Care Act is a law that has made strides toward mental health parity and expanded civil healthcare rights (Dawes, 2018), it has not supported a change in how nurses and other professionals work with communities to ensure equitable healthcare and positive outcomes for all.

# EXPANDING THE CIRCLE OF LEADERSHIP THROUGH CARING SOCIAL JUSTICE, SACRED ACTIVISM, EQUITY, DIVERSITY, AND INCLUSION

Our world is seeing the importance of community and the impact of communities' well-being on the health of the community members and the world. The COVID-19 pandemic demonstrated that each of us is connected not only to each other but also to our local and global communities, as the actions of one community had direct impacts on the health of another. This truth of interconnection is at the root of Unitary Caring Science as "an evolved view of science located in a unitary world view of Oneness of all" (Watson, 2020, p. 700).

As minoritized groups have experienced the pandemic differently than groups that hold more political and social capital, the racial disparities in COVID-19 positivity rates and death rates are complex and systematic (Chowkwanyun & Reed, 2020). This is especially apparent in how Black Americans have experienced the pandemic to date (Chowkwanyun & Reed, 2020; Reed, 2020) and in global disparities related to how countries with less financial and scientific resources have experienced the pandemic (Kumar & Chander, 2020).

When we approach health inequity issues through a lens and scope of Unitary Caring Science Theory, nurses have an opportunity to re-envision how care is provided as we change how professional, legal/regulatory, financial/economic, scientific, and ethical systems interact when caring theory is applied (Koithan et al., 2017). When nurses recognize that vulnerable populations and their needs are not "others," rather viewing them as interconnected beings with infinite consciousness and the capacity for evolution, nurses can strive for the best opportunities to be created for all beings. Nurses must recognize that the healthcare system must work for all people across socioeconomic, cultural, and developmental needs (Koithan et al., 2017). Nurses can then undertake comprehensive assessments of populations facing health disparities, determine the populations' unique needs and strengths, and recognize our potential to act as advocates for change in policies and healthcare systems.

This disparity phenomenon is not unique to the COVID-19 pandemic but can be seen globally, across multiple illnesses minoritized groups experience. This difference between groups with power and those excluded from power has historically been labeled *health disparities*. While there are numerous potential explanations for this difference, systematic, structural barriers that exclude some population sectors are a key component to understanding this difference (Churchwell et al., 2020).

This difference in the experience of health and well-being between those in power and those who are not leaves us with a moral imperative to create space for all people to pursue health and well-being as a human right. This call for equity often manifests as social justice. Nursing has a sacred calling to advance humanity's health and well-being, manifesting Unitary Caring Science as sacred activism (Watson, 2020).

*Social justice* is the ethical and moral action towards an ideal that all members of society should have the same basic rights, protection, opportunities, and social benefits (National Association of Social Workers, 2017). This sacred obligation is the manifestation of caring for a community and society (Watson, 2020). Loving a community or society is embracing its strengths and areas to improve. By working to better a community or society in pursuit of a sacred duty to acknowledge the humanity in every member, we raise the higher consciousness of our community and ourselves.

In the context of health, social justice approaches can manifest as action to remove barriers to health and SPDH for all groups, including those historically disadvantaged and those who have had access to more resources and care. This might look like hiring nurse case managers to work with minoritized populations with chronic illness to navigate how to obtain services and care in a healthcare system. The nurse case manager works with each individual to help address SPDH barriers to managing chronic illness. This can also manifest in larger systematic public health interventions. For example, moving chemical plants from a socioeconomically disadvantaged neighborhood to a more industrial area of town would be a system-level intervention to address social justice issues. Nurses can take action as political advocates for change when they identify patterns of SPDH that serve as barriers to populations, maximizing their health potential.

The American Association of Colleges of Nursing (AACN) outlined their position that the values of diversity, inclusion and equity are central to their mission (AACN, 2017). The AACN defines *equity* as "the ability to recognize the differences in the resources or knowledge needed to allow individuals to participate in society fully" (2017, p. 1). This operationalizes healthcare to recognize the differences in access to certain types of healthcare benefits or opportunities to pursue health and well-being. *Equality* provides the same resources to every group without considering the different needs or structural barriers for certain populations that are often historically oppressed. *Equity* acknowledges the different needs and historical experiences of minoritized or BIPOC populations in their pursuit of health and well-being.

*Inclusion* is defined by the AACN (2017, p. 1) as "environmental and organizational cultures in which faculty, students, staff, and administrators thrive." Inclusive healthcare systems and nursing leadership allow for diversity of backgrounds with minoritized groups and welcome and encourage diversity of thought and experience. Complex problems and systems require diverse thoughts and experiences to find real-world solutions. Inclusion does not happen in a vacuum but requires an intentional practice of nursing leadership and education to move the profession and science of nursing into the future. Acknowledging the caring-moral imperative to include diverse voices and perspectives moves humanity towards wholeness and higher consciousness. Nursing has an ethical and caring-moral obligation to pursue healing, caring, and wholeness for all of humanity (Watson, 2020).

AACN (2017, p. 1) defined *diversity* as "a broad range of individual, population, and social characteristics including but not limited to age; sex; race; ethnicity; sexual orientation; gender identity; family structures; geographical locations, national origins, immigrants and refugees; language; physical, function, and learning abilities; religious beliefs; and socioeconomic status." Understanding diversity beyond racial or ethnic categories expands our understanding of inclusion and creates the framework for intentionality needed to build an environment of inclusion. To build a truly inclusive community, nurses must operationalize loving-kindness and interconnection in our organizations, systems, and communities.

The manifestation of loving-kindness of community-level systems calls each of us to take action to pursue the ideals of social justice. We are called to increase equity, inclusion, and diversity across healthcare systems (Watson, 2020). This practice of loving-kindness is not only directed towards our patients and community but lives in the pursuit of loving-kindness towards ourselves and our colleagues. Diversity of thought is not related to the patients we care for but to the education of our practitioners and our leadership. Inclusion and diversity of thought, people, and ideas improve our nursing education, research, and philosophy. It is only in pursuing the inclusion of all voices that we can move healthcare and ourselves towards higher consciousness. It is only through diversity that we can begin to identify and address the foundations of systemic racism that impacts the SPDH.

Understanding the true interconnection of humanity requires a realization and acknowledgment of all of our inclusion in the undivided wholeness. If we are all part of the Oneness of life, we are all ourselves and each other (Watson, 2018). Our sense of division between our existence and the existence of others is only an illusion created by our embodiment and not the truth of our humanity. The French philosopher, Emmanuel Levinas, described how each of us is called to be face-to-face with others, acknowledge their humanity, and see our own humanity in the face of the other (Levinas, 1996). I am you, and you are me. We cannot be separated and divided, for we are the same.

While we are interconnected and even part of the Oneness (Watson, 2018), it is important to acknowledge that this concept does not mean we understand the experience of others or that we can ignore the differences between us. Instead, this interconnection allows us to understand the importance of our differences and how the diversity of our experiences creates space for us to connect in innovative and evolving ways, striving to expand our science, philosophy, and understanding further than we could have done alone.

Living this understanding of Oneness through the practice of Unitary Caring Science (Watson, 2018) makes it imperative to create space for the voices of all people and experiences. As nursing opens more opportunities for BIPOC populations who have been historically marginalized to share their voice and their leadership, we not only improve the quality of our teams and leadership, but we begin to represent the populations of people that we serve and create a space for healing.

The COVID-19 pandemic provided nursing a recent lived experience of the complex dynamics that impact health and well-being worldwide; it became evident how power structures can exclude or empower different groups, impeding or facilitating their pursuit of health and well-being. Complex problems require more innovative, dynamic, and unique solutions that can only come from diverse groups fostering inclusive ideas and thought. The intentionality of action can increase nursing's inclusion of historically disadvantaged groups, ensuring the profession's relevancy and creating diverse nursing leadership for the future of health and healthcare.

# SOCIAL JUSTICE ISSUES AND CARING-MORAL JUSTICE ISSUES

Nursing leaders have a call to address not only the differences in health across marginalized and nonmarginalized groups but also to address social justice issues within the nursing profession. This includes creating space for BIPOC populations and others who have been historically excluded by an intentional practice of invitation, encouragement, and support. Nurses and healthcare professionals in positions of power have a caring-moral calling to use their privilege to create spaces for diverse voices and ideas. This action supports the philosophy and values of nursing and improves the systems in which diverse voices are included.

Unitary Caring Science drives nursing to address social injustices through a multitude of approaches. Advocacy for policy change, funding social programs, healthcare reform, outreach, and support for diverse future nursing leaders can all address social and political determinants of health. Inequity in policies can look like the placement of a chemical plant in a disadvantaged community or one school system offering more laptop computers for their students to use than one in a minoritized neighborhood. These policies and practices benefit the group in power while leaving behind the historically oppressed groups who need advocates willing to engage in community action to change local, national, and global policy.

Community and public health can only be implemented effectively through working relationships with community members. How can nursing leaders build relationships with community members if they are excluding members of the community? Nursing leaders cannot lead a community if they exclude members of the community and do not welcome diverse viewpoints and ideas. It's only through building interconnected, caring relationships that we can begin to uncover the inequities that structural racism has created.

All of us benefit when inequity is addressed and diversity becomes an intentional practice. None of us alone have access to the richness and depth of ideas, innovation, and understanding of others' experiences when certain groups are excluded or marginalized. Creating spaces for some groups while excluding others is a detriment to our societal and moral growth. By only including voices from our groups, we reinforce old beliefs and ideas instead of moving science and philosophy into the future. Nursing leadership has a caring-moral imperative to lead the way, including diverse voices, ideas, experiences, and backgrounds to make healthcare and the world better and more inclusive. Nurses can consider the caring ethics and morals that guide our social justice efforts.

# UNITARY CARING-BASED ADVOCACY FOR NURSE LEADERS

> "It is time to transform the healthcare system through policy initiatives that support praxis that honors nursing's unitary paradigm, clearly recognizing that it is challenging to change nursing practice until all relevant systems (legal/regulatory, financial, scientific, professional, ethical) re-envision health and wellbeing and the actions that support its attainment." (Koithan et al., 2017, p. 262)

When nurses enact Watson's Caritas Process using a Unitary Caring Science approach within a context of SPDH, they come to know the population's stories, contexts, and aspirations as we reflect on their needs and health concerns. This creates a platform for creative advocacy based in caring-moral justice approaches to emerge so that we can create a public healthcare system that employs nurses who can establish meaningful relationships with diverse populations in their socio-cultural environments. Nurses need to be activists who "recognize that whole person well-being is intimately tied to the food security, the safety of communities, respect and personal freedom for individuals as well as the sovereign rights of Indigenous nations, and the sense of place and space" (Koithan et al., 2006, p. 265). Nurses can also acknowledge the evidence that supporting relationship-building within and among a community, supporting the strength of families and their affectional ties, and the presence of external support systems may indeed help to support the growth of resilience needed for vulnerable populations to best manage their health (Werner, 1989).

Nurses are obligated to listen to the populations we serve. Using Watson's Unitary Caring Science approach, we can examine systemic issues through reflective processes and community assessments, incorporate Caring Science and one's whole being, and identify the biases that emerge from structural racism constructs, so that together along with those we serve, we can form a mutually satisfactory interpretation of what the community's health strengths and needs are (Falk-Rafael, 2005). Nurses can note that environmental determinants of health are multifactorial and complex. They become inseparable from other health risk factors such as genetics and lifestyle concerns so that social justice issues and policy change driven by political action become the work of the nurse (Falk-Rafael, 2005).

As Watson (2006) stated, caring, healthcare economics, and administrative practices are often viewed as conflicting with one another, which may be in part due to the separation of unitary human caring as the underlying foundation and moral-ethical framework of all we do in nursing and healthcare. Indeed, many policies and short-term efforts toward addressing larger systemic issues overlook the need to care deeply for the humanity we serve. Watson (2006) suggests a shift toward basing our healthcare practices, economics, and policies on humanity's moral framework and caring. Through a lens of caring, we are motivated to create changes that address the social and moral justice issues that impact SPDH. Nurses can enact a sense of the sacred as they undertake their political advocacy efforts.

Watson's (2006) principles can easily be applied to policy development and sacred-caring political advocacy when addressing SPDH, including (pp. 49–50):

- Developing professional healthcare and public health policies, practices, and decision-making processes based on morality, ethics, and sacred-caring values versus strictly economic and cost-driven interventions

- Moving from a purely mechanical cure-based approach to healthcare to incorporating spiritual health and healing. This is our moral imperative to return to caring being the core of the nursing practice, as we create connections with the vulnerable populations we serve who suffer from the effects of systemic racism

- Creating authentic caring- healing environments in hospitals (vs. hospitality environments)

- Moving away from corporatization and the for-profit nature of health and toward a "public covenant for health citizenry," including BIPOC populations

- Recognition of the importance of caring-healing values, ethics, and the holistic knowledge of nurses as underutilized resources in our current healthcare systems

- Calling for the cost of healthcare and economics that drive policy formation to include the cost-benefit and cost-effectiveness of human caring–based approaches

Applying critical race theory (CRT) components can further help us examine racialization issues that contribute to BIPOC populations' health inequity issues and support the sacred-caring work of advocating for populations (Ford & Airhihenbuwa, 2010). Racial inequalities are often attributed to nonracial causes, such as socioeconomics. Nurses must remain focused on discovering the integral, relevant, and antecedent ways that racial factors continue to condition disease distributions within communities. CRT addresses social isolation and social hierarchy positions (privileged versus marginalized, minority versus majority) to help nurses focus on moving marginalized groups and BIPOC populations to a caring-centered position for consideration around addressing health inequities. CRT aims to move beyond understanding inequities and toward eliminating them.

Ford and Airhihenbuwa (2010) took CRT to the next step by creating a Public Health Critical Race (PHCR) Praxis Model that calls for us to first examine contemporary patterns of racial relations as social constructs. As nurses applying a Unitary Caring Science lens, we must be committed to identifying the patterns of systemic racism in our communities with the impacted populations to determine how transpersonal human caring-based nursing interventions can create a sacred grounding framework for addressing inequities.

# IMPLICATIONS FOR PRACTICE

The following are implications for nurses and the future of nursing practice:

- SPDH must be addressed by nurses from a caring or Unitary Caring Science perspective. This holistic approach of identifying patterns and working directly with communities to address their health disparities is key to create meaningful change in our current systems.

- Nurses should be obligated to enhance their political advocacy skills, as they recognize the suffering that SPDH create and that moving beyond that suffering requires political action.

- Critical race theory is a tool that nurses can use to uncover the roots of systemic racism in healthcare that underlie SPDH. When coupled with Unitary Caring Science approaches, the nurse has the tools they need to create meaningful change for BIPOC and vulnerable populations.

- All of our work as nurses should be infused with loving-kindness and recognition of our Oneness.

# SUMMARY

Nurses can consider Watson's (2006) concept that the nurse's intentionality and caring-healing consciousness transcends time, space, and physicality and informs future practices and interactions. All of the nurse's work, including political advocacy, can emerge from a platform of the sacredness of Unitary Caring Science. Watson (2006) made it clear that caring intention and consciousness energetically affect the whole field. This caring intention and consciousness would also apply to nurses developing or implementing policy. They assess for patterns and consider the structural, social, and political shifts needed to create transformative changes with the SPDH. When nurses are motivated to advocate for change through a foundation of caring-based theory such as the Unitary Caring Science approach, we create a worldview where *all* human beings deserve health equity and have value, we create a world where nurses can care for vulnerable and diverse populations with an emphasis on the community's needs, inclusive of love, faith, compassion, caring, and a higher power (Falk-Rafael, 2005). We must acknowledge that when acting from a place of caring and using Unitary Caring Science approaches, all nurses become ethically obligated to identify and address the structural racism and biases in their workplaces. As we strive to address the social and caring-moral justice issues before us, which are also often the very things that stand in the way of our creating transpersonal caring moments, the scared nature of our political advocacy roles becomes clear.

# REFLECTIVE QUESTIONS

1. Review the CDC website around Social Determinants of Health. https://www.cdc.gov/socialdeterminants/index.htm

2. What SDOH effects have you seen regularly in your professional role? What are some current federal, state, or local healthcare policies that might address the issue?

3. How are political determinants of health different from social determinants of health? Why is it important to address both?

4. Why is it important for nurses to infuse loving-kindness as they use Unitary Caring Science approaches in their advocacy work?

5. Reflect on your own structural racism experiences and biases in healthcare that you have experienced or witnessed as a patient, a family member, or a provider. How can we begin to dismantle structural racism?

6.  Create a visual representation of the intersection of SPDH, Unitary Caring Science, and political advocacy. Prepare to discuss this or create a narrative around it.

---

# NARRATIVE

A Black 47-year-old man living with heart failure (whom we will call Al) was enrolled in a research study at the local safety-net hospital. Al was hesitant to be involved with his cardiology team, and at enrollment into the research study with the research nurse and social worker, he talked about how he didn't trust healthcare. He shared that a family member of his was experimented on in the Tuskegee airmen experiments. Al felt his family had been experimented on enough throughout their history by healthcare professionals who were supposed to help him.

Al talked about how the historical impact of healthcare's inequitable treatment of minoritized groups like his family had made him so fearful of healthcare that he didn't get help for his severe edema, shortness of breath, and chest pain until he could no longer work because of the severity of his symptoms. He wasn't willing to have his heart failure more actively managed by his cardiology team. Because of his passive response to his illness, he had only ended up accessing care when he was in an emergency state. Al shared that he had joined the research study only to share his experience and wanted to make sure people weren't being experimented on as they had been in the past.

This is an example of how healthcare and policy created situations that exploited minoritized groups and destroyed trust with people who needed to be included and welcomed. This patient's historical experience with systematic oppression directly impacted his relationship with his healthcare providers in the current day.

---

# AUTHOR BIOGRAPHIES

**Carey S. Clark, PhD, RN, AHN-BSC RYT, FAAN,** Professor of Nursing, Pacific College of Health and Science, has been interested in healthcare policy for over 20 years. From her experience as an American Nurses Advocacy Institute fellow to developing healthcare policy courses to advocating for cannabis legislation reform, Clark has advocated for change in policy that supports social justice reforms. She is the immediate past president of the American Cannabis Nurses Association and the editor of the textbook *Cannabis: A Handbook for Nurses.* She has taught across the levels of nursing education, and she developed an award winning holistic-caring nursing curriculum for RN-BSN students at University of Maine at Augusta. She currently teaches for Pacific College of Health and Science. Clark has a wide background in professional nursing experience, including in the medical-surgical, pediatrics, psychiatric, camp, hospice, and parish nursing settings, and she strives to support students and nurses as they apply nursing theory in their practice settings and advocacy efforts.

**Rachel Johnson-Koenke, PhD, LCSW,** Assistant Professor, University of Colorado, College of Nursing, VA Eastern Colorado Healthcare System, is a licensed clinical social worker and health science researcher. She is currently an assistant professor at the College of Nursing, University of Colorado where her research interest is around the use of narratives and Unitary Caring Science to help people living with chronic illness. Johnson-Koenke conducts research at the Eastern Colorado Healthcare System, VA Medical Center exploring narratives and Unitary Caring Science. She also mentors, supervises, and supports clinician researchers and nursing students to conduct research from their unique, important, and insightful disciplinary lens.

# REFERENCES

American Association of Colleges of Nursing. (2017). *Diversity, equity, and inclusion in academic nursing.* https://www.aacnnursing.org/News-Information/Position-Statements-White-Papers/Diversity

The Aspen Institute. (2016). *Eleven terms you should know to better understand structural racism.* https://www.aspeninstitute.org/blog-posts/structural-racism-definition/

Braveman, P. (2014). What are health disparities and health equity? We need to be clear. *Public Health Reports, 129,* 5–8. doi: 10.1177%2F00333549141291S203

Centers for Disease Control. (2021). *Social determinants of health: Know what affects health.* https://www.cdc.gov/socialdeterminants/index.htm

Chowkwanyun, M., & Reed Jr, A. L. (2020). Racial health disparities and Covid-19—Caution and context. *New England Journal of Medicine, 383*(3), 201–203.

Churchwell, K., Elkind, M. S., Benjamin, R. M., Carson, A. P., Chang, E. K., Lawrence, W., Mills, A., Odom, T. M., Rodriguez, C. J., & Rodriguez, F. (2020). Call to action: Structural racism as a fundamental driver of health disparities: A presidential advisory from the American Heart Association. *Circulation, 142*(24), e454–e468.

Dawes, D. E. (2018). The future of health equity in America: Addressing the legal and political determinants of health. *Journal of Law, Medicine, and Ethics, 46,* 838–840.

Dawes, D. E. (2020). Health inequities: A look at the political determinants of health during the COVID-19 pandemic. *American Journal of Health Studies, 35*(2), 77–82.

Drevdahl, D. J. (2018). Culture shifts: From cultural to structural theorizing in nursing. *Nursing Research, 67*(2), 140–160. doi: 10.1097/NNR.0000000000000262

Falk-Rafael, A. (2005). Advancing nursing theory through theory-guided practice. The emergence of a critical caring perspective. *Advances in Nursing Science, 28*(1), 38–45.

Ford, C. L., & Airhihenbuwa, C. O. (2010). The public health critical race methodology: Praxis for antiracism research. *Social Science and Medicine, 71,* 1390–1398.

Jones, D. (2019). Political participation in the least healthy place in America: Examining the political determinants of health in Mississippi Delta. *Journal of Health, Politics, Policy, and Law, 44*(3), 506–531. doi: 10.1215./03616878-7367048.

Kickbusch, I. (2015). The political determinants of health – 10 years on. *BMJ, 350*, h81. https://doi.org/10.1136/bmj.h81

Koithan, M. S., Krietzer, M. J. & Watson, J. (2017). Linking the Unitary Paradigm to policy through a synthesis of Caring Science and integrative nursing. *Nursing Science Quarterly, 30*(3), 262–268. doi: 10.1177/0894318417708415

Kumar, P., & Chander, B. (2020). COVID 19 mortality: Probable role of microbiome to explain disparity. *Medical Hypotheses, 144*, 110209. https://doi.org/10.1016/j.mehy.2020.110209

Levinas, E. (1996). *Emmanuel Levinas: Basic philosophical writings*. Indiana University Press.

National Association of Social Workers. (2017). *NASW Code of Ethics*. https://www.socialworkers.org/About/Ethics/Code-of-Ethics/Code-of-Ethics-English

Reed, D. (2020). Racial disparities in healthcare: How COVID-19 ravaged one of the wealthiest African American counties in the United States. *Social Work in Public Health*, 1–10.

Reich, M. R. (2019). *Editorials: Political economy analysis of health*. World Health Organization. https://www.who.int/bulletin/volumes/97/8/19-238311/en/

Taylor, J. (2019). *Racism, inequality, and healthcare for African Americans*. The Century Foundation. https://tcf.org/content/report/racism-inequality-health-care-african-americans/?session=1

US Department of Health and Human Services. (n.d.-a). *Healthy People 2030. Increase the proportion of adults who get recommended evidence-based preventative health care*. https://health.gov/healthypeople/objectives-and-data/browse-objectives/health-care-access-and-quality/increase-proportion-adults-who-get-recommended-evidence-based-preventive-health-care-ahs-08

US Department of Health and Human Services. (n.d.-b). *Healthy People 2030. Education: Access and quality*. https://health.gov/healthypeople/objectives-and-data/browse-objectives/education-access-and-quality

US Department of Health and Human Services. (n.d.-c). *Healthy People 2030. Social and community context*. https://health.gov/healthypeople/objectives-and-data/browse-objectives/social-and-community-context

US Department of Health and Human Services. (n.d.-d). *Healthy People 2030. Economic stability*. https://health.gov/healthypeople/objectives-and-data/browse-objectives/economic-stability

US Department of Health and Human Services. (n.d.-e). *Healthy People 2030. Neighborhood and built environment*. https://health.gov/healthypeople/objectives-and-data/browse-objectives/neighborhood-and-built-environment

Watson, J. (2006). Caring theory as an ethical guide to administrative and clinical practices. *Nursing Administration Quarterly, 30*(1), 48–55.

Watson, J. (2018). *Unitary Caring Science: Philosophy and praxis of nursing*. University Press of Colorado.

Watson, J. (2020). *Nursing's global covenant with humanity – Unitary Caring Science as sacred activism*. Wiley Online Library.

Werner, E. E. (1989). High-risk children in young adulthood: A longitudinal study from birth to 32 years. American Journal of Orthopsychiatry, 59(1), 72–81. https://doi.org/10.1111/j.1939-0025.1989.tb01636.x

Viens A. M. (2019). Neo-Liberalism, austerity and the political determinants of health. *Health Care Analysis: Journal of Health Philosophy and Policy, 27*(3), 147–152. https://doi.org/10.1007/s10728-019-00377-7

Young, R., Hinnant, A., & Leshner, G. (2016). Individual and social determinants of obesity in strategic health messages: Interaction with political ideology. *Health Communication, 7*, 903-910. https://doi.org/10.1080/10410236.2015.1018699

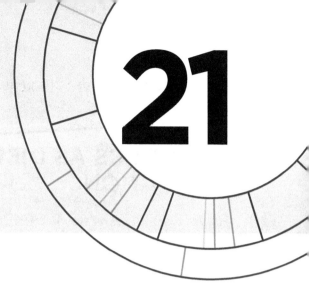

# CREATING A CONNECTED WORLD: A CALL TO ETHICS OF FACE AND BELONGING

Mark D. Beck, DNP, MSN, BS, RN
Stephanie Wilkie Ahmed, DNP, NP-BC
Sara Horton-Deutsch, PhD, RN, PMHCNS, FAAN, ANEF

## LEARNING OBJECTIVES

After completing this chapter, the learner will be able to:

- Manifest a shared vision for nursing leadership as a foundation for all endeavors (service and academic partnerships)

- Remain open to solutions that honor multiple sides and perspectives

- Explain the Ethics of Face and Belonging for creating an environment where everyone wants to belong

- Use silence, listening, reflection, seeing and accepting each person as a whole, and other principles and practices of emergent strategies to hold space for change

# PANDEMICS AS DISRUPTIVE INNOVATIONS

*"Humanity has but three enemies: fever, famine, and war; of these, by far the greatest, by far the most terrible is fever."*

–Sir William Osler, "The Study of the Fevers of the South" (1896)

*"You cannot solve a problem with the same consciousness that created it."*

–Albert Einstein

A pandemic is a natural phenomenon that commands the full attention of humanity whenever it has raised its ugly head. The pandemic of 2020 is no different. Historical pandemics from the distant and not-so-distant past had to contend with the pace of transportation and the "right environments" that were favorable to the infectious agent (A Boire, 2014; Leach et al., 2021; Loresto et al., 2021; Pan et al., 2020). From a chaos theory perspective, pandemics have created three important aspects to consider what the "new normal" looks and feels like: 1) appreciation of white space, 2) invitation to "the unusual suspects," and 3) allowing for serendipity (Brafman & Pollack, 2013).

Following the decimation of the population in 1348–1350 from the Bubonic Plague, life was completely upended, with entire towns depopulated and abandoned. The calamity left many with a lack of purpose or meaning in their lives. This need was so great that within 50 years, out of the devastation of the plague-ravaged population, a compendium of essays was collected and compiled into what became known as *Ars Moriendi* or "The Art of Dying" (Dugdale, 2020; Galvan & Todres, 2009). Within the next hundred years, Europe would begin the movements of the reformation, the founding of universities associated with the Renaissance (1348 University of Prague; 1350 University of Florence; between 1348-1372 universities in Vienna, Krakow, and Heidelberg were created along with four new colleges at Cambridge and two at Oxford), and the Renaissance itself (Brafman & Pollack, 2013). The loss of what was then considered "normal life" led to the creation of "white space." This lack of structure created a "silence" where people could begin to reimagine the role of and need for the displaced segment of society. The ranks of the clergy were decimated in the plague due primarily to the administration of the sacraments to the affected populations. The clerical ranks, including the cloistered monastics, were hit hard by the plague. The ferocity and swiftness of transmission of the plague, and their minimal knowledge of their enemy (germ theory was not discovered until the 19th century), left the population with a feeling of being punished by God for something. With the clerical ranks depleted, the laity (unusual suspects) did not have the clergy to interpret the Word of God for them nor to administer the sacraments (a requirement for salvation and the hereafter), as was the custom of the day. The *Ars Moriendi* thus was created to fill in that gap of the comfort of the laity that the clergy once had occupied (Dugdale, 2020; Maykut & Wild, 2019). The *Ars Moriendi* met the need for sense making or meaning making, which is a fundamental requirement for being a human being (B. Brown, 2017; Hofmann et al., 2009; Lanham et al., 2013; Madsbjerg, 2017).

The need for a new, updated version of *Ars Moriendi* for healthcare providers in the 21st century is now (Dass & Bush, 2018; Dugdale, 2020; Ostaseski, 2017). The issue that healthcare has now is that the pandemic is not over and will not be in the traditional sense of that word for some time to come. Scientists are still studying and learning about the virus and how it is mutating and becoming an adaptable lifeform (Christakis, 2020). From a Darwinian perspective, it's not the survival of the fittest that endures and thrives; it is the organism that is most adaptable to change (Darwin, 1859). As introduced in Chapter 2, Hindsight provides a perspective of how we arrived at this point; Insight provides the current currency for Foresight thinking and planning. "Creating the future requires transformational rather than transactional leadership. Transformation is influenced by anticipation" (Pesut, 2019, p. 197). Foresight transformation is fueled by imagining a future utilizing full-spectrum thinking (Johansen, 2020).

Serendipity does have a neurobiological foundation to what has been termed the default network mode (DNM; Brafman & Pollack, 2013; Cabane & Pollack,

2017; Siegel, 2010, 2018). The brain constantly gathers information even when we are seemingly daydreaming and not utilizing our executive function (focused work). Neuroscience has discovered that when the brain is seemingly "offline," it gathers and processes information, forming new relationships and connections. This recently discovered phenomenon is what has been theorized as sudden insight or the "aha" moment (Cabane & Pollack, 2017). Serendipity has a function, after all. Engaging the brain in seemingly "mindless" tasks such as knitting, crocheting, playing the piano from memory, doodling, and playing with fidget toys allows the DNM to work in the background, making new connections and solving problems. This phenomenon explains the Archimedes "eureka" moment and the stories of Einstein's insights into relatively (bathtubs and working at the Swiss Patent Office are optional; Brafman & Pollack, 2013; Cabane & Pollack, 2017). Taking a walk to "clear your head" takes on a new perspective and gives credence to mindfulness practices. Creating white space for issues to emerge with clarity, seeking out unusual suspects with different perspectives on an issue, and allowing for serendipity all help the brain to process and make new connections—requisites for transformational leadership.

# LEADING IN AN ERA OF DIVERGENCE: CHALLENGES AND OPPORTUNITIES

*"Every system is perfectly designed to get the results it gets."*

–W. Edwards Deming

*"Full-spectrum thinking is the ability to seek patterns and clarity across gradients of possibility—outside, across, beyond, or maybe even without any boxes or categories—while resisting false certainty."*

–Bob Johansen, Full-Spectrum Thinking

# "NORMAL-FOR-NOW" FROM A VOLATILITY, UNCERTAINTY, COMPLEXITY, AND AMBIGUITY (VUCA) PERSPECTIVE

After the terrorist attacks of September 11, 2001, a new acronym was coined by the US Army War College to describe the new normal environment that the world was experiencing: Volatility, Uncertainty, Complexity, and Ambiguity (VUCA; Bennett & Lemoine, 2014; Lawerence, 2013; Stretton, 2021; Yoder-Wise, 2021). Each concept requires a definition, strategy, and intervention and can often be conflated to a single concept that gets lost in the translation to action. VUCA is a critical ingredient for any leadership development program in any discipline but is especially critical in healthcare and within the discipline of nursing. VUCA has become a critical conceptual approach now, given the disruption of the pandemic and the new "normal-for-now" and information overload that the world and healthcare are currently experiencing. VUCA 2.0 has been proposed to help provide clarity (Yoder-Wise, 2021):

- **Volatility to *Vision*** helps to clarify and refine what is future is envisioned

- **Uncertainty to *Understanding*** focuses on deep listening to understand the nuances of the issues

- **Complexity to *Clarity*** focuses on the big picture: the goal to be achieved and the commitment required

- **Ambiguity to *Agility*** reveals where the pivot points reside within the current system and where it may need resources and support

Crises of any ilk have two inherent qualities: danger if nothing changes, and opportunity if the operating assumptions reveal a new direction. The key to understanding the concept of crisis is that these seeming opposites are inextricably entangled (paradoxical relationship); it is not either/or but both/and (B. Brown, 2017; Govaerts et al., 2019; Sabetzadeh et al., 2011; Wesorick, 2016). Imagine yin without yang; what would that symbol look like or even mean? VUCA, if left unattended, can wreak havoc on the best strategic plans.

Crafting VUCA 2.0 requires resources to understand what assumptions the current business model is impacting and how often. The graveyard of businesses is littered with the corpses of organizations that recognized their VUCA insights too late; examples within living memory are Blockbuster and Kodak (McGrath, 2019). Both companies were once thought invincible and the top of their industry, until technology in the form of broadband (streaming), digital film (Fuji Film), and home convenience (Netflix) changed the market, and thus the underlying assumptions of their business models. These are *inflection points*, where enough subtle changes happening on the periphery of the business, slowly at first, then suddenly, changes the operating assumptions of the model. The leadership challenge is identifying what information needs gathering, analyzing, and evaluating for congruence with the business model assumptions. Changes to these assumptions may indicate an inflection point that needs attention (McGrath, 2019).

This pandemic has created inflection points across industrial sectors on a global scale. The healthcare industrial complex was brought to its knees, as was most every other interdependent sector of the economy. The supply chain has been constructed to be lean with few redundancies; excellent on inventory, supply, and cashflow management except when it is interrupted with no backup. This very scenario played out on the world stage regarding acquiring medical-grade personal protective equipment (PPE). The evening news was replete with video of healthcare providers wearing garbage bags and reusing a mask for an entire shift or until deemed non-usable (Christakis, 2020). Once the world went into a pandemic mode, trade was disrupted globally. The world is now so complex and interdependent that when one giant cargo ship gets grounded in the Suez Canal, shipping and product delivery are disrupted globally for an indeterminant period.

# INFLECTION POINTS

A pandemic is a VUCA event on steroids. Many Cassandra scientists predicted this event was coming (Garrett, 1994, 2000; Osterholm, 2017). While we had epidemics within our lifetime (SARS, MERS, H1N1, Ebola, AIDS), few have mobilized and completely captured the world's attention like COVID-19 (Christakis, 2020; Nundy, 2021). A few survivors of the Great Influenza of 1918 are alive to remember that event, and it is only a footnote in the history books; more people died of influenza than were killed in WW1. The divisions and misinformation campaigns were similar in both pandemics (Barry, 2018).

"An inflection point is a change in the business environment that dramatically shifts some element of your activities, throwing certain taken-for-granted assumptions into question. Someone, somewhere, see the implications, but all too often they are not" (McGrath, 2019, p. 1).

Inflection points begin at the peripheral edge of the encounter with the customer, the point farthest from the decision-making structures of an organization. These changes most often are subtle encounters. These changes can be overlooked or not seen as important nor even of interest to those working on the front line (McGrath, 2019). They have metrics to meet, satisfaction scores to keep elevated, and may not even know that those changes are relevant to their survival. Inflection points resulting from VUCA events present a real danger if the assumptions of the business model are not given a stress test to explore weaknesses in processes, resource allocation, and synergy with all the other aspects of the business venture; a stress test is an opportunity to refine, reevaluate, and recommit to the assumptions of their working model. Pandemic pivots might have some situations carry on after the pandemic is officially over. Examples of such pivots are the move for massive investment into telehealth visits and hospital-at-home programs (Nundy, 2021). Many of these pivots will have long-lasting research and investment strategies. Healthcare delivery will change in response to organizations and sectors changing assumptions; the patient-provider relationship has become more vital and central to the delivery of healthcare. As technology advances into every aspect of care delivery, organizations and providers need to invest in the human-to-human connections at the core of the healing relationship (Charon, 2001; Holmgren et al., 2011; Ragan & Kanter, 2017). Human-to-human connections fall within the affective domain of learning; the affective domain is the integrating domain for the Conceptual Age (Pink, 2005).

# LEADERSHIP PRACTICES AND MICROPRACTICES

*"The professions will survive only if they are versatile, focusing not only on knowledge and skills—which will undoubtedly change—but also on the overarching purpose of healthcare. Compassion and human connection are central to that purpose."*

–Brian Hodges, *Without Compassion, There Is No Healthcare*

*What Does Human Being Mean?*

*"How do you measure the expense of an erosion of effort and engagement, or waning of agency and autonomy, or a subtle deterioration of skill? You can't. Those are the kinds of shadowy, intangible things that we rarely appreciate until after they are gone, and even then, we may have trouble expressing the losses in concrete terms. But the costs are real. The choices we make, or fail to make, about which tasks we hand off to computers and which we keep for ourselves are not just practical or economic choices. They are ethical choices. They shape the substance of our lives and the place we make for ourselves in the world. Automation confronts us with the most important questions of all: What does human being mean?"*

–Nicholas Carr, *Utopia Is Creepy*

# A WHOLE NEW MIND AND THE AFFECTIVE DOMAIN

There is no language to describe the wild and crazy rollercoaster ride the world has been on since 9/11. During this time, we have seen the rise of technology giants such as Google, Microsoft, Apple, the social media giants Facebook, Instagram, TikTok, Twitter, and a host of others. All these firms have promised customers seamless integration and were touted as time-saving revolutions to enhance our lives. While machines have certainly automated much of what nurses do and how they document and deliver care, these "applications" have also come between the nurse and the patient; the electronic health record (EHR) is an apotheosis of these applications (Khairat et al., 2020).

Pink wrote about the coming of what he has termed as "the conceptual age," where high concept and high touch, characterized by creators and empathizers, is the next stage of the world's development (Pink, 2005). He predicates this pattern is predicated upon the presence of affluence from the abundance of cheap and affordable goods, mostly manufactured in Asia, from the globalization and automation of markets. He suggests we have gone from the Agricultural Age in the 18th century, to the Industrial Age in the 19th, to the Information Age in the 20th, and are entering the Conceptual Age in the 21st. He postulates this based on three questions: 1) Can someone overseas do it cheaper? 2) Can a computer do it faster? and 3) Is what I'm offering in demand in an age of abundance? (Pink, 2005, p. 51). He asserts how someone answering these questions will determine what kind of jobs are in demand. In the 1980s, MBAs were all the rage and commanded high salaries.

The market for MBAs is waning given the advent of automation and the availability of cheaper outsourcing in Asia; MFAs are now the sought-after degree. Understanding the experience of the product and its effect on the end-user requires an understanding of EQ. Emotional intelligence (EQ) has superseded intelligence (IQ) as a predictor of job satisfaction and job demand. While IQ is still important, EQ and social intelligence (SI) are the new currency of job satisfaction and demand (Koya et al., 2017; Shanta & Gargiulo, 2014). Why? Much of the IQ work is now automated or done cheaper elsewhere (Pink, 2005). This is evident in health-care, where we have a shortage of radiologists in this country. With the advent of high-speed internet, this function can be done on the other side of the world at a fraction of the cost of recruiting, hiring, and retaining a board-certified radiologist. What cannot be outsourced is the patient contact and delivery of hands-on care to the patient (Susskind & Susskind, 2015). That requires a human. The pandemic has accelerated this process exponentially as it has become an inflection point (Christakis, 2020; Nundy, 2021). What might a primary visit be like if an MFA and design thinking principles were utilized to design the experience?

Pink postulates the human attributes required in the Conceptual Age are six: 1) Design, 2) Story, 3) Symphony, 4) Empathy, 5) Play, and 6) Meaning. All these skills are contextual, right-brain-directed functions that require human interaction. These six attributes fall within the affective domain of Bloom's taxonomy. While cognitive knowledge and psychomotor skills will still be required, many of these tasks will become more automated with machine learning or artificial intelligence (AI), and remote monitoring devices will become more ubiquitous and user-friendly in creating a more patient-centered healthcare environment (Nundy, 2021).

The affective domain is where institutional values are learned, communicated, and disseminated (Neumann & Forsyth, 2008; Ondrejka, 2014; Valiga, 2014). The affective domain is where patient satisfaction scores that are tied to value-based reimbursement algorithms reside. The affective domain connects the cognitive and psychomotor domains and imparts meaning. The cognitive domain is the head, psychomotor the hands, and what connects and strengthens both is the affective domain, that being the heart.

## DESIGN

Design is about making products, services, or lifestyles an experience. Design thinking is no longer the domain of engineers exclusively but a collaboration with design thinking skills. Design goes beyond function to create an experience or feeling in the form. Design thinking is also needed in process improvement and education (Barrett, 2017; Beaird et al., 2018; Hamington, 2017; Su & Osisek, 2011; Ziegler et al., 2020). The new 4th edition of the Scope and Standards of Practice for Nursing emphasizes this skill set (American Nurses Association [ANA], 2021). An example of design thinking in the curriculum is to have nurses co-create an info-graphic for a target audience on a targeted topic. This assignment requires that the group research their targeted audience and utilize design principles to engage the learner in the informational activity for long-term health effects.

## STORY

The story has been the human medium of education and identity for millennia (Armstrong, 2005; Mangino, 2014; Mitty, 2010; Mokhtar et al., 2011; Pellico & Chinn, 2007; Ragan & Kanter, 2017; Smith & Liehr, 2005). Understanding the patient's story is key to diagnosis, treatment, and the healthcare relationship with all providers. Sir William Osler, recognized as the father of modern medicine, is quoted as saying, "Listen to the patient, he is telling you the diagnosis" (Osler quotes, n.d.). The story is how humans connect. The dialogical relationship is transformational for both the patient and the nurse (Garno, 2010). Listening with authentic presence (bearing witness) to the patient's story is a healing environment experience (Campbell & Davis, 2011; Cody, 2001, 2007; Drought, 2002). The narrative medicine movement has brought medicine back to its ancient roots; the provider-patient relationship is its focus (Alicea-Planas, 2016; Charon, 2001; Mangino, 2014; Ragan & Kanter, 2017). Nurses have attended to the story of another since time immemorial (Mitty, 2010; Timbrell, 2017). Learning what "bearing witness" means and how to attend to that story is a key skill to know and adopt in the healthcare arena (Djkowich et al., 2019; Hall, 2003; Naef, 2006; Schroeder, 2016).

## EMPATHY

*Empathy* is a human ability, "the action of understanding, being aware of, being sensitive to, and vicariously experiencing the feelings, thoughts, and experience of another of either the past or present without having the feelings, thoughts, and experience fully communicated in an objectively explicit manner" (Merriam-Webster, n.d.). The pandemic has tested the ability of organizations, patients, families, and providers to empathize. The news is replete with stories of their continuous struggle to provide meaningful empathy and worthiness. These stories are reminiscent of those in the *Ars Moriendi* (Dugdale, 2020). All providers are struggling with maintaining some semblance of equilibrium. The activation of the "Wounded Healer" archetype is key to this connection and belonging (Conchar & Repper, 2014; Niven, 2008).

## PLAY

Play, an integral part of the socialization process, involves learning to cooperatively work together for the common good and is a key element in brain development. Stuart Brown, a pediatric psychiatrist, has studied play as part of his practice. His research emphasizes the essential role of play in human development, social cohesion, accelerated learning, creativity and innovation, and the health benefits of laughter and humor on humans (Brown & Vaughn, 2010). Play is an essential component of high-functioning and resilient teams. How might game theory be employed to accelerate and deepen learning in the classroom? How might game theory help students or patients learn about health literacy (Orwoll et al., 2018)?

## SYMPHONY

Symphony is the ability to see the big picture from a complex lens. A symphony is a collection of instruments that create harmonies greater than the sum of any of the individual instruments (Pink, 2005). A conductor is trained to understand and interpret a score to harmonize the various instruments, creating a sound experience, one that is greater than the sum of its constituent instruments. The science of living systems, systems thinking, complexity science would be analogous to the symphony (Paley, 2007; Weberg, 2012; Wheatley, 2017). How might the science of living systems be incorporated into healthcare education to improve coordination and delivery of care (Bird & Strachan, 2020; Kiviliene & Blazeviciene, 2019; Lanham et al., 2013; Rowe & Hogarth, 2005)?

## MEANING

Meaning, sense making, or having a purpose is a fundamental element of being human (Frankel, 1984; Madsbjerg, 2017). This aspect of the affective domain is a defining attribute of being human. The pandemic response has challenged this aspect of being in healthcare and a human being perhaps as much as any event since the last world wars. The shared trauma of this pandemic has challenged some providers to question their value, meaning, and purpose for being. The PTSD experienced for some will be life-altering (Christopher et al., 2020; Goulston & Hendel, 2020). The broadcast news is replete with stories of people completely changing their livelihoods to find new meaning and purpose. Many in the healthcare profession have done the same (Hofmann et al., 2009). Many leaders have also found their opportunity to dig deep and find new meaning and purpose in leadership (April & Chimenya, 2019). Inherent within each crisis humanity encounters are dangers and opportunities. The global pandemic response may well determine the future of humanity as viruses are apolitical lifeforms and do not respect boundaries. E. O. Wilson summed this thought up succinctly, "If all mankind were to disappear, the world would regenerate back to the rich state of equilibrium that existed ten thousand years ago. If insects were to vanish, the environment would collapse into chaos" (E. O. Wilson Quotes, n.d.). The same can be said for viruses and bacteria.

# HOLDING SPACE FOR PARADOXES/ POLARITIES

Paradoxes are a part of life; they can bring immense joy or pain depending on how they are processed into the narrative of lives and their subsequent outcomes.

Brown asserts that "in its Greek origins, a paradox is the joining of two words, *para* (contrary to) and *doiken* (opinion). The Latin *paradoxum* means 'seemingly absurd but really true'" (B. Brown, 2017, pp. 40–41). Healthcare providers—like their patients, families, and communities—encounter paradoxes in their daily work. Where in the healthcare curriculum are students taught to hold space for ideas, concepts, or feelings that appear to be in opposition? The culture of healthcare is about science and finding the answer to any given issue or problem. Nevertheless, healthcare is about being present with human beings who bring all their feelings, joys, sorrows, and misunderstandings of what it means to be human into that exam room. The "business" of healthcare is about input, output, and outcomes. Each of these is a line item on a spreadsheet. That is the paradox of today's healthcare delivery. Yet, those who can stand in that space, and hold that paradox, often create the healing environment where humans, both patient and provider, experience healing, even if there is no pill, procedure, or remedy available. It can be a place of profound healing and meaning for all participants (Manderscheid & Freeman, 2012; Peterson, 2017; Sabetzadeh et al., 2011). The ontology of nursing, the "being," needs parity with the "doing" or task-based aspects throughout the curriculum. Serendipity and emergent strategies arise in this paradoxical space.

# LEADING CHANGE: RESTORING CARE TO HEALTHCARE

*"It is often thought that medicine is the curative process. It is no such thing; … nature alone cures. … And what [true] nursing has to do … is to put the patient in the best condition for nature to act upon him."*

–Florence Nightingale, *Notes on Nursing*

One of the most posited questions in Shakespearian literature is, "To be, or not to be?" Considered more appropriate perhaps as academic discourse rather than a philosophical question to be contemplated by the discipline, achievement of nursing's highest aspirational ideal, health for all, does require such understanding.

With its first provision for nursing practice based upon compassion and respect for the inherent dignity and worth of all, *The Code of Ethics for Nursing with Interpretive Statements* (The Code) makes explicit the values of the profession (ANA, 2015). Beckoning nurses beyond the bedside practice is reconceptualized for the future, evolving to include population health and telehealth. With the integration of social justice into nursing and health policy, The Code restates and restores the caritive and emancipatory underpinnings of the discipline (ANA, 2015).

Nursing affirms and holds health as a fundamental human right (ANA, 2015). Seeking to make the health system safer, organizations have heeded the counsel promoted by the National Academies of Practice's "To Err is Human" (1999) and "Crossing the Quality Chasm" (Institute of Medicine, 2001), implementing quality programs and measuring healthcare outcomes. With the enactment of the Affordable Care Act, healthcare reimbursement models shifted toward value-based payments was implemented, and ostensibly, with recognition of collective efforts, Americans should be among the healthiest. However, nationally, rates of hospitalizations from preventable causes and the rates of avoidable deaths remain higher than those of global peers (Commonwealth Fund, 2020). While allocating 16.9% of the nation's GDP for healthcare and further shifting higher out-of-pocket expenses to the consumer, the life expectancy rates of Americans are lower than those experienced by other countries that spend far less (Commonwealth Fund, 2020). In such circumstances, the universal achievement of health seems unlikely.

While a variety of factors, both individual and societal, contribute to understanding what constitutes health, it is broadly recognized that its advancement requires both access and equity. Because contemporary models of health and healthcare have been so strongly influenced by reimbursement drivers, *social determinants of health* (SDOH)—those nonmedical factors such as low literacy, housing, income disparities, access to nutrition, and the experience of discrimination (National Academies of Sciences, Engineering, and Medicine, 2021)—have been historically under-recognized as influential to health status, leaving those who live along society's margins both unseen and with unmet needs.

*"The face presents itself and demands justice."*

–Emmanuel Levinas (2013)

Through the lens of Levinasian ethics, nursing is empowered to move beyond society's established separatist ontology and the associated medical-technical model of healthcare that deconstructs those it encounters into the sum of their parts (the kidney in room 601), procedures (the total hip), diagnoses (the diabetic), social status (the homeless man or woman), or the pejorative related to the regularity by which one seeks care (the frequent flyer). Such depersonalization of humanity within the healthcare system is representative of a biocidic (life-destroying) environment.

The concept of alterity is central to Levinasian ethics. However, based upon the primacy of another, Levinas sought to develop the first philosophy, and his interest in such occurred via a seemingly innocuous and recurring event—the face-to-face encounter with *"the Other."*

In *Totality and Infinity*, Levinas (2013, p. 198) states that "the face speaks thereby inviting one into relation," and through this encounter, one's inherent obligation to *the Other* is revealed. Conceptually the Ethic of Belonging is the antecedent to being. As it is with those individuals living on the margins, one who is not seen does not exist and therefore can neither be nor belong. This gap must be addressed if the healthcare system is to impact SDOH. It is why the affective domain of learning must be reintegrated into nursing education and practice.

Dismantling of factors that contribute to barriers for healthcare access and equity requires nursing to innovate and influence society by advancing the values of the discipline. Through encountering *the Other*—in this instance, those who are vulnerable and/or marginalized—there is an opportunity to reconnect with the moral "ought." In this way, the praxis of nursing is advanced in the form of sacred activism that holds the Ethic of Face and the Ethic of Belonging as a value.

# PRAXIS: MOVING TOWARD SACRED ACTIVISM AND INFORMED MORAL ACTIONS

*"This evolved unitary consciousness of shared humanity requires our awareness to attend to how we are touching others and the planet earth; how we give voice and action toward human caring as perhaps a form of sacred activism within a larger cosmology."*

–Jean Watson (2018, p. 19)

With a recommendation that hospitals and health systems support community-level policy actions, Castrucci and Auerbach (2019) have designed a model to address SDOH using the representation of a stream, where influencing upstream strategies creates downstream effects.

- **Upstream** strategies seek to impart a broad community impact, improving conditions via such tactics as law, policy, and regulations, thereby fostering health for all.

- **Midstream** strategies seek to impart a singular impact by addressing individual social needs via tactics that include screening for social factors (e.g., access to food or housing), providing referrals and direct support via social workers, and other community health–based resources.

- **Downstream** strategies provide clinical care and medical interventions.

The systematic dismantling of the nation's public health system focuses nursing's effort most frequently downstream, working within the health system engaged in delivering direct clinical care or, to some degree, midstream managing resources at the individual level.

How does our current inflection point allow us to:

- Reconceive what nursing practice and population health could look like upstream—what new roles would be conceived or restored?

- Imagine how the power paradigm could be redistributed to strengthen the leadership and role of those in the community to self-define needs?

- Define how contributions would be measured?

- Develop and foster cross-discipline, community-based relationships?

- Evolve novel partnerships when solving homelessness or food scarcity?

*"The nurse owes the same duties to self as to others including the responsibility to promote health and safety, preserve wholeness of character and integrity, maintain competence and continue personal and professional growth."*

–Provision 5, *The Code of Ethics for Nurses with Interpretive Statements* (ANA, 2015)

The ability for healthcare organizations to achieve overarching goals has largely been credited with the employment of a staff who possess the appropriate knowledge and expertise to meet patient care demands, coupled with an organizational ability to deploy them. Care needs are appropriately at the forefront of organizational priorities; however, beyond a benefits package inclusive of health insurance, somewhat surprisingly, few have focused on the wellness of those employees who are called to care for others.

Working within a complex environment with a high degree of unpredictability and rapidly shifting demands, nurses and other members of the interprofessional team frequently report feeling dissatisfied (Halcomb et al., 2018) in their roles. In response, and broadly addressed in the literature, healthcare organizations began shifting focus toward building a resilient workforce (Manomanidis et al., 2019). In doing so, however, the inherent resilience of the nursing workforce seems to have gone unrecognized, and the responsibility to adapt and cope has been placed upon the staff. Shifting the discussion from resilience to wellness reframes the issue.

Organizational culture has a strong influence on nurse wellness. To this end, nurse leaders have an important role in transforming both the culture of the healthcare organization and the unit to support the wellness of staff. This responsibility to foster wellness and balance is clearly addressed in the *Code of Ethics for Nurses with Interpretive Statements* (ANA, 2015, p. 19) and was further recognized in the updated report, *The Future of Nursing 2020-2030: Charting a Path to Achieve Health Equity* (National Academies of Sciences, Engineering, and Medicine, 2021), where a salvo was issued calling for the prioritization of the health and well-being of nurses by academe, licensing boards, and employers.

Most often considered in the context of the body physical, wholistically, wellness must allow for the interconnectedness of both physical and mental health (Boston University Center for Psychiatric Rehabilitation, 2020) and conceptually in its fullness encompass eight dimensions: emotional, environmental, financial, intellectual, occupational, physical, social, and the spiritual. When guided by Human Caring Theory, such an approach to nurse wellness would provide a moral, ethical, and theoretical framework upon which nurse leaders could advance culture change, thus aiding healthcare organizations to evolve toward being more humane and caring communities. Furthermore, and as discussed in earlier chapters, a foundation for an authentic caring-healing environment can only be advanced where the well-being of staff is prioritized along with caring for patients.

How does our current inflection point allow us to:

- Reconceptualize staffing models and/or schedules to promote nurse wellness?

- Explore what lifestyle interventions can be implemented in the workplace to foster healthy, risk-reducing behaviors among nurses?

- Discover what types of techniques can be taught organizationally to promote positive adjustment to adversity and/or changing dynamics?

# IMPLICATIONS FOR PRACTICE: INSPIRING ACTION

According to the National Nursing Workforce Study (Smiley et al., 2021), nursing will be one of the highest professional growth areas in the next decade, and the global pandemic has only accelerated this trend. Nurse leaders who value the Ethic of Belonging and uphold a caring ontology aim to lead from a sacred place. They are poised to create and regenerate healthy and healing environments that focus on wellness. Adrienne Marie Brown's work on *Emergent Strategies* (2017) and *Holding Change* (2021) provides a road map for navigating a future together, a path toward a more plentiful and flourishing world. *Emergence* is how complex systems and patterns arise out of multiple and straightforward interactions (Obolensky, 2014). Emergent strategies embrace complexity systems and focus on the neglected affective domain of learning. They are about getting in the right relation with change by realigning with intrinsic values, an indigenous worldview that appreciates the relationality of all things. Brown (2021, p. 13) states, "At the intersection of an ancient understanding, science, the sacred, and science fiction sits a set of principles that helps us practice shaping change." Again, the essence of emergent strategies is shaping and generating complex systems and patterns through simple interactions. For example, Brown explains that if we attend to nature's lessons and recognize that we are part of nature, we can unveil our organic gifts and our way toward collective opportunity.

In her study and practice of emergent strategies, A. M. Brown (2017, 2021) identifies core principles to guide the use of the method to navigate change:

- Small is good (large is a reflection of the small)

- Change is constant (be like water)

- There is always enough time for the right work

- There is a conversation in the room that only these people can have. Find it.

- Never a failure, always a lesson.

- Trust the people.

Building on emergent strategies, Brown (2021) describes "holding change" as her variation of "holding space" and how leaders can sacredly hold collective work. Ultimately, the purpose of holding change is to make it easy for people with shared intentions to be together, move toward their vision and values, and navigate conflict in a way that is generative and accountable. As many of our structures in healthcare are crumbling, we are at the moment in human history when we need courageous nurse leaders to shift away from competitive and directive leadership. We need leaders who are focused on listening deeply, accepting each other, and seeing each other as a whole. Viewed in this way, nursing leadership is sacred work.

# SUMMARY

The pandemic of 2020 caught the world by surprise even though it was predicted and planned for during the transition between US administrations in 2017 (Toosi et al., 2020). Lessons from this pandemic will be ongoing and iterative until the pandemic has been declared over. Having shared language (VUCA) assists with creating shared mental models for strategic intervention (VUCA 2.0; Sullivan & Yoder-Wise, 2019; Yoder-Wise, 2021). The leadership challenges for this VUCA time will be devising what information from the periphery of the core business needs to be curated to stress test the assumptions of their business model. Intentionally seeking early signs and warnings of subtle changes from the periphery can illuminate inflection points. Understanding these inflection points helps leadership evaluate the data for any course corrections, resource reallocation, and strategic planning changes needed for VUCA 2.0 implementation.

The Conceptual Age prioritizes the high-tech, high-touch attributes of the affective domain (Pink, 2005). The advent of AI into healthcare will shift many routine, mundane monitoring to machine learning, redefining roles and jobs (Susskind & Susskind, 2015). The interface with technology will only grow more pervasive, and some will characterize it as intrusive. A prime example is utilizing robots in rendering some caring functions (Locsin & Schoenhofer, 2019; Wolf et al., 2019). Humans are a social species, which means they rely on forming connections for feelings of safety, meaning, purpose, and the sense of belonging (Ashktorab et al., 2017; Beattie et al., 2018; Page et al., 2021; Theede, 2018; Udah, 2019; Vogel, 2016; Wiklund Gustin & Wagner, 2013). Fostering the attributes of the affective domain is primarily about connection, safety, and co-creating a sacred space of belonging (Jefford et al., 2021; Maslow, 1998; Wei et al., 2021).

At times in rendering healthcare, occasions arise where conflicting values come into play. Examples include wanting hospice patients to have as much lucid time with their loved ones while meeting conflicting pain management goals. These occasions require that the care team hold polarities or paradoxes in the same sacred space of healing. As AI becomes ubiquitous in delivering care, holding space for seemingly paradoxical concepts or initiatives is seemingly absurd but true (B. Brown, 2017). Patients and families need that sense of meaning and belonging, that they are not alone in this journey. This is part of the art of nursing and an aspect of nursing's unique nature (ANA, 2021; Sims et al., 2020). This is the intersection where service and academia can meet current and future inflections points. The new American Association of Colleges of Nursing (AACN) *Essentials of Nursing*, with its focus on relational coordination and competencies, coupled with the ANA *Scope and Standards of Practice* with its reaffirmation of the "art and science" of nursing; the reaffirmation of caring as a key element of nursing as possessing disciplinary-unique knowledge sets the stage for a co-creating healthcare of the future (AACN, 2020; ANA, 2021).

Moving beyond medicalized, industrialized healthcare delivery based in the 19th century industrial model of production can be transformed with Conceptual Age values and connections; strengthening the need for human connections, a basic need for connection and safety, securing a sense of belonging (Watson, 1990, 2021; Wiklund Gustin & Wagner, 2013). Holding paradoxical space invites white space to assist with clarity, seeks unusual suspects for alternative perspective-taking, and invokes serendipity in emerging strategies. These strategies show us that adaptation and evolution depend on critical, deep, and authentic connections. The cure is not the aim; healing is, love is. The archetype of the Wounded Healer is powerful when claimed and exercised (Conti-O'Hare, 2002; Hall, 1997; Loaganathan, 2002; Quinn, 2014). Academia and service can create a new paradigm of the Wounded Healer, where connection and belonging are the keys to health. The inflection point is here.

# REFLECTIVE QUESTIONS

1.  How does the concept of an inflection point in business inform leaders' decision-making moving forward?

2.  What role/function do white space, unusual suspects, and serendipity play as aspects of chaos theory?

3.  How might learning "to hold opposites or paradoxical concepts in the same space" help with decision-making in the delivery of healthcare?

4.  The affective domain is often called the "soft skills" domain. How has the pandemic affected healthcare providers' sense of purpose and meaning with the work they perform? Support your position.

5.  How do the concepts of white space, unusual suspects, and serendipity support diversity, equity, and inclusion initiatives?

## NARRATIVE

A large, vertically integrated health system with a Unitary Caring Science (UCS) affiliation identified a business need to increase the number of BSN-prepared nurses within their organization as part of the journey toward Magnet status. After conducting a review of the nursing workforce, the organization realized that their nursing workforce had a retention rate that remained relatively constant over the study period. Given that these nurses would remain with the organization until retirement replacing them with BSN-prepared nurses was not going to accomplish the 80% target goal for the Magnet journey during their projected timeline. The organization had a longstanding academic-service partnership with a private local health sciences university. A proposal to create an RN-to-BSN program with a UCS foundation was made to this university. The proposal included significant tuition support for their working nurses who wished to return to school to complete this degree. The program's stated ultimate objective was to change the nursing culture at this organization. How can the six human attributes of the 21st Century Conceptual Age be integrated into both the educational and practice settings of these organizations to engage and ultimately retain nurses in the organization and/or profession?

# AUTHOR BIOGRAPHIES

**Mark D. Beck, DNP, MSN, BS, RN, Caritas Coach, HeartMath Trainer,** Assistant Professor and Interim Program Director, Samuel Merritt University, has held various roles within inpatient and academic education for over 30 years. He has established departments of inpatient education, been a clinical instructor, created new graduate training programs, implemented a hospital-wide theory-based model of care, and help multiple academic roles in a variety of academic institutions. He is a Caritas Coach, certified HeartMath Trainer, and has completed a post-doctorate with Jean Watson. He has published on his experience with designing, implementing, and evaluating a theory-based curriculum. His passion is helping nurses to understand their role in "being present" with patients and families while they accomplish their many tasks.

**Stephanie Wilkie Ahmed, DNP, NP-BC,** Associate Chief Nursing Officer, University of Miami Health System & Watson Caring Science Scholar in Residence, University of Miami Health System, is a Watson Scholar and Caritas Coach. Seeking to advance a healthcare system that fosters inclusivity and addresses social determinants of health, Her post-doctoral work is underpinned by Watson's Human Caring Theory and Levinassian ethics, *The Ethic of Face* and *The Ethic of Belonging*. She presently serves in the capacity of Associate Chief Nurse Executive at the University of Miami Health System. An executive nurse leader with over 20 years of progressive healthcare experience, Ahmed is passionate about nursing's role to address contemporary healthcare challenges, including access, quality, and the human experience of care. An innovative thinker, Ahmed brings experience in advanced nursing practice, care redesign, and clinical effectiveness. She has served in the capacity of Magnet Program Director and has held key roles advancing practice, professional development, and quality. A clinician and scholar, Ahmed is editor and contributing author to *DNP Education, Practice, and Policy: Mastering the DNP Essentials for Advanced Nursing Practice.*

**Sara Horton-Deutsch, PhD, RN, PMHCNS, FAAN, ANEF,** is a Caritas Coach and a Professor and the Director of the Kaiser Permanente/USF Partnership at the University of San Francisco, where she mentors the next generation of nursing leaders through the lens of Caring Science and values-based leadership. She also serves as a Faculty Associate with the Watson Caring Science Institute. In 2021, she co-created and initiated the Caritas Leadership Program, a uniquely customized six-month program guiding participants through executive Caring Science leader dialogues, interactive circles, and participant transformation projects. She is also a founding partner of Better Together Healing, LLC, a holistic practice partnership specializing in an integrative approach to heal the self, build collaborations, and create healthy and bounded communities. As a therapeutic practitioner and Caritas leadership coach, she collaborates with healthcare professionals and organizations seeking balance and growth who are open to engaging in innovative approaches to healing. Her comprehensive approach includes certifications in professional coaching and training through the Leadership Circle and Working with Resilience, providing comprehensive profiles and assessments to raise the conscious practice of leadership and build regenerative success at work.

# REFERENCES

A Boire, N. (2014). Lessons learned from historic plague epidemics: The relevance of an ancient disease in modern times. *Journal of Ancient Diseases & Preventive Remedies, 02*(02). https://doi.org/10.4172/2329-8731.1000114

Alicea-Planas, J. (2016). Listening to the narrative of our patients as part of holistic nursing care. *Journal of Holistic Nursing, 34*(2), 162–166.

American Association of Colleges of Nursing. (2020). *Draft 2021 AACN Essentials.*

American Nurses Association. (2015). Provisions of the code of ethics with interpretive statements. In *Code of ethics for nurses with interpretive statements* (pp. v–xii). Author.

American Nurses Association. (2021). *Nursing: Scope and standards of practice.* Author.

April, K., & Chimenya, G. (2019). Leader sensemaking in times of crisis. *Effective Executive, 22*(3), 14–41.

Armstrong, K. (2005). *A Short history of myth.* Canongate Books, Ltd.

Ashktorab, T., Hasanvand, S., Seyedfatemi, N., Salmani, N., & Hosseini, S. V. (2017). Factors affecting the belongingness sense of undergraduate nursing students towards clinical setting: A qualitative study. *J Caring Sci, 6*(3), 221–235. https://doi.org/10.15171/jcs.2017.022

Barrett, D. (2017). Rethinking presence: A grounded theory of nurses and teleconsultation. *J Clin Nurs, 26*(19–20), 3088–3098. https://doi.org/10.1111/jocn.13656

Barry, J. (2018). *The great influenza: The story of the deadliest pandemic in history*. Penguin Random House.

Beaird, G., Geist, M., & Lewis, E. J. (2018). Design thinking: Opportunities for application in nursing education. *Nurse Educ Today, 64*, 115–118. https://doi.org/10.1016/j.nedt.2018.02.007

Beattie, J., Innes, K., Griffiths, D., & Morphet, J. (2018). Healthcare providers' neurobiological response to workplace violence perpetrated by consumers: Informing directions for staff well-being. *Appl Nurs Res, 43*, 42–48. https://doi.org/10.1016/j.apnr.2018.06.019

Bennett, N., & Lemoine, G. (2014). What VUCA really means for you. *Harvard Business Review* (Jan-Feb).

Bird, M., & Strachan, P. H. (2020). Complexity science education for clinical nurse researchers. *J Prof Nurs, 36*(2), 50–55. https://doi.org/10.1016/j.profnurs.2019.07.007

Boston University Center for Psychiatric Rehabilitation. (2020, October 21). *Eight dimensions of wellness*. https://cpr.bu.edu/resources-and-information/eight-dimensions-of-wellness/

Brafman, O., & Pollack, J. (2013). *The chaos imperative: How chance and disruption increase innovation effectiveness and success*. Crown Business.

Brown, A.M. (2017). *Emergent strategies*. AK Press.

Brown, A.M. (2021). *Holding change*. AK Press.

Brown, B. (2017). *Braving the wilderness: The quest for true belonging and the courage to stand alone*. Penguin/Random House.

Brown, S., & Vaughn, C. (2010). *Play: How it shapes the brain*. Avery.

Cabane, O., & Pollack, J. (2017). *The net and the butterfly*. Penguin Random House.

Campbell, M., & Davis, L. (2011). An exploration of the concepts of bearing witness as a constituent of caring practice. *International Journal for Human Caring, 15*(1), 7–12.

Castrucci, B. J. C., & Auerbach, J. (2019, January 1). *Meeting individual social needs falls short of addressing Social Determinants of Health*. Health Affairs. https://www.healthaffairs.org/do/10.1377/hblog20190115.234942/full/

Charon, R. (2001). Narrative medicine: A model for empathy, reflection, profession, and trust. *Journal of the American Medical Association, 286*(15), 1897–1902.

Christakis, N. (2020). *Apollo's arrow*. Little Brown Spark.

Christopher, R., de Tantillo, L., & Watson, J. (2020). Academic caring pedagogy, presence, and communitas in nursing education during the COVID-19 pandemic. *Nursing Outlook*. https://doi.org/10.1016/j.outlook.2020.08.006

Cody, W. (2001). Bearing witness-not bearing witness as synergistic individual-community becoming. *Nursing Science Quarterly, 14*(2), 94–100.

Cody, W. (2007). Bearing witness to suffering: Participating in cotranscendence. *International Journal for Human Caring, 11*(2), 17–21.

The Commonwealth Fund. (2020). *U.S. health care from a global perspective, 2019: Higher spending, worse outcomes?* https://www.commonwealthfund.org/publications/issue-briefs/2020/jan/us-health-care-global-perspective-2019.

Conchar, C., & Repper, J. (2014). "Walking wounded or wounded healer?" Does personal experience of mental health problems help or hinder mental health practice? A review of the literature. *Mental Health and Social Inclusion, 18*(1), 35–44. https://doi.org/10.1108/mhsi-02-2014-0003

Conti-O'Hare, M. (2002). *The nurse as wounded healer*. Jones & Bartlett Learning.

Darwin, C. (1859). *Origin of the species*. John Murray.

Dass, R., & Bush, M. (2018). *Walking each other home*. Sounds True.

Djkowich, M., Ceci, C., & Petrovskaya, O. (2019). Bearing witness in nursing practice: More than a moral obligation? *Nursing Philosophy*, *20*(1), e12232. https://doi.org/10.1111/nup.12232

Drought, T. (2002). The privilege of bearing witness. *Nurs Ethics*, *9*(3), 238–239. https://doi.org/10.1191/0969733002ne505xx

Dugdale, L. (2020). *The lost art of dying: Reviving lost wisdom*. HarperCollins.

E. O. Wilson quotes. (n.d.). BrainyQuote.com. https://www.brainyquote.com/quotes/e_o_wilson_176373

Frankel, V. (1984). *Man's search for meaning*. Washington Square Press.

Galvan, K., & Todres, L. (2009). Embodying nursing openheartness: An existential perspective. *Journal of Holistic Nursing*, *27*(2), 141–149.

Garno, M. (2010). Transforming nursing through dialogical relationship: A pedagogy of connectedness. *International Journal of Human Caring*, *14*(1), 21–26.

Garrett, L. (1994). *The coming plague*. Hyperion.

Garrett, L. (2000). *Betrayal of trust*. Hyperion.

Goulston, M., & Hendel, D. (2020). *Why cope when you can heal?* HarperCollins.

Govaerts, M. J. B., van der Vleuten, C. P. M., & Holmboe, E. S. (2019). Managing tensions in assessment: moving beyond either-or thinking. *Medical Education*, *53*(1), 64–75. https://doi.org/10.1111/medu.13656

Halcomb, E., Smyth, E., & McInnes, S. (2018, August 7). Job satisfaction and career intentions of registered nurses in primary health care: an integrative review. *BMC Family Practice*. https://bmcfampract.biomedcentral.com/articles/10.1186/s12875-018-0819-1

Hall, J. (1997). Nurses as wounded healers. *The Australian Journal of Holistic Nursing*, *4*(1), 11–16.

Hall, V. P. (2003). Bearing witness to suffering in AIDS: the testing of a substantive theory. *J Assoc Nurses AIDS Care*, *14*(4), 25–36. https://doi.org/10.1177/1055329003252050

Hamington, M. (2017). Integrating care ethics and design thinking. *Journal of Business Ethics*, *155*(1), 91–103. https://doi.org/10.1007/s10551-017-3522-6

Hofmann, D. A., Lei, Z., & Grant, A. M. (2009). Seeking help in the shadow of doubt: the sensemaking processes underlying how nurses decide whom to ask for advice. *Journal of Applied Psychology*, *94*(5), 1261–1274. https://doi.org/10.1037/a0016557

Holmgren, L., Fuks, A., Boudreau, D., Sparks, T., & Kreiswirth, M. (2011). Terminology and praxis: clarifying the scope of narrative in medicine. *Lit Med*, *29*(2), 246–273. https://doi.org/10.1353/lm.2011.0323

Institute of Medicine (US) Committee on Quality of Health Care in America. (1970, January 1). *Crossing the quality chasm*. National Center for Biotechnology Information. https://www.ncbi.nlm.nih.gov/books/NBK222274/

Jefford, E., Nolan, S., Munn, J., & Ebert, L. (2021). What matters, what is valued and what is important in mentorship through the Appreciative Inquiry process of co-created knowledge. *Nurse Educ Today*, *99*, 104791. https://doi.org/10.1016/j.nedt.2021.104791

Johansen, B. (2020). *Full spectrum thinking*. Berrett-Koehler Publishers, Inc.

Khairat, S., Xi, L., Liu, S., Shrestha, S., & Austin, C. (2020). Understanding the association between electronic health record satisfaction and the well-being of nurses: Survey study. *JMIR Nursing*, *3*(1), e13996. https://doi.org/10.2196/13996

Kiviliene, J., & Blazeviciene, A. (2019). Review of complex adaptive systems in nursing practice. *Journal of Complexity in Health Sciences*, *2*(2), 46–50. https://doi.org/10.21595/chs.2019.21169

Koya, K., Anderson, J., & Sice, P. (2017). The embodied nurse: Interdisciplinary knowledge exchange between compassionate nursing and recent developments in embodied leadership studies. *Journal of Advanced Nursing*, *73*(12), 3028–3040. https://doi.org/10.1111/jan.13363

Lanham, H. J., Leykum, L. K., Taylor, B. S., McCannon, C. J., Lindberg, C., & Lester, R. T. (2013). How complexity science can inform scale-up and spread in health care: Understanding the role of self-organization in variation across local contexts. *Social Science & Medicine, 93*, 194–202. https://doi.org/10.1016/j.socscimed.2012.05.040

Lawrence, K. (2013). Developing leaders in a VUCA environment. In University of North Carolina (Ed.), *Kenan-Flagler Business School*. University of North Carolina.

Leach, M., MacGregor, H., Scoones, I., & Wilkinson, A. (2021). Post-pandemic transformations: How and why COVID-19 requires us to rethink development. *World Dev, 138*, 105233. https://doi.org/10.1016/j.worlddev.2020.105233

Levinas, E. (2013). *Totality and infinity: An essay on exteriority*. Duquesne University Press.

Loaganathan, L. (2002). The journey into healership: Chiron the wounded healer and recovery in mental health. *A Day in the Life, 6*(3), 5–11.

Locsin, R. C., & Schoenhofer, S. O. (2019). Robots, caring, and nursing in a world of advancing technology. *International Journal for Human Caring, 23*(2), 109–111. https://doi.org/10.20467/1091-5710.23.2.109

Loresto, F. L., Jr., Nunez, L., Tarasenko, L., Pierre, M. S., Oja, K., Mueller, M., Switzer, B., Marroquin, K., & Kleiner, C. (2021). The nurse COVID and historical epidemics literature repository: Development, description, and summary. *Nursing Outlook, 69*(3), 257–264. https://doi.org/10.1016/j.outlook.2020.12.017

Madsbjerg, C. (2017). *Sensemaking: The power of the humanities in the age of the algorithm*. Hachette Book Group, Inc.

Manderscheid, S. V., & Freeman, P. D. (2012). Managing polarity, paradox, and dilemma during leader transition. *European Journal of Training and Development, 36*(9), 856–872. https://doi.org/10.1108/03090591211280937

Mangino, H. (2014). Narrative medicine's role in graduate nursing curricula: Finding and sharing wisdom through story. *Creative Nursing, 20*(3), 191–193. https://doi.org/10.1891/1078-4535.20.3.191

Manomomidis, G., Panagopoulou, E., & Montgomery, A. (2019, January 27). Resilience in nursing: The role of internal and external factors. *Journal of Nursing Management*. https://pubmed.ncbi.nlm.nih.gov/30066352/.

Maslow, A. (1998). *Toward a psychology of being* (3rd ed.). Wiley & Sons LTD.

Maykut, C., & Wild, C. (2019). Relational comportment: Embodying caring as a contemplative journey. *International Journal for Human Caring, 23*(4), 295–301. https://doi.org/10.20467/1091-5710.23.4.295

McGrath, R. (2019). *Seeing around corners: How to spot inflection points in business*. Houghton Mifflin Harcourt.

Merriam-Webster. (n.d.). *Empathy*. In Merriam-Webster.com dictionary. https://www.merriam-webster.com/dictionary/empathy

Mitty, E. (2010). Storytelling. *Geriatric Nursing, 31*(1), 58–62.

Mokhtar, N. H., Halim, M. F. A., & Kamarulzaman, S. Z. S. (2011). The effectiveness of storytelling in enhancing communicative skills. *Procedia - Social and Behavioral Sciences, 18*, 163–169. https://doi.org/10.1016/j.sbspro.2011.05.024

Naef, R. (2006). Bearing witness: A moral way of engaging in the nurse-person relationship. *Nursing Philosophy, 7*, 146–156.

National Academies of Practice (1999). *To err is human: Building a safer health system*. https://www.nap.edu/resource/9728/To-Err-is-Human-1999--report-brief.pdf.

National Academies of Sciences, Engineering and Medicine. (2021). *The future of nursing 2020 – 2030: Charting a path to achieve health equity*. The National Academies Press. https:doi.org/10.17226/25982

Neumann, J., & Forsyth, D. (2008). Affective domain for institutional values. *Journal of Continuing Education in Nursing, 39*(6), 248–252.

Nightingale, F. (1946). *Notes on nursing: What it is, and what it is not.* Lippincott, Williams & Wilkins.

Niven, E. (2008). The wounded healer concept in nursing. *Nursing Ethics, 15*(3).

Nundy, S. (2021). *Care after Covid: What the pandemic revealed is broken in healthcare and how to reinvent it.* McGraw Hill.

Obolensky, N. (2014). *Complex adaptive leadership: Embracing paradox and uncertainty.* Gower.

Ondrejka, D. (2014). *Affective teaching in nursing.* Springer Publishing Co.

Orwoll, B., Diane, S., Henry, D., Tsang, L., Chu, K., Meer, C., Hartman, K., & Roy-Burman, A. (2018). Gamification and microlearning for engagement with quality improvement (GAMEQI): A bundled digital intervention for the prevention of central line-associated bloodstream infection. *American Journal of Medical Quality, 33*(1), 21–29. https://doi.org/10.1177/1062860617706542

Ostaseski, F. (2017). *The five invitations.* Flatiron.

Osterholm, M. (2017). *The deadliest enemy.* Hachette.

Page, M. B., Bishop, K., & Etmanski, C. (2021). Community belonging and values-based leadership as the antidote to bullying and incivility. *Societies, 11*(2). https://doi.org/10.3390/soc11020029

Paley, J. (2007). Complex adaptive systems and nursing. *Nursing Inquiry, 14*(3), 233–242.

Pan, X., Ojcius, D. M., Gao, T., Li, Z., Pan, C., & Pan, C. (2020). Lessons learned from the 2019-nCoV epidemic on prevention of future infectious diseases. *Microbes Infect, 22*(2), 86–91. https://doi.org/10.1016/j.micinf.2020.02.004

Pellico, L., & Chinn, P. L. (2007). Narrative criticism: The power of storytelling. *Journal of Holistic Nursing, 25*(1), 58–67.

Pesut, D. J. (2019). Anticipating disruptive innovations with foresight leadership. *Nursing Administration Quarterly, 43*(3), 196–204. https://doi.org/10.1097/NAQ.0000000000000349

Peterson, G. R. (2017). Polarity management: A functional way to handle your team's dysfunction. *Kappa Delta Pi Record, 53*(1), 24–27. https://doi.org/10.1080/00228958.2017.1264817

Pink, D. (2005). *A whole new mind: Why right-brainers will rule the future.* Riverhead Books.

Quinn, J. F. (2014). The integrated nurse: Way of the healer. In M. Kreitzer & M. S. Koithan (Eds.), *Integrative Nursing* (pp. 33–46). Oxford University Press.

Ragan, S. L., & Kanter, E. (2017). Learning the patient's story. *Semin Oncol Nurs, 33*(5), 467–474. https://doi.org/10.1016/j.soncn.2017.09.003

Rowe, A., & Hogarth, A. (2005). Use of complex adaptive systems metaphor to achieve professional and organizational change. *Journal of Advanced Nursing, 51*(4), 396–405.

Sabetzadeh, F., Tsui, E., & Tsui, E. (2011). Social motives polarity and its impact on knowledge sharing. *Vine, 41*(1), 76–88. https://doi.org/10.1108/03055721111115566

Schroeder, R. (2016). Bearing witness: The lived experience of sitting with patients. *Archives of Psychiatric Nursing, 30*(6), 678–684. https://doi.org/10.1016/j.apnu.2016.03.005

Shanta, L., & Gargiulo, L. (2014). A study of the influence of nursing education on development of emotional intelligence. *J Prof Nurs, 30*(6), 511–520. https://doi.org/10.1016/j.profnurs.2014.06.005

Siegel, D. (2010). *Mindsight: The new science of personal transformation.* Bantam Books.

Siegel, D. (2018). *Aware: The science and practice of presence.* Penguin Random House.

Sims, S., Leamy, M., Levenson, R., Brearley, S., Ross, F., & Harris, R. (2020). The delivery of compassionate nursing care in a tick-box culture: Qualitative perspectives from a realist evaluation of intentional rounding. *International Journal of Nursing Studies, 107*, 103580. https://doi.org/10.1016/j.ijnurstu.2020.103580

Smiley, R. A., Ruttinger, C., Oliveria, C. M., Hudson, L. R., Allgeyer, R., Reneau, K. A., Silvestra, J. H., & Alexander, M. (2021). The 2020 national nursing workforce survey. *Journal of Nursing Regulation, 12*(1). https://www.journalofnursingregulation.com/article/S2155-8256(21)00027-2/fulltext

Smith, M., & Liehr, P. (2005). Story theory. *Holist Nurs Pract*, 19(6), 272–276.

Stretton, A. (2021). Accelerating global and local VUCA-related disruptors as drivers for organisational strategic responses. *PM World*, X(IV), 1–15.

Su, W. M., & Osisek, P. J. (2011). The Revised Bloom's taxonomy: Implications for educating nurses. *J Contin Educ Nurs*, 42(7), 321–327. https://doi.org/10.3928/00220124-20110621-05

Sullivan, L., & Yoder-Wise, P. S. (2019). Disrupt now for future focus. *Nurs Adm Q*, 43(4), 333–336. https://doi.org/10.1097/NAQ.0000000000000378

Susskind, R., & Susskind, D. (2015). *The future of the professions: How technology will transform the work of human experts*. Oxford University Press.

Theede, M. (2018). Polyvagal theory affirms the importance of nursing. In S. Proges & D. Dan (Eds.), *Clinical applications of the polyvagal theory: The emergence of polyvagal-informed therapies* (pp. 149–167). W.W. Norton & Co.

Timbrell, J. (2017). Instructional storytelling: Application of the clinical judgment model in nursing. *J Nurs Educ*, 56(5), 305–308. https://doi.org/10.3928/01484834-20170421-10

Toosi, N, Lipman, D., & Diamond, D. (2020). Before Trump's inauguration, a warning: 'The worst influenza pandemic since 1918.' *Politico*. https://www.politico.com/news/2020/03/16/trump-inauguration-warning-scenario-pandemic-132797

Udah, H. (2019). Searching for a place to belong in a time of othering. *Social Sciences*, 8(11). https://doi.org/10.3390/socsci8110297

Valiga, T. M. (2014). Attending to affective domain learning: Essential to prepare the kind of graduates the public needs. *J Nurs Educ*, 53(5), 247. https://doi.org/10.3928/01484834-20140422-10

Vogel, C. (2016). *The art of community: Seven principles for belonging*. Berrett-Koehler Publishers.

Watson, J. (1990). Caring knowledge informed moral passion ANS. *Advances in Nursing Science*, 13(1), 15–24.

Watson, J. (2018). The philosophy of science: Starting point/inverting the paradigm. In *Unitary Caring Science: The philosophy and praxis of nursing*. University Press of Colorado.

Watson, J. (2021). *Caring Science as sacred science*. Lotus Library.

Weberg, D. (2012). Complexity leadership: A healthcare imperative. *Nursing Forum*, 47(4), 268–277.

Wei, H., Hardin, S. R., & Watson, J. (2021). A Unitary Caring Science resilience-building model: Unifying the human caring theory and research-informed psychology and neuroscience evidence. *Int J Nurs Sci*, 8(1), 130–135. https://doi.org/10.1016/j.ijnss.2020.11.003

Wesorick, B. (2016). *Polarity thinking in healthcare: The missing logic to achieve transformation*. HRD Press.

Wheatley, M. (2017). *Who do we choose to be?* Berret-Koehler Publishers, Inc.

Wiklund Gustin, L., & Wagner, L. (2013). The butterfly effect of caring - clinical nursing teachers' understanding of self-compassion as a source to compassionate care. *Scand J Caring Sci*, 27(1), 175–183. https://doi.org/10.1111/j.1471-6712.2012.01033.x

Wolf, Z. R., Boykin, A., Bulfin, S., Groebbel, C., Packard, M., Ray, M. A., & Schoenhofer, S. (2019). Guiding principles for transforming curriculum through integration of technology as expression of caring. *International Journal for Human Caring*, 23(4), 338–348. https://doi.org/10.20467/1091-5710.23.4.338

Yoder-Wise, P. S. (2021). From VUCA to VUCA 2.0: Surviving today to prosper tomorrow. *Nurs Educ Perspect*, 42(1), 1–2. https://doi.org/10.1097/01.NEP.0000000000000774

Ziegler, E., Carroll, B., & Shortall, C. (2020). Design thinking in nursing education to improve care for lesbian, gay, bisexual, transgender, queer, intersex and two-spirit people. *Creat Nurs*, 26(2), 118–124. https://doi.org/10.1891/CRNR-D-20-00003

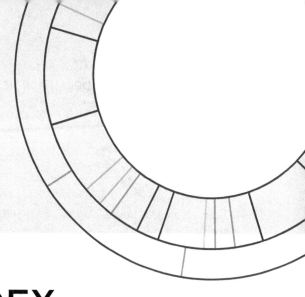

# INDEX

NOTE: Page references noted with an *f* are figures; Page references noted with a *t* are tables.

## A

academic Caritas Leadership Program, 267–77

accessing: healthcare, 327, 528–29; policymaking processes, 498–502

acculturative stress, 479

achievement-oriented leadership, 16

actions: concepts lost in translation of, 553; inspiring, 55–56; planning, 512; in population health, 325–27

activism, 399, 534–38; sacred, 565–68

Adams, Virginia, 466

adaptable elements, 65*t*

adaptive systems, 312–14; community health as, 315–16

Adopt the Appreciative Inquiry 4-(D) cycle of improvement, 452

adult cognitive development theory, 444

adult development, 447, 448

advocacy, 52; for policy changes, 539; Unitary Caring Science, 540–43

advocates: history of U.S. nurse policy, 492–94

affective domain, 556–62

Affordable Care Act (2010), 494, 528, 533, 534

Africa, 392; Centers for Disease Control and Prevention, 402; leadership challenges in, 399–401. *See also* global health

African Americans: discrimination against, 478–79; in education, 466–74; health insurance and, 528, 529; male students, 469; women, 346, 480 (*see also* women)

African Union, 402

agenda setting, 495, 500

agents, political change, 510–12

aggression, 181

agility, 553

aging populations, 392

Agricultural Age, 557

AI (artificial intelligence), 302*f*; patient care and, 300–303

ailments, collective, 213

# F

# I

# M

# T

# U

# V

# W–X

# Y-Z